Bioethics and Armed Conflict

Basic Bioethics

Glenn McGee and Arthur Caplan, editors

Bioethics and Armed Conflict

Moral Dilemmas of Medicine and War

Michael L. Gross

The MIT Press
Cambridge, Massachusetts
London, England

MIT Press books may be purchased at special quantity discounts for business or sales promotional use. For information, please e-mail special_sales@mitpress.mit .edu or write to Special Sales Department, The MIT Press, 55 Hayward Street, Cambridge, MA 02142.

This book was set in Sabon by SNP Best-set Typesetter Ltd., Hong Kong and was printed and bound in the United States of America. Printed on recycled paper.

Library of Congress Cataloging-in-Publication Data

Gross, Michael L., 1954–
Bioethics and armed conflict : moral dilemmas of medicine and war / Michael L. Gross.
    p.   cm.   (Basic bioethics)
Includes bibliographical references and index.
ISBN 0-262-07269-6 (alk. paper)—ISBN 0-262-57226-5 (pbk. : alk. paper)
1. Medical ethics. 2. Military ethics. 3. War. 4. Medicine, Military—Moral and ethical aspects. I. Title. II. Series.

R724.G76   2006

                                                              2005056158

10 9 8 7 6 5 4 3 2 1

For my brother, Larry, who fought disease valiantly

Contents

Series Foreword

We are pleased to present the twentieth book in the series Basic Bioethics. The series presents innovative works in bioethics to a broad audience and introduces seminal scholarly manuscripts, state-of-the-art reference works, and textbooks. Such broad areas as the philosophy of medicine, advancing genetics and biotechnology, end-of-life care, health and social policy, and the empirical study of biomedical life are engaged.

Glenn McGee
Arthur Caplan

Basic Bioethics Series Editorial Board
Tod S. Chambers
Susan Dorr Goold
Mark Kuczewski
Herman Saatkamp

Preface

I am neither a physician nor a full-time, professional soldier, but, like many throughout the world, a one-time conscript, some-time reservist, and occasional patient. That should answer many readers' first question. While some may regard this as a disadvantage, it affords, instead, a measure of objective distance from which to study the interplay of medicine and war. It is one of the great virtues of modern bioethics to admit, indeed encourage, all those with an interest in medicine, philosophy, politics, law, and religion to enter and to explore the field. There are no insiders or outsiders. Everyone in bioethics (or almost everyone) comes from somewhere else, and these interdisciplinary crosscurrents offer a stimulating environment for inquiry.

Geography also provides objective distance. Many contemporary issues confronting bioethics and armed conflict now plague the Middle East: torture, terrorism, violations of neutrality, low-intensity warfare, nonlethal weaponry, and armed intervention. Viewed from up close, it is often difficult to free oneself from the raw emotion the daily news evokes. But leave Haifa for Florence, and things look slightly different. Italy offers a sweeping historical view of medicine and war, as casual trips through the once blood-soaked but now peaceful countryside bring the visitor face to face with those who laid the foundation for the practice of medicine during war. In Turin, the first great military surgeon, Ambrose Paré, witnesses and vigorously condemns the mercy killing of seriously wounded soldiers in 1537. Leaving Milan in 1797, Napoléon's chief medical officer, Dominique Larrey, puts his mind to the organization of "flying ambulances," which will, for the very first time, dedicate troops and equipment to evacuate wounded soldiers from the battlefield.

But Larrey's efforts will prove inadequate to care for the great number of sick and injured soldiers associated with modern warfare. And so, after witnessing the horrors of the battle of Solferino near Verona in 1859, it remained for Henry Dunant to envisage the radical idea of employing volunteer medical workers to care for the wounded. His efforts saw the establishment of the International Committee of the Red Cross and with it the foundation of modern humanitarian law.

As evocative as the Italian countryside is, however, it lacks a suitable English-language library. For want of a library, I'd have faced endless delays but for the dedication of Sara Lazar, who worked tirelessly to provide material from the books and journals of the University of Haifa and other local libraries and institutes in Israel. I could not have managed without her assistance.

I am also indebted to colleagues who helped me work through the many questions this book raises. Jonathan Moreno, Tony Rogers, Saul Smilansky, and Daniel Statman read through chapters that proved particularly vexing, offering insight, support, and good cheer. Chapter 7 raises a particularly sensitive issue and I have to thank Stuart Charmé for making invaluable suggestions for taking the ragged edges off a contentious, but now hopefully balanced and convincing discussion. I am also grateful for the opportunity to present some of these ideas publicly at the International Bioethics Retreat now organized in memory of the late David Thomasma. Dave's articles on torture and human rights first drew my attention to the complex questions of bioethics and war, and the retreat provides an ideal venue to thrash out these contentious issues. My sincere thanks to David Bennahum, Tomi Kushner, Rosamond Rhodes, and all the other participants for their constant probing and stimulating discussions.

While many sources for this book draw on Western accounts of medicine and war, I was fortunate to gain access to several descriptions of medical care in North Vietnam during the Vietnam War. James G. Zumwalt allowed me to quote from his working manuscript *Bare Feet, Iron Will* and from the interviews he conducted with former North Vietnamese medical personnel. Lady Borton was kind enough to send me an advance copy of her translation of the memoirs of Dr. Le Cao Dai, *The Central Highlands: A North Vietnamese Journal of Life on the*

Ho Chi Minh Trail 1965–1973. I also wish to thank Cambridge University Press for permission to reprint portions of "Physician Assisted Draft Evasion: Civil Disobedience, Medicine and War" that appear in chapter 9. This first appeared in the *Cambridge Quarterly of Healthcare Ethics* 14, no. 4 (2005).

My appreciation for my family's patience and encouragement goes without question. My special thanks to Daphna and Saul for their proofreading and valuable suggestions and to Elisheva for her probing questions about euthanasia and war.

Finally, a word to those who may think that this book is politically charged and too polemical. Bioethics, as I noted, is a marvelously adaptive and tolerant discipline that thrives on the hard moral questions that drive life and death. Politics, peace, medicine and war are no different.

Michael L. Gross
Florence, Italy
Haifa, Israel
August, 2005

1

Setting the Stage

Two prevailing attitudes set the stage for the discussion of bioethics and armed conflict. The first, affirmed by the World Medical Association, declares that "medical ethics in times of armed conflict is identical to medical ethics in times of peace" (WMA 2004). A brief glance at the table of contents of this book should be sufficient to seriously question, if not belie, the WMA's declaration. But if it is so obviously mistaken, how does the WMA assert itself with such certainty in the first place? The answer to this question lies in another prevailing attitude about the medical profession vigorously defended in recent years by Edmund Pellegrino and David Thomasma. "The physician," they write, "has ethical obligations that transcend self-interest, exigency and even social, political and economic forces" (1993, 36). By emphasizing a transcendent obligation, they wish to shield the doctor-patient relationship from competing interests that sometimes overwhelm modern medical care, and may threaten a patient's trust and jeopardize his or her well-being. While Pellegrino and Thomasma do not discuss war, one cannot imagine confronting greater social, political, and economic forces than those that accompany armed conflict. Should medicine transcend these forces as well? The WMA seems to believe so. For only then can one conclude that a physician's moral obligations remain absolutely constant, so that medical ethics in time of war is, indeed, identical to medical ethics in time of peace.

Yet, as physicians try to save lives in an endeavor dedicated to taking them, they confront hard dilemmas. It is the nature of these dilemmas to question, if not recast, a physician's moral obligations. Bioethical dilemmas arise when fundamental moral principles conflict, and during war competing bioethical principles must not only contend with one another but with the overriding principles of military necessity and reason of state that animate any issue of military ethics. Actors and interests multiply during war. Combatants and noncombatants, enemies and allies, states and individuals, citizens and soldiers, prisoners of war, the wounded and the dying, those who can return to combat duty and those who cannot, all litter the battlefield. Medicine is called on to cure and, sometimes, to kill. A patient's right to life and self-determination shrinks, human dignity strains under the barrage of military necessity, and calculations of expected utility move beyond a patient's or patients' welfare to embrace the interests of the nation-state and the political community it represents. War transforms, contracts, and subordinates the traditional doctor-patient relationship, but rarely preserves it intact, as in peacetime. Medicine is not above the fray; medical ethics in time of war is not identical to medical ethics in time of peace.

This chapter opens with an account of the role medicine plays in armed conflict, a role never as magnanimous or as benevolent as it sometimes seems in Western nations today. Soldiers and sailors fared poorly, the sick and wounded poorer still. Yet, in spite of the appalling conditions in the field, intellectual development continued apace. The war convention, those rules of humanitarian law and just war that the international community adopted to regulate armed conflict between sovereign states, reached its apex in The Hague just before World War I. And, by some accounts, it was a great success: adversaries slaughtered one another like gentlemen, and civilians enjoyed significant protection. But these accomplishments, however dubious, did not hold in the Second World War. The war made fair game of enemy civilians on both sides and brought unspeakable horrors upon prisoners of war, partisans, and unprotected noncombatants. After the war, the international community tried again, hoping for conventions to regulate war out of existence. They might have succeeded had not substate actors—insurgents, guerrillas, and terrorists—picked up where the nation-state left off.

Postwar interest in humanitarian law, combined with technological progress, changing social norms, and soaring medical costs, also gave birth to bioethics, a discipline that attempted to reconcile traditional medical duties with the demands of a liberal consumer society. Benign paternalism was pushed aside in favor of respect for autonomy, universal health care (at least in most developed nations), and economic efficiency. Technology forced the issue of brain death, offered the gravely ill an extended life span, often at the expense of its quality, and brought medicine firmly into the public arena as critical issues left the confines of the physician's office to become the purview of social movements, private corporations, legislatures, and the courts.

Both the ethics of war and the ethics of medicine generate overarching principles to steer medical care and guide political behavior. The principles of each discipline run parallel, conflicting with and complementing one another under the broad categories of the right to life, self-determination, dignity, and utility. Each of these principles is the subject of detailed discussion in the next chapter. In this chapter, following a discussion of medicine's role in war, they set the stage for the dilemmas of bioethics and armed conflict.

The Role of Medicine in Armed Conflict

Physicians have been regular fixtures in armed conflict since ancient times but, for the most part, were unable to offer wounded soldiers little more than comfort, splints, bandages, and, if necessary, rudimentary surgery. Seriously wounded soldiers died of their wounds, leaving physicians to treat those who survived the hours or sometimes days it took the injured to reach medical care. While battlefield care was primitive and amputation the only surgical method of choice, warfare in the sixteenth and seventeenth centuries did not approach the destructiveness or ferocity it would reach after the French Revolution. War was endemic, but armies were expensive to maintain, thereby leading the great powers to fight with a certain restraint born of economic necessity. Technology also tempered destruction. Most premodern weaponry did not inflict fatal injury. Instead, wounded soldiers most often died of infection, gas gangrene, sepsis, and tetanus, while a great many more uninjured soldiers succumbed to disease—dysentery, typhoid fever, typhus, plague, and smallpox (Gabriel and Metz 1992, vol. 1, 30–32; Porter 1997, 372). Infection and disease presented major challenges to military medicine, making preventive medicine rather than acute care its overriding priority.

In ancient times, defeat was also a leading cause of death. As lines of infantry collapsed under the pressure of battle, defeated troops retreated with abandon. Until the invention of the chariot, retreating troops were largely unmolested. With mobility, however, came slaughter as victors mercilessly hunted down retreating troops and often killed them to the last man. Medical intervention for these unfortunates was unheard of. Defeated armies could easily suffer 70 percent killed and wounded, while the casualties among the victors might barely exceed 10 percent (Dupuy 1995, 28). In modern times, the gap between winners and losers closed. Since the U.S. Civil War (1861–1865), for example, nearly 60 percent of engaged American forces, and far fewer of all troops, have suffered death or injury in action.[1] Ancient wars might have been relatively bloodless except for the impulse to annihilate one's enemies.

The scope and destructiveness of warfare increased drastically with the Napoleonic Wars (1799–1815). The size of opposing forces was unprecedented. Six hundred thousand French troops participated in Napoléon's ill-fated invasion of Russia (1812). Casualty rates increased dramatically. One-third of the 150,000 soldiers present at Gettysburg were killed, wounded, or captured as military technology introduced rifled muskets and cannons, and breech-loading, repeating rifles. The enormous deployment of troops, increased numbers of casualties, and complex logistics posed unprecedented problems and would lead Napoléon's medical staff, for example, to develop "flying" ambulances to evacuate the injured, dedicate trained personnel to provide care, and institute triage to effectively utilize scarce medical resources. While physicians throughout the nineteenth century adopted these innovations, old problems remained. Disease continued to take more lives than combat injuries until the First World War, when improved sanitation decreased the death rate from disease and improved armaments increased death from injuries sustained in battle.

Military tactics, like the laws of armed conflict, are slow to change in the wake of galloping military technology. While the U.S. Civil War saw rifled breech-loading guns that could deliver firepower more accurately than anything previously used on the battlefield, military commanders continued to assemble troops to mass firepower in the same way they had when muskets were wildly inaccurate. Soldiers on both sides were easy targets for the new long-range and more accurate rifles. Similarly, commanders in World War I mounted frontal assaults against well-entrenched positions defended by machine guns and artillery, and suffered casualties not seen on the battlefield before or since.

Yet, in spite of scientific progress, particularly in the nineteenth century, medical care lagged behind military innovation. Despite burgeoning knowledge about infection and disease transmission, physicians could still provide little more than rudimentary care for gunshot and shrapnel wounds. Soldiers suffering from head, chest, and abdominal injuries usually died despite medical efforts. Infection remained difficult to control until the invention of antiseptic techniques late in the nineteenth century and, even then, doctors were slow to adopt Lister's new techniques. Surgery was confined largely to amputation and while improved care increased survival rates, recovery was long and few of these soldiers could return to battle. As a result, economics alone would dictate greater emphasis on preventive care and on maintaining the health of battle-ready soldiers rather than on acute care that could do little more than salvage the lives of men who could no longer contribute to the war effort.

Nevertheless, the resources devoted to medical care were insufficient to perform either task. In spite of advances in hygiene, surgery, and antiseptics, few armies were willing to commit the necessary personnel and resources to bring these advances to their soldiers. Death from disease and infection reached unprecedented levels during the Crimean War (1854–1856). Yet it took nothing more than the dedicated efforts of a few volunteer nurses and the clamor of public opinion to significantly improve survival rates and bring care to a level commensurate with midcentury British medical standards. Prior to World War I, no industrialized, democratic nation could wage war without losing more men to disease than to armed combat. Yet the Japanese, fighting the Russians from 1904 to 1905, did. Emerging from centuries of isolation, Japanese doctors not only adopted European medicine with a vengeance but, more significantly, were willing to bring it to the battlefield, shipping sufficient medicine to vaccinate soldiers against infectious disease, providing adequate personnel and supplies to evacuate and care for the wounded, and disciplining their soldiers to rigorously follow military procedures for sanitation and hygiene (Gabriel and Metz 1992, vol. 2, 226–233).

Following the First World War, the state of military medicine improved dramatically. Advances in medical technology, together with the introduction of motorized transport to evacuate the wounded, increased survival rates for the seriously injured. At the same time, the ideological nature of world war and the existential threat posed by Nazism (and, for some, Communism) elevated war from a tool of state to one of apocalyptic proportions. World War II, Korea (1950–1953), and Vietnam (1961–1975) brought an unprecedented enthusiasm for military medicine as part of a national effort to rid the world of one scourge or another. The Western nations fighting in these conflicts left a legacy of superb military medical care. Improved care was the result of several interrelated factors: the military benefits medical treatment could provide, the availability of sufficient medical resources to care for the injured, and the obligation these nations felt to those willing to give their lives. Yet, in many respects, the grounds for providing medical care to the wounded are more apparent than real, an argument I take up in detail in chapter 3. Nor does comprehensive care typify the care other parties to the conflict could offer. Not surprisingly, Western medical care dominates modern military medical historiography. After Korea and Vietnam, the history of military medicine turns its eye toward the Falklands (1982), the Persian Gulf (1991, 2003), and the Middle East (1967, 1973, and 1982). We know little of military medicine in North Vietnam or pre–World War II China, for example, but anecdotal evidence suggests that neither the North Vietnamese nor the Communist Chinese could provide more than rudimentary care. And, even with rudimentary care, they did not always devote the resources they might have toward evacuating and caring for their wounded, an attitude characterizing medical care in many advanced nations prior to the advent of humanitarian law.

Military Ethics and Humanitarian Law

While one often looks to military organizations to provide professional care for wounded combatants, nonmilitary, volunteer personnel were the first to bring adequate care to the battlefield. This was true during the

Crimean War, and the idea to enlist civilian personnel to provide care during war guided the early activities of the International Committee of the Red Cross (ICRC). Moved by the horrors he witnessed at the battle of Solferino, Italy, in 1859, Henry Dunant led the world community to organize the Red Cross and ratify international conventions that would protect *volunteer* medical personnel during war. Medical care was not a constant feature or a particularly high priority of armies engaged in war. Dunant ([1862] 1986) was moved not only by the horror of war and the terrible wounds soldiers suffered, but also by lack of sufficient resources to bring mid-nineteenth-century medical expertise to the battlefield to care and comfort the wounded. Armies lacked, whether by accident or design, trained medical personnel, adequate supplies of bandages, chloroform, clean water and bedding, and any semblance of an efficient means to evacuate the wounded from the battlefield and bring them to aid stations and hospitals. The evacuation techniques developed by Napoléon's medical officers, perfected by the Union army, and adopted by Bismarck did not consistently find their way to European battlefields. Dunant realized this and did not waste his time appealing to military authorities for more medical personnel. Instead, he conceived of an organization of volunteers to tend the wounded.

In the early days of the Red Cross two groups of personnel provided care to the wounded: military medical personnel, whose ranks slowly grew with the development of humanitarian law, and members of volunteer committees such as the Red Cross. Early international resolutions and conventions in 1863 and 1864 placed the latter under the authority of the former and extended neutrality to each as both ministered to the wounded (Geneva Convention, 1864; Geneva Conference, 1863). Emerging humanitarian law to protect the wounded and those caring for them formed an integral part of contemporary just-war theory.

Contemporary Just-War Theory

While "just-war theory" commonly describes the broad field of ethics and war, its roots are religious and premodern. War, anathema to early Christian theologians, was nevertheless an increasingly important feature of political life as Christianity assumed the reins of political power. Faced with the need to combat armed adversaries bent on destroying the

Christian state and to regulate war among Christian princes, early thinkers were compelled to justify war and bloodshed. This they accomplished with aplomb, coining the terms and developing the concepts that would later infuse international and humanitarian law.

The law of armed conflict, extant in one form or another since antiquity, protected combatant rights and interests and made significant strides throughout the entire modern era, particularly as the major European states consolidated their power by 1500 and found it necessary to equip and control larger armed forces. In earlier periods, wars engaged relatively small armies and while reciprocal agreements often protected the rights of knights and nobles, the lives of common soldiers were of little consequence. The growth of the European powers in the sixteenth and seventeenth centuries brought significant change to the newly emerging laws of armed conflict. During this period, conventions protecting and repatriating prisoners of war, guaranteeing the neutrality of medical personnel, and safeguarding the lives and property of noncombatants gained support (Parker 1994; Green 1998, 59–98).

At the same time, the spirit of the Enlightenment transformed fundamental ideas underlying the nature of war. If the ancients took great pains to exterminate their enemies as they fought in the service of God, and premodern monarchs fought chivalrous wars as they pursued honor and self-interest, modern war evolved as an instrument of state policy. Although armies grew steadily larger and casualties increasingly horrendous, war, as a tool of state policy, is inherently self-limiting. Its goal is not to annihilate an enemy but to disable, disarm, and force one's adversary to surrender. "The fighting forces must be *destroyed*," writes Clausewitz ([1832] 1976, 90; original emphasis), "that is, they must be *put in such a condition that they can no longer carry on the fight.*" A similar view received formal international support in St. Petersburg (1868) as delegates to an International Military Commission considered the use of new and dangerous forms of warfare. "The only legitimate object which States should endeavor to accomplish during war," declared the delegates, "is to weaken the military forces of the enemy. . . . For this purpose it is sufficient to disable the greatest possible number of men." Annihilation may have served the glory of God, but it did little to further the interests of the modern nation-state. Bismarck fought his wars of necessity to gain resources for Prussia; he would have gained little had he destroyed the people and possessions of the lands he conquered.

As the law of armed conflict developed, it banned certain forms of weaponry, prohibited perfidious practices of warfare, and moved to protect the lives of combatants and noncombatants. Early examples of banned weaponry included "dumdum" bullets and poison gas. Perfidy or "treacherous" forms of warfare that abused the protections afforded by fledging international law and convention were equally reprehensible. Only a convention of surrender that protected combatants who laid down their arms could stem the "unnecessary effusion of blood" that some theorists, like Grotius ([1625] 1901, 364), hoped would distinguish modern, rational, and enlightened war from its ancient and barbaric precursor. Surrender depended entirely on trust and the assurance that one's enemy would not feign surrender to gain a tactical advantage. International conventions are essential if the fragile trust that must bind adversaries is ever going to take hold. Absent trust and convention, war would be impossible to end short of extermination.

Humanitarian Law

In contrast to conventions that regulate the conduct of war, humanitarian law emphasizes the immunity of noncombatants, a category that includes civilians as well as captured or wounded combatants. War designed to disable rather than annihilate has no cause to kill wounded or captured enemy soldiers on the condition, of course, that they remain incarcerated for the duration of hostilities. As prisoners of war and no longer a threat to their enemy, wounded soldiers should enjoy the basic rights ordinary civilians enjoy: the right to life and respect for dignity. These were not new concepts, ingrained many years previously in the founding ideology of revolutionary America and France, but they did not always find their way to the battlefield. Francis Lieber, who codified the rules of war for the Union Army in 1863, was among the first to extend protection to prisoners of war on the grounds that they were not criminals but "lawful enemies," "subject to no punishment . . . nor revenge wreaked upon [them] by the intentional infliction of any suffering, or disgrace, cruel imprisonment, want of food, by mutilation, death or any barbarity" (Lieber Code, 1863, Article 49). Nor were wounded soldiers criminals either and, for this reason, were equally entitled to humane treatment at the hands of their captors.

More vulnerable than combatants, civilians were not lawful enemies and should, therefore, enjoy greater protection from the horrors of war. This proved easier to accomplish in theory than in practice. If nineteenth-century European armies hoped that local citizens would remain passive during war, watching with disinterest as armies crisscrossed their land and violently locked horns, they were often disappointed. Citizen armies became the watchword following the French Revolution, and civilian populations formed an increasingly integral part of any nation's war effort. As a result, civilians often found themselves the target of looting, requisitions, blockades, bombardment, and reprisal. The international community sought to curb the worst of these excesses and, with this in mind, the Hague Conventions prohibit bombardment of undefended cities, the destruction of nonmilitary structures, and pillage. The laws of armed conflict direct occupying armies to maintain public property, avoid collective punishment, and respect "family honours and rights, individual lives and private property, and religious convictions" (Hague Convention, 1899, Articles 46, 47).

If the British blockade of Germany in World War I tested the limits of these prohibitions, World War II put them to flight. Both the Allied and Axis powers indiscriminately and intentionally bombed civilian populations, while the Nazis and Japanese brutalized occupied peoples beyond description. Trying to pick up the pieces of noncombatant immunity after the war, the 1949 Geneva Conventions, and later the 1977 Protocols to the Geneva Conventions, dedicated an entire convention, the Fourth, to the protection of civilians. The convention moves beyond the Hague Conventions by protecting civilians in either enemy or occupied territory from pillage, reprisals, indiscriminate destruction of property, torture, and kidnapping. The conventions further enjoin occupying powers to maintain public order, preserve personal property and the natural environment, provide medical treatment, and take special care to protect the lives and well-being of women and children. These conventions form the cornerstone of humanitarian law today. While many may point to abuses of humanitarian law to discredit its importance, there is no doubt that international humanitarian law guides the actions of any number of nations, shapes international public opinion, and provokes indignation against rogue actors. Humanitarian norms and the conventions of war also regulate the provision of medical care during war, a goal they share with bioethics.

Contemporary Biomedical Bioethics

Contemporary bioethics is more recent than contemporary just-war theory and rose to distinction in the post–World War II period. That period, also synonymous with the final and most advanced codification of humanitarian law and laws of armed conflict, saw tremendous technological progress. Wartime development of penicillin, medicine's first "golden bullet," placed, for the first time, medical science's dream of eradicating disease from the face of the earth within reach.

As medical science accumulated scientific knowledge with remarkable speed, a very strong paternalistic relationship developed between doctors and patients. During this period doctors acquired their "godlike" stature, a position unknown in previous times as doctors could offer little beyond comfort, bandages, and primitive surgery while "curing," as Roy Porter (1997, 680) notes, "remained a subordinate consideration." The great strides in medicine prior to World War II came in the field of public health as sanitation, hygiene, and vaccinations greatly improved the lives of immeasurable individuals by controlling such infectious diseases as malaria, tuberculosis, smallpox, typhoid, typhus, and cholera.

The development of antibiotics, on the other hand, brought a therapeutic revolution. Now doctors could cure disease, an achievement investing them with near supernatural status. Patients were only too glad to place themselves in their doctors' hands, ask few questions, and do what they were told. The provision of medical care was changing, as well, reinforcing the trend toward "medicalization" of life. Increasing numbers of physicians cared for their patients in clinics, surgeries, and hospitals rather than in the patient's home. Health expenditures increased across the industrialized world as patients could not seem to get enough of modern medical care. The changes came fast and furious:

If the half century after 1880 was marked by the doctor's ability to diagnose disease scientifically while remaining therapeutically powerless, the post World

War II era was characterized by the ability to triumph over the classic killers and relieve suffering. But though doctors became therapeutically more potent, in large measure they ceased to give the patient what they want. With effective weapons against organic disease, they tended to forget the psychological significance and benefits of the doctor-patient relationship. The new generation of physicians was filled with therapeutic self-confidence: a display of humanity had become therapeutically unnecessary and risked being forgotten. (Porter 1997, 686)

This trend, however, did not last long. By the 1950s and early 1960s medical self-confidence, what some may even call arrogance, was undermined by the limits of its own technology, consumer consciousness, and the burgeoning cost of medical care. These changes brought the birth of modern bioethics. It is common to tie the emergence of modern bioethics to two phenomena: technological development and social change. Technological progress saw the development of life-sustaining equipment, particularly ventilators and dialysis machines. Social change and upheaval brought the steady emergence of consumer, ethnic, and gender consciousness and the empowerment of minority groups fighting for civil rights and an end to the war in Vietnam.

If dialysis machines could sustain the life of chronically and desperately ill patients, ventilators offered medicine the unusual prospect of keeping a dead patient alive. Artificial respiration, developed to maintain cardiopulmonary functioning in a patient who would have otherwise died, raises novel questions. In some cases, intervention is temporary, necessitated by certain kinds of cardiac surgery and discontinued once a patient recovers. In other cases, however, a patient cannot live independently of life support. Should a chronically ill patient with decreasing quality of life enjoy expensive medical treatment? New technology raised this question for the first time and it remains largely unanswered today. At the same time, respirator-dependent patients often suffered damage to the whole or upper brain, leading doctors to speculate whether these patients might serve as a source of organs for transplantation. This raised a host of medical, ethical, religious, and legal questions that were to preoccupy bioethics in its early years. By traditional standards of cardiopulmonary activity, ventilated patients were very much alive. In some cases, however, they showed no signs of brain function and the congruence of brain death, respiration, and a working heart was unprecedented, never before possible without the aid of machines. Was the patient dead or alive? The question was important for many obvious reasons, but not the least because only a dead patient could donate vital organs. This extraordinary state of affairs led the medical community to develop a new standard of death: brain death, defined as the cessation of all brain activity in the lower and upper brain. Once brain dead, a patient could relinquish his or her vital organs for transplant. The brain-death standard earned widespread acceptance in the late 1960s, and while it solved one problem, it created others when patients were not brain dead. A non-brain-dead patient was clearly alive but entirely dependent on ventilator support. Did this mean that one had to treat this patient indefinitely with or without the patient's consent? At first blush, the answer seemed to be yes, for to do otherwise would be to kill the patient.

Answering these questions required philosophical as well as medical tools. Then existing codes of medical ethics prohibited harming patients or accelerating their deaths in any way, thereby suggesting that respirator-dependent patients require artificial ventilation until they no longer breathe or show definitive signs of brain death. Engaging these issues, the growing bioethics community developed an impressive repertoire of moral principles to evaluate many questions in a new light. First among these was an emerging concept of patient self-determination that supplemented traditional medical concerns for patient welfare. If physicians thought themselves capable of making decisions conducive to their patient's benefit and without patient approval, the idea of patient self-determination undermined this authority.

The emergence of patient self-determination coincided with the rising level of consumer, ethnic, gender, and racial awareness that was to dominate American civic consciousness in the 1960s. Both the Vietnam War and the civil rights movement encouraged minority groups to oppose the status quo. And, to various degrees, many successfully transformed public policy. About this time patient rights movements emerged, not with the express purpose of controlling life and death but with the more general goal of influencing medical policy for the poor and underprivileged. The National Welfare Rights Organization, for example, focused on crucial aspects of basic health care such as primary and acute medical care, informed consent, confidentiality, privacy, and community representation on hospital boards (Annas 1978). At the same time, patient self-determination made it impossible to resolve the question posed by artificial respiration solely as the prerogative of the medical community. Doctors had to consider a patient's wishes in some way. Over time, and with the assistance of the courts, physicians, philosophers, and theologians, lawmakers in the United States and other industrialized nations would consider and approve nearly every possible permutation of withholding or withdrawing life-sustaining treatment, food, or fluids, from terminal, nonterminal, competent, once-competent, and never-competent patients (see Steinbock and Norcross 1994). These developments questioned, in a way previously unimaginable, the state's traditional duty to protect life and the physician's long-standing obligation to protect the welfare and life of patients. Patient self-determination, medicine's duty to do no harm and provide benevolent care, and the state's duty to protect the lives of its citizens coalesced to shape the fundamental principles of contemporary bioethics. Multiple fundamental principles create fertile ground for moral dilemmas, all the more difficult to resolve as bioethics confronts the reality of war.

Moral Dilemmas of Medicine and War

Dilemmas arise when deep-seated moral principles conflict and dictate at least two mutually exclusive actions, which are both obligatory but are not attainable in tandem. Many bioethical dilemmas, for example, set respect for autonomy against the duty to protect life, and leave the state to square off against individuals who seek to end their own life. In other cases, the duty to tell the truth, divulge medical information, control costs, or efficiently distribute limited resources may conflict with a physician's concern for a patient's welfare. While there are any number of central dilemmas to the practice of medicine, some easily resolved and others not, it is important to remember that the most crucial element of any dilemma is behavioral. Dilemmas, by their very nature, compel a person to decide and act in a certain way. These are not theoretical exercises. At the end of the day one must choose a definitive course of action.

Choosing to act in one way or another often requires one to rank conflicting principles so one choice is ethically more compelling than the other. This is a complicated process whereby one tries to weigh the relative significance of each principle at stake and, at the same time, consider the costs and benefits that each course of action provides. Alternatively, one may defuse a dilemma entirely by constructing an option that is not morally problematic. Creative solutions are just as much a part of modern bioethics as dilemma resolution. Modern warfare presents a different array of dilemmas for medicine than those found during times of peace, but the structure remains the same. Exacerbating military medical dilemmas is a greater assortment of competing principles and interests. These multiply during armed conflict as the ethical principles of war augment those of medicine.

The Ethical Principles of Medicine and War

Resolving dilemmas of medicine and war first demands an understanding of the principles at stake. Chapter 2 clusters the principles of bioethics and military ethics under four related concepts: the right to life, autonomy or self-determination, dignity, and utility. In bioethics, these four categories yield such familiar principles as the right to life, informed consent, confidentiality, privacy, nonhumiliation, beneficence, and nonmaleficence (do no harm). In military ethics and contemporary just-war theory these concepts yield principles in many ways similar. Unlike bioethical principles, however, the principles of contemporary just war often reach beyond the welfare of a single individual—that is, the patient—to consider instead the aggregate interests of combatants and noncombatants, and the collective interests of the state. At the same time, they must also contend with military necessity.

Many of these principles, largely inchoate prior to World War II but the subject of increasing interest since then, collide during armed conflict. Medical ethics in peacetime is not identical to medical ethics during war for two reasons. First, the hallmark principles that drive bioethical decision making in ordinary clinical settings are largely absent. Military personnel do not enjoy a right to life, personal autonomy, or a right of self-determination to any degree approaching that of ordinary patients. Second, the principles of contemporary just war may simply override many bioethical concerns. Military necessity grants paramount authority to reason of state, proportionality limits but does not eliminate

Table 1.1
Bioethical dilemmas during armed conflict

Caregiving dilemmas		Noncaregiving dilemmas
Conventional warfare	Unconventional warfare	
Caring for the wounded	*Medical neutrality*	*Torture and ill-treatment*
Preserving manpower	Of medical personnel	Interrogational torture
Maintaining morale	Of medical installations	Passive torture
State's duty	Of medical care	
Patient rights		*Unconventional*
Informed consent		*weapons development*
Confidentiality		Chemical weapons
Battlefield euthanasia		Biological weapons
		Nonlethal weapons
Distributive justice and triage		
Scarce medical resources		
Scarce medical knowledge		

excessive harm, and the doctrine of double effect permits unintentional harm to noncombatants. As the ethical principles governing medicine and war converge during armed conflict, difficult dilemmas inevitably raise their head.

During armed conflict, dilemmas of medical ethics arise in several distinct settings as medical expertise is used for either healing (caregiving) or nonhealing (noncaregiving) purposes and in the context of conventional and unconventional war (table 1.1).

The Right to Medical Care

The first category of dilemmas that medical personnel face arises in the context of individual care and during conventional warfare. Every caregiving dilemma presupposes both a physician's duty to provide care and a patient's right to receive it. But what is axiomatic in peacetime is not always obvious during war. "Why," we might ask, "should we treat wounded soldiers, particularly those seriously injured?" This is the subject of chapter 3 and the answer is not immediately apparent. One cannot invoke a soldier's right to life, for military service severely compromises this right. One cannot appeal to utility, for the tragic fact remains that those soldiers requiring the most medical care and resources will not return to duty or contribute in any meaningful way to the war effort. While one might consider the effect of medical care on the morale of healthy soldiers, it is not clear whether soldiers fight any better or worse if medical care is rudimentary or technologically advanced. Perhaps the state owes its fighters a special debt of gratitude for risking their lives, whether they can return to duty or not. While some nations do, in fact, treat their injured soldiers significantly better than those suffering similarly serious injuries from birth or accident, one wonders whether military service is not a morally arbitrary criterion for distributing scarce resources among the critically ill. In the end, one must consider that if military necessity is an overriding consideration during wartime, then there might be good grounds for simply letting some wounded soldiers die or, at best, offering them no more care than remains available to others. Military necessity plays no less havoc with other patient rights.

Informed Consent, Confidentiality, and the Right to Die

If a soldier's right to medical care is suspect, then war may certainly compromise other patient rights central to bioethics. Such basic rights as informed consent, confidentiality, and the right to die anchor the discussion in chapter 4. Informed consent is the hallmark of bioethics, yet allowing soldiers to decide medical care for themselves might be chaotic. Where does one draw the line? May one compel soldiers to accept standard medical care but allow them to choose experimental care that might protect them against novel biological and chemical agents? The answer is not clear. If soldiers have but limited autonomy, on what basis may they refuse experimental or investigational drugs? This issue turns partly on acceptable risk during war and on the difference between military risk and medical risk. If a commander may expose his soldiers to significant military risk to gain an important military objective, may he not accept a similar level of medical risk when treating them? One would think that the risks are commensurable.

War confounds and compromises traditional concern for confidentiality if and when medical personnel must denounce injured enemy soldiers to the authorities. What principles govern a physician's conduct in these situations? Are enemy soldiers akin to dangerous criminals, so that the public good permits one to violate confidentiality? However much one might think so, one cannot forget that the principle underlying all aspects of humanitarian treatment for wounded soldiers lies in just the opposite direction: enemy soldiers are not criminals and may not suffer for their actions. International instruments pondering justifications for violating confidentiality leave the question open, permitting physicians to decide for themselves based on prevailing norms of medical ethics. Yet bioethical norms offer no obvious answer without considering the competing norms of military ethics.

Finally, patient rights raise the question of battlefield euthanasia. Military personnel retain little of their right to life; do they have the right to die? As critically ill patients, do they have the right to refuse life-sustaining treatment if appropriate medical care can salvage them for active duty? There is no question that ordinary patients command this right, but it is entirely uncertain that soldiers do. If soldiers are not allowed to die by their own choosing, may others allow them to die? Consider a soldier wounded behind enemy lines while any attempt to evacuate him will either jeopardize a mission or threaten the welfare of others. May his commanding officer abandon a wounded soldier and let him die and, if so, may he kill him as well? Each of these questions, like those surrounding informed consent and confidentiality, push well beyond the parameters of medical ethics during peace and arise, again, as bioethical principles confront the necessity of war.

Triage and Distributive Justice

Dilemmas of distributive justice (chapter 5) are particularly acute as physicians face the question of distributing scarce medical resources to the wounded. Principles governing triage during war often conflict with one another. On the one hand, the principle of medical need requires medical personnel to treat those in greatest need first, "without regard to rank or distinction," as Dominique Larrey ([1814] 1987, vol. 2, 142)—the pioneer of military triage—famously phrased it. Yet we often forget that Larrey's facilities, while primitive, were generally sufficient for his needs. When supplies are short and medical facilities overrun with casualties, however, a different principle takes hold. Rather than provide need-based treatment, medical care turns to distributing resources to salvage the greatest number of soldiers and return them to active duty. Military necessity repudiates any distributive principle defined by medical need and discriminates against nonmilitary personnel and enemy civilians and soldiers, in favor of one's own combatants.

Nor does triage pertain only to scarce medical resources. World War II, for example, saw the rapid and secret development of penicillin. Aside from the dilemmas of penicillin triage and the question of who merits prior claim to a scarce resource, one wonders about the ethics of classifying medical research during war. Allied scientists took great pains to censor public information vital to the development of penicillin, claiming that it might benefit their enemies. Similar questions arise today with regard to the secrets of genetic engineering. Does military necessity demand that one withhold medical information from the enemy in the same way it might limit their access to medical resources? This, too, is a question of distributive justice that arises primarily during armed conflict and that is not easily resolved by the established principles of bioethics.

Unconventional Warfare and Military Medical Ethics

All the dilemmas described above arise easily enough in the context of conventional warfare. But warfare has changed dramatically since World War II, and the post–World War II attempt to contain conventional warfare by universal enforcement of the 1949 Geneva Conventions would slowly unravel as warfare assumed a form that was increasingly unconventional. Unconventional war is any form of war that is not conventional—that is, armed conflict between sovereign states fielding modern armies and fighting according to the conventions of modern warfare. At one end of the spectrum, unconventional warfare describes nuclear, chemical, or biological warfare—wars waged with weapons of mass destruction that often require biological and medical expertise to be fully effective. While the international community now prohibits the development and deployment of these weapons, they remain the object of intense interest among some third-world nations and insurgent groups.

At the other end of the spectrum, unconventional warfare is decidedly low-tech and embraces low-intensity conflict and guerrilla warfare that often flout the accepted rules of war. As described earlier, the conventional laws of armed combat first gained ascendancy in the wake of the Enlightenment, when it became clear to most observers that war was primarily a means to secure the political goals of sovereign states. These states fielded professional armies, hierarchically controlled and easily identified. They fought to disable their enemy, and this credo became the guiding force behind limiting the destruction of war in the early modern period. This misplaced sense of restraint was first exposed in the First World War and thoroughly repudiated in the Second. Yet the aversion to fighting wars of obliteration remained and sovereign states hoped that international humanitarian law grounded in the authority of an international body would serve to brake the aggressive tendencies of mankind. The law, however, remained the purview of sovereign states, and while it has kept many sovereign states from fighting one another in the aftermath of World War II, belligerent actors of another sort appeared in their stead.

Among the first substate actors to appear in the twentieth century were the remnants of vanquished forces of nations that surrendered to the Germans in World War II and took up arms as partisans in the service of their defeated army. Only once the war ended did the international community extend combatant protections to partisans. By then, however, partisans had disappeared, replaced by guerrillas, insurgents, and lately terrorists. These forces do not represent sovereign or formerly sovereign nations or the remnants of conventional forces. Rather, they are insurgent or revolutionary movements representing nonstate actors and engaging in asymmetrical conflict against an occupying or colonial state. Decisive conventional warfare did not dominate the post–World War II period. Instead, major conflagrations continued for long periods, as adversaries not easily cowed by enormous firepower fought the great powers to a standstill. In recent years, the focus has been shifting further from conventional warfare as fierce ethnic rivalries break up formerly sovereign states. Paramilitary groups and militia fight one another in a throwback to ancient wars of annihilation. They no longer seek to defeat their enemy by disabling sufficient numbers of soldiers, but to oust one's adversary entirely, soldiers and civilians alike, from the land each side covets. These conflicts continue to confound international law, because the conventional forces insurgents face are bound by a conventional law and morality that their opponents often repudiate.

Medical Neutrality and Unconventional Warfare

The changing climate of contemporary warfare creates new challenges for bioethics. Medical neutrality, firmly entrenched by the middle of the nineteenth century and largely respected by belligerents ever since, is increasingly problematic. Although international law protects medical personnel, medical installations, and the wounded, grave problems arise when adversaries practice terror or abuse the rights and protections that combatants, noncombatants, and medical facilities enjoy. Acute dilemmas arise when wounded combatants turn themselves into suicide bombers, when terrorists harm rescue workers coming to aid the wounded, and when guerrillas use hospitals or ambulances for hostile purposes. These exigencies, the subject of chapter 6, may force military planners to defer the care and evacuation of wounded combatants or civilians, impede the work of medical personnel, or compromise the status of hospitals and ambulances.

Similarly, one may consider that using medical facilities for military purposes conflicts with medical neutrality. During the Vietnam War the U.S. Army established the Medical Civic Action Program (MEDCAP) to provide medical care to "win the hearts and minds" of the South Vietnamese and distance them from the influence of North Vietnamese guerrillas. While the program brought medical care to millions of South Vietnamese, MEDCAP was part of "medical stability operations" designed to pacify the countryside and generate political support for the South Vietnamese government. Medicine became an important tool of war, immediately raising the question whether and how medicine is a legitimate tactic of counterinsurgency warfare. Programs like MEDCAP test the limits of medical neutrality in novel ways unforeseen by bioethics or international law.

Unconventional warfare also forces noncaregiving dilemmas as it tests the willingness of medical personnel to lend their expertise to interrogation or weapons development. These are among the most intractable dilemmas health-care professionals may have to face. Noncaregiving dilemmas are unique to war because they upend the conventional paradigm that guides medical practice within which some aspect of a patient's welfare is always a primary consideration. When confronted with torture and ill-treatment or chemical- and biological-weapons development, the overriding bioethical principle at stake is not beneficence but "do no harm" as medical personnel are called on to use their expertise in a way that causes injury and harm. During armed conflict, however, harm is relative to the legitimate aims of war. Although international conventions prohibit ill-treatment and restrict the development of chemical and biological weapons, difficult questions arise as modern states confront terrorism, battle insurgents and militants fighting among civilians, or attempt to deter other nations wielding nuclear and other unconventional weapons.

Torture and Interrogation

International law categorically prohibits torture and ill-treatment. Nevertheless, some states, particularly those facing the threat of terror, do not always honor the prohibition and physicians continue to find themselves called on to assist in interrogations. While they may not inflict torture directly, physicians play an instrumental role without which investigators could not proceed. At various times, medical personnel verify the health of suspects, certify fitness for extreme forms of interrogation, and treat prisoners following questioning. In violation of humanitarian law, these physicians facilitate "interrogational" torture. Distinct from "terroristic" forms of torture that repressive regimes inflict on their political opponents and ordinary citizens, interrogational torture aims to elicit the information necessary to prevent deadly terror attacks and save innocent lives. Interrogational torture may be "active" and employ various forms of "moderate physical pressure," or "passive" and deny medical care to injured suspects until they provide the information that interrogators seek. As officials in democratic nations push the limits of acceptable interrogation, some observers fear for civil liberties while other are prepared to acknowledge the need for "aggressive" interrogation in exceptional circumstances. Are these attempts to justify ill-treatment defensible? And, if so, may physicians ever participate in any form? These questions anchor the discussion in chapter 7. While medical ethics condemns ill-treatment, physicians may sometimes ask themselves whether they can refuse to participate in activities they may condone for other individuals. A similar difficulty arises as one considers medical involvement in the development of chemical and biological warfare.

Chemical and Biological Warfare

International agreements prohibit the use and development of most kinds of chemical and biological weapons. The World Medical Association, too, declares it unethical for physicians to lend their expertise to the development of unconventional weapons. While most states are destroying their stockpiles of chemical and biological weapons, a significant minority continue to maintain their arsenals of unconventional weapons. This leads some nations to develop deterrent capabilities and forces physicians to face demands that they contribute their expertise to unconventional weapons development.

At the same time, the armed forces in many Western nations weigh the advantages of employing nonlethal chemical weapons in the low-intensity conflicts that increasingly characterize contemporary geopolitics. Unable to bring the force of conventional weapons to bear in built-up urban areas without causing overwhelming devastation, many nations now find it necessary to consider nonlethal, incapacitating alternatives to reduce civilian casualties as they battle insurgents or militants in "military operations other than war." Can medical personnel unilaterally and unequivocally withdraw from weapons development? This question dominates chapter 8 and turns on the ethics of biological and chemical weapons, the history of their development and deployment, and the efforts of the international community to limit their use. Like nuclear weapons, chemical and biological weapons are devastating, imperil the environment, overtax health services, and create unpredictable long-term harm. Nevertheless, many nations maintain their nuclear arsenals if only for deterrent purposes. Increasingly, officials are asking whether they may also develop chemical weapons for their deterrent and/or nonlethal capabilities.

Bioethics and Peace

The international medical community confronts many of the dilemmas just described with the conviction that physicians' duties to care for and serve their patients are absolute and inviolable. As a result, international norms prohibit medical workers from participating in interrogational torture and the development of chemical and biological weapons, affirm the absolute protection due medical personnel and facilities on the battlefield, forcefully assert the right of informed consent, and demand strict neutrality as medical resources are distributed to wounded soldiers.

Is, then, medical ethics in time of war identical to medical ethics in time of peace? The dilemmas at the center of this book clearly suggest that it is not. Medical ethics alone does not offer the tools necessary to resolve the dilemmas described here unless, of course, medicine ignores the exigencies of war. Sometimes it is difficult to escape this conclusion once medicine assumes a "higher calling" that places it beyond the norms and mores of society and reaches instead to a class of higher moral duties not necessarily incumbent on every person. The World Medical Association fails to see a difference between the bioethics of war and the bioethics of peace because it firmly believes that medical personnel are neutral in every sense of the word, not only "protected" but "above the fray" and "foreign" to the practice of war. While they may tend the wounded, their primary concern is their patient's well-being.

Is medicine a pacifist vocation? Should physicians do everything they can to embrace peace and distance themselves from the practice of war? These questions highlight potential difficulties for medicine during war. On the one hand, overriding concern for a patient's interest seems to push medicine toward pacifism and a repudiation of anything remotely connected with taking rather than preserving life. Alternatively, the idea of a "higher calling" may suggest a double standard: abridged patient rights, utilitarian triage, aggressive interrogation, or the development of nonlethal chemical weapons may be necessary practices of war, but those that medical personnel must shun.

Neither implication is appealing. Rather, every citizen, regardless of profession, bears the obligation to assess the morality of war. The idea of a higher calling, if by this one means an appeal to moral principles anchored in dignity and human rights, is the purview of every citizen. But humanitarian law and human dignity do not repudiate war. On the contrary, they justify war when these principles are threatened and regulate the conduct of war when it is necessary. Clearly, there are just wars and unjust wars. When there are good grounds for war, every citizen has an obligation to lend support. When there are no good grounds for war, every citizen bears the responsibility to disobey. In between, we are all compelled to work toward peace. Ordinary citizens struggle hard and long with these conflicting obligations, and the dilemmas medical personnel face are part and parcel of those we all face as we confront the horrors of war and limits of human endurance.

2

The Ethics of Medicine and the Ethics of War

Patient rights, neutrality, distributive justice, interrogational torture, and unconventional warfare pose fundamental dilemmas for medicine during wartime. Attempts to resolve these dilemmas using prevailing principles of biomedical ethics, such as respect for autonomy or beneficence, fail to account for the exigencies of war and often lead observers to advise physicians to wage their war on sickness and injury as if there was no war against an armed adversary. This leads medicine to universally condemn medical participation in torture and the development of unconventional weapons and, at the same time, leaves little patience for violating norms of informed consent, confidentiality, and distributive justice. During war, however, the specter of military necessity raises its head, tempered only by the familiar principles of proportionality and utility. While the bulwark of human dignity may hold fast against torture, military necessity quickly undermines traditional concern for informed consent, confidentiality, justice, and, indeed, the duty to safeguard human life that drives medicine in the first place. In short, it appears that the ethics of medicine and the ethics of war are at odds with one another, utilize conflicting principles, and reach vastly different conclusions about medical practice during wartime.

I suggest that this is not the case. Instead, the ethics of medicine and the ethics of war rest on similar philosophical foundations, and rather than considering each discipline separately, it is more fruitful to view them as representative of a shared set of principles. Both disciplines grew in the shadow of rapidly advancing liberal ideas, staggering technological change, and social upheaval. Each discipline enunciates central principles that draw directly from the Enlightenment: the state's duty to protect an individual's right to life, the paramount place of autonomy, self-determination, and human dignity, and the dictates of utility that constrain the duty to protect life or dignity at any cost. Nevertheless, the primary actors and their concerns differ. In bioethics, two actors dominate moral decision making as physicians and patients consider the duty of one to protect the life and well-being of the other. However, three sets of actors—the state, combatants, and noncombatants—characterize military ethics, and their life, well-being, autonomy, and dignity are incommensurable and often conflict. Ordinary bioethical dilemmas, sufficiently vexing in their own right, become considerably more complex when superimposed on those of medicine during war.

Life, Dignity, and Utility

Table 2.1 describes the range of principles that animate bioethics and contemporary just-war theory.

Four broad sets of principles—the right to life, respect for autonomy, human dignity, and utility—underlie the ethics of medicine and war. As such, there is a rough symmetry between the underlying principles of contemporary just war and bioethics. The duty of a physician or of the state to protect an individual's right to life infuses both disciplines. Whether the right to life is grounded in natural law, contract, or utility is a question to take up shortly, but whatever its source, it generates a concomitant duty on the part of others to protect individual and/or collective life. In most cases, this duty falls to the state as it protects its citizens' right to life together with the collective life and security of the political community. In medicine, a physician's obligation to save life is more narrowly focused and generally puts aside collective or third-party interests to concentrate exclusively on a patient's needs.

War jeopardizes the right to life of both individuals and states. Soldiers enjoy but a conditional right to life that they will lose once they don a uniform and take up arms against one another. During war, civilians only retain a limited right to life. Noncombatant immunity—the state's obligation to protect the lives of enemy noncombatants—falls to the doctrine of double effect. Humanitarian law protects noncombatants from wanton harm, but not from unintentional death and destruction

Table 2.1
Ethical principles of medicine and war

Ethical principles / Subject of concern	Medicine — Patients	War — Individuals — *Noncombatants*	War — Individuals — *Combatants*	War — Collectives — *State/Community*
Right to life (RTL) / *Related principles*	**Full RTL** / Right to medical care / Quality of life	**Abridged RTL** / Noncombatant immunity / Doctrine of double effect	**Conditional RTL** / Right to kill	**National RTL** / Sovereignty / self-defense
Autonomy — Medical autonomy / Political autonomy	**Full** / **Full**	**Full** / **Abridged**	**Abridged** / **Abridged**	**Full political autonomy** / Territorial integrity / Self-determination
Related principles	Informed consent, privacy, confidentiality, the right to die	Freedom of movement, assembly, representation		
Dignity / *Related principles*	**Patient dignity** / Respect for personhood / Non-humiliation	**Human dignity** / Humanitarian law / Freedom from torture, servitude, and degradation		**National dignity** / National honor / Nonhumiliation
Utility / *Related principles*	**Individual utility** / Patient's best interest / Beneficence, nonmaleficence	**Aggregate utility** / Maximum lives / Proportionality	**Aggregate utility** / Maximum salvageable lives / Salvage, return to duty	**Superaggregate utility** / Reason of state / Military necessity

during essential military operations. But aside from the interests of soldiers and civilians, state interests are the first casualty of war. A state's
right to life, solidly enshrined in the idea of "reason of state," often drives
military decision making to the exclusion of all else.

Autonomy and human dignity, two lynchpins of medical and military
ethics, augment the right to life. Autonomy underscores the paramount
role that individuals play as they seize hold of their own destiny by
molding the religious, political, and scientific forces that shape their
lives. In bioethics, respect for autonomy emphasizes the patient's role
in medical decision making. Patients are free to accept or reject medical advice in the same way citizens shape their political destiny as
they choose representatives, vote on policy, and engage in political
activism. Autonomy, however, breaks down during war. Soldiers are
doubly disadvantaged, enjoying marginal autonomy and little of their
right to life as they engage in war. If noncombatants, on the other hand,
enjoy greater protection from harm and continue to retain modest measures of autonomy, they often find their lives less valued than able-bodied
soldiers, who will command a greater share of scarce medical resources
during war.

If war endangers lives and circumscribes autonomy, it should not affect
the protections that human dignity affords. Dignity turns on respect for
the inherent worth of a person qua human being and applies to all individuals equally, a goal yet unrealized but certainly set in motion by the
religious, philosophical, and scientific upheavals of the Enlightenment.
Human dignity is not synonymous with the right to life, for soldiers lose
their right to life while retaining their human dignity. Instead, dignity is
an acknowledgment of an intrinsic value of humanness that should, for
example, prevent torture and ill-treatment at the hands of the enemy.
Nor is dignity the same as autonomy, as medical ethics readily exemplifies. While incompetent patients, for example, lose autonomous decision-
making capacity, they can and should be treated with dignity. Dignity
and autonomy do coincide when patients are competent, for it is difficult, if not impossible, to respect the dignity of competent patients
without allowing them a central and overriding voice in medical decision making. In these ways, respect for human dignity, as distinct from
the right to life and respect for autonomy, is central to both military and

medical ethics. Bioethics and humanitarian law enshrine these three deontological principles: life, autonomy, and dignity.

Finally, one must consider questions of utility that come from trying to preserve life, autonomy, and dignity at any costs. Physicians, for example, must provide beneficent care and "do no harm." Ordinarily, the precept *do no harm* (nonmaleficence) means no more harm than necessary *to a patient*. Because the traditional doctor-patient relationship is dyadic, third-party interests do not, indeed should not, ordinarily affect a physician's obligation to care for patients. Increasingly, however, we are seeing how health-care providers look beyond their patients to consider the interests of both family members and the community at large, particularly as medical costs soar.

The state finds itself in a similar position as it goes about its business of protecting its citizens. The state bears two responsibilities. First, it must consider aggregate utility as it pursues policies to benefit the greatest number of discrete individuals. For noncombatants, aggregate utility is a function of the lives the state can save; for combatants, it is a measure of the number of salvageable soldiers that return to duty. But state interests also transcend aggregate utility to include indivisible collective interests—that is, *super*aggregate utility sometimes defined as "reason of state" or a "way of life." When threatened, states weigh the option of waging war to preserve their citizens' lives or their territorial integrity or national honor. But war is not without costs that may easily impair civil liberties or bring harm to the very citizens whose lives the state purports to defend. As policymakers, military planners, and commanders in the field weigh these costs, they will find that necessity, proportionality, and noncombatant immunity impose strict constraints. One does not pursue war at any cost. Necessity, together with the need to avoid excessive harm, limits the ends and means of armed conflict. The imperative *do no harm*, understood as either avoiding harm on balance or minimizing harm, is as central to bioethics as it is to military ethics.

The right to life, respect for autonomy and dignity, and utility often collide, and when they do the challenge of contemporary bioethics and contemporary military ethics remains to sort out competing principles so that medical or military personnel may act justly and secure the goals each holds dear. This is the essence of resolving any dilemma. However, the problem is considerably more complex when it becomes necessary to compare and contrast principles across two disciplines, as the dilemmas of bioethics and armed conflict demand. This requires a closer look at the fundamental ethical principles of medicine and war.

The Right to Life

If war is ultimately an act of self-defense, a last resort albeit violent attempt to save one's life or the lives of one's compatriots, then medicine and war share at least this common goal: both, ultimately, strive to preserve human life. This includes the lives of patients, soldiers, and civilians.

The health-care professional's duty to save a patient's life is the easiest to understand. Medicine does not need a natural or contractual right to life nor a religiously inspired doctrine of sanctity of life to understand its duty to save life at nearly any cost. It operates under a far different assumption. Death, although inevitable, is a grievous harm. To avert or mitigate death, pain, and suffering, health-care professionals choose to acquire the tools and knowledge of medicine. Their duty is a professional one, imposed by a covenant or "sacred trust" between the profession and the members of society that doctors care for. "The existence of genuine medical need," write Pellegrino and Thomasma (1993, 36), "constitutes a moral claim on those equipped to help." At no time is this need greater than when a person faces avoidable death.

The right to medical care is not yet a political claim right anchored in an individual's civil liberties and incumbent on the welfare state to respect. Rather, it is, as Pellegrino and Thomasma suggest, a right bound up in the moral relationship between doctor and patient. Only later would many modern states step in and assume an obligation to provide the means for universal medical care. Both physicians and the state would also cooperate to limit a patient's right to life as galloping technology forced the medical and legal community to realize that it is neither medically desirable nor respectful of a patient's other rights to assume an absolute obligation to keep a patient alive at any cost. Until the invention of sophisticated life-support systems, medicine fought death with a certain equanimity and resignation born of a desire to prolong life and reduce suffering as best it could. For the most part, their best efforts would accomplish both these ends simultaneously.

With the advent of advanced life support and medical care, however, it became possible to prolong life without necessarily reducing suffering or improving a person's quality of life. As questions of end of life and beginning of life mounted, the medical community turned to the state to define the limits of a person's right to life and a physician's concomitant obligation to preserve life and provide medical care. The liberal state, for the most part, deferred to patient self-determination, allowing competent patients—or physicians and family when patients were not competent—to limit their right to life when its quality deteriorated. This process progressed slowly, demanding not only the cooperation of the medical community, but also the assent of the political community together with its courts and legislature to alter the traditional obligation of the state to protect the lives of its citizens.

The State's Duty to Protect Life

The state's duty to protect life is the centerpiece of modern political theory, spanning both theories of natural rights and utilitarianism. Contract theory made the first and boldest claim to an individual's natural right to life and the state's concomitant duty to protect it. The *right* to life was a new idea and not at all identical to the *sanctity* of life of earlier times. Sanctity of life acknowledged God's ownership of life; people were merely entrusted with their living bodies until God decided differently. Scientific advances, however, rapidly made Creators out of men and women, undermined religious and feudal authority, and emboldened individuals to shape political society in their image rather than God's. The Enlightenment endowed people with a certain omnipotence and absolute freedom that they would then exchange for security and other goods that only a well-organized state could provide.

Absolute freedom was the starting point for the Enlightenment's thinkers. But it was not their end point. Instead, absolute freedom marked the beginning of a theoretical exercise to justify the coercive power of the state necessary for domestic and international order. Assuming that absolute freedom characterized the natural state of all human beings, the puzzle turned on how to move from an absolutely free state of nature to the less-than-free state in which one finds oneself in political society. The social contract provided an answer as individuals freely relinquished some of their basic freedoms in return for the state's promise to provide security. Unlike the sacred trust between physicians and patients born of the knowledge of the one and need of the other, the political "trust," to use Locke's term, was the product of an agreement that obligated the state to safeguard every individual's rights and vital interests. To do so, states enact and enforce laws to preserve law and order. They may also go to war.

War presents special problems for contract theory. How does an individual safeguard his vital interests by laying down his life in defense of the state? What could possibly justify war, as it destroys the lives, liberty, and property of those the state was founded to protect? One answer turns to utilitarianism. The state considers the lives and interests of all its members equally. The state makes war to save its citizens' lives and property from foreign aggressors on the assumption that natural rights and civil liberties *in the aggregate* will suffer more at the hands of invaders than from the ravages of war. But is this always the case? It is an often-noted paradox of war that surrender to an invading force will generally spare more lives than it costs. Yet few states, particularly in modern times, ever surrender for this reason. On the contrary, no nation freely gives itself over to another, and common sense dictates that when one nation threatens another, the victimized nation has the right to defend itself. The state responds to this threat by raising an army and making war. Measured only by lives lost and property destroyed, few wars could meet the demand of utility if aggregate welfare was the only criterion of success. Instead, states and their citizens must be fighting for something else beyond their rights and property. And, indeed, they are.

The State's Duty to Safeguard Collective Life and Interests

Wars protect more than the aggregate lives of a state's citizens. They also protect the state and the political community. The state encompasses the formal trappings of sovereignty: institutions of government, law enforcement, and security; international recognition; and clearly delineated borders. A political community may be of prior construction and denotes the framework of cultural, educational, linguistic, and social traditions that allow individuals to formulate and pursue a common vision of the good life. The interests of the state and the community (or communities) it nurtures and protects through its political institutions are more than the sum of those of its individual members. These are superaggregate interests and speak to the welfare of the community as a personality in its own right.

The idea of a superaggregate, collective personality is often attributed to Rousseau's idea of the General Will. Contrasting the General Will with the Will of All, Rousseau was convinced that a contracted state generated more than the aggregate interest of all its members. Rather, it created a new, corporate interest that served the moral life of each and every member. This idea of the state harks back to the ancient city-state that not only saw to the interests of each of its members but also developed a common, communal life that *transformed* the interests of its members. Individuals altered and adapted their preferences, desires, interests, and, indeed, their very political consciousness to conform to those of the General Will. Rousseau's General Will does not represent the majority or aggregate of private interests but a different level of moral consciousness that embraces a shared and communal life plan.

As the modern state evolved, national honor replaced the glory of kings or gods that motivated men to fight in earlier times. Intense, national patriotism along with great armies of conscripted citizen-soldiers fueled Napoléon's contribution to the ferocity of modern warfare and enabled him to put hundreds of thousands of men in the field. Growing civic consciousness, particularly on the Continent, energized collectivist or organic theories of state that ascribe an intrinsic value to the modern state beyond the interests of its individual members. Not bald economic growth, but only the formative cultural spirit (Volksgeist) of the nation-state would contribute to humankind's greater purpose, its Weltgeist. But one need not raise the ghosts of German Romanticism to see that the state, for most individuals, embodies significant value beyond the aggregate welfare of its members. The state assumes a superpersonality with moral interests of its own.

During war, this vision takes hold in any state, no matter how liberal, as men and women not only fight to preserve their lives, rights, and property but are often willing to sacrifice these interests to preserve the integrity of their state and community. Ethnic and national groups clamor for statehood to protect the narrow interests of their members but, more importantly, to leave their mark on the world community without which their national "self" is irreversibly crippled. National self-determination—a state's right to express and defend its superaggregate interests—ranks as high, if not higher, than its duty to protect the lives of its citizens. During armed conflict, the overwhelming desire to preserve state and collective interests jeopardizes the lives of the very citizens the state is sworn to protect, to say nothing of those on the other side. What, then, remains of the individual's right to life? If bioethics respects every person's right to life without exception and without qualification, war abridges the rights of combatants and noncombatants alike.

Combatants and Noncombatants

A firm distinction between combatants and noncombatants is essential to ascribe rights and duties to each. The 1949 Geneva Conventions (Article 3) enshrine a parsimonious but increasingly difficult-to-sustain distinction: noncombatants are "persons taking no active part in the hostilities" and include prisoners of war and the wounded, while civilians are simply "people who do not bear arms." Combatants, on the other hand, bear arms and take an active part in the hostilities as members of opposing armed forces. Combatants must be "commanded by a person responsible for his subordinates, have a fixed distinctive sign recognizable at a distance, carry arms openly and conduct their operations in accordance with the laws and customs of war" (Rogers 1996, 8; also Geneva Convention (I), 1949a, Article 13 (2); Green 2000, 102–122).

While this includes irregular soldiers, volunteer corps, partisans, and members of militias, it excludes "illegal combatants": common criminals, freelance fighters, and terrorists. While many difficulties plague our attempt to cogently define an "active part in the hostilities" (below), one generally thinks in terms of two discrete groups of actors, combatants and noncombatants, each with its own set of rights and obligations.

There are interesting changes afoot, however. By 1977, it was clear that the nature of war was rapidly changing. Guerrillas and insurgents fighting wars of national liberation replaced partisans fighting as a remnant of the defeated conventional forces of a sovereign state. Civilians, in turn, found themselves entangled with combatants far more intensely in the postwar period than in previous conflicts. Guerrillas operated from, and trained within, civilian areas, vigorously and sometimes violently recruiting material aid and labor from noncombatants. Civilians now found themselves actively a part of hostilities in way that did not characterize previous conflicts.

To address the newly emerging and more precarious position of both combatants and noncombatants, the international community updated the 1949 Geneva Conventions. The 1977 Protocols, ratified by all but a handful of nations, expand the definition of *combatant* to include guerrillas fighting wars of national liberation against "colonial, alien and racist regimes" (hence "CAR" conflicts) and broaden the protections that the war convention accords to civilians.[1] Legal combatants must serve as part of a military organization that enforces compliance with international law, but they need not wear distinctive insignia or carry their arms openly at all times. This denies combatant status to criminals, terrorists, freelance fighters, and rogue militia. Guerrillas, militants, and insurgents, however, enjoy the status of combatants and the rights of prisoners of war (POWs) (Protocol I, 1977a, Article 44).[2]

In all this, one's "active" role in the hostilities remains crucial. If uniforms no longer distinguish combatants from noncombatants, the essential defining feature remains one's active participation in acts of war. Apart from those who bear arms, whether in uniform or not, there are always those who take a more active part in war than others. How are these individuals to be treated? Ordinarily one tries to distinguish between those who contribute to the threat war poses and those who do not. Gordon Graham (1997, 67), for example, makes a simple distinction: "Combatants are those people the purpose of whose activity is to contribute to the threat; noncombatants are those people who do not actively contribute in this sense, although they may constitute part of the relevant causal chain."

Graham's purpose is clear: enemy civilians will inevitably contribute to the war effort in one way or another. However, unless they expressly contribute to the threat war presents to others, then they retain their status as noncombatants. The threat, in most cases, is an armed threat. Those who contribute to an armed threat are those who are themselves armed, those who arm them, and those who command them. Munitions workers lose their immunity; bakers and tailors do not. During insurgency, civilians may contribute directly to the war effort by storing arms or by sheltering, hosting, or transporting insurgents and/or terrorists. But drawing a firm line is difficult. While noncombatants may not bear arms, they provide their soldiers with succor, food, and clothing. As they do so, many civilians who support guerrillas would probably argue that they cannot effectively resist opening their homes to insurgents. Inasmuch as most occupied civilians are vulnerable to some measure of coercion, however "friendly," denying them noncombatant status would effectively gut the concept. As a result, the combatant-noncombatant distinction does not always signify two discrete groups but rather ends on a continuum. At its extremes, the distinctions and respective rights of each group are clear. Nevertheless, there are those gray cases that muddy any clear distinction and ascription of rights. These problems are especially acute during insurgency warfare and raise a number of problems for bioethics and humanitarian law that did not arise in earlier forms of warfare. I will consider these in detail in chapter 6.

Combatants' Right to Life   During war, a state no longer has an overriding duty to preserve the lives of all its citizens. The state may not wantonly harm its own soldiers or jeopardize their lives needlessly, but it will certainly place many of its young men and women in harm's way. Faced with an armed adversary, soldiers suddenly find that they command the right to kill but no longer retain an unconditional right to life. Innocent of any wrongdoing, many will be shot and killed. Soldiers, therefore, lose their right to life conditionally in armed combat and only insofar as the risk of death serves broad, usually very broad, military goals.

How does this happen? By what right may a state sacrifice the lives of some of its citizens in order to protect the lives of others? One answer suggests that soldiers *agree* to give up their right to life to protect others or to protect the integrity of the state. This reflects the contractual nature of political obligation. While enlisting soldiers agree willingly, conscripts consent tacitly, either because they choose to remain where they live or fail to object to military service. Tacit consent, however, is a thin basis on which to ground such a weighty obligation. Most citizens have no realistic option of emigrating or refusing conscription during wartime. Instead, one might see young conscripts as rational beings who will consent to a hypothetical contract akin to Rawls's original position. Assuming a fair system of distributing the burden of national defense, most individuals would buy in when war is necessary to protect the common good. But this is not always so. Fighting in a war and endangering oneself for the common good poses a classic collective-action problem. Yossarian put it best in Joseph Heller's novel *Catch-22* (1996, 113):

Yossarian I don't want to be in the war anymore.
Major Major Would you like to see our country lose?
Y We won't lose. We've got more men, more money and more material. There are ten million men in uniform who could replace me. Some people are getting killed and a lot more are making money and having fun. Let somebody else get killed.
MM But suppose everybody on our side felt that way?
Y Then I'd certainly be a damned fool to feel any other way. Wouldn't I?

Yossarian's self-interested logic is impeccable, and to avoid calamity, the state must coerce individuals into risking their lives so the state can fulfill its duty to protect the lives of its citizens and the integrity of its community. A contract, real or hypothetical, does not bind individuals to defend one another in times of crisis. Instead, they contract with one another in order to impose a sovereign who will coerce them into risking their lives when it is in their rational interest to avoid fighting. Otherwise, there can be no security. Hobbes recognized this dilemma very clearly.[3]

In the absence of any clear contractual commitment to give up one's life, perhaps the logic of self-defense offers soldiers the right to kill and endangers their right to life? Paradigm cases of self-defense pit two individuals against one another, an attacker (A) and a victim (V). Additional players include bystanders (B) who can intervene at relatively little cost. To justify V's right to kill A, as well as B's obligation to intervene, A must pose a "material threat"—that is, an immediate and otherwise unavoidable grave or mortal threat that less violent means cannot eliminate. In addition, A's action must be morally unjustified and without cause, A must intend to kill or gravely injure V, and A must be responsible for his action (uncoerced and without diminished mental capacities). Under these circumstances V may kill A because A is "morally noninnocent," so that A's right to life is lost, suspended, or overridden by either V's right to life and/or his right to self-defense (see Montague 1981; McMahan 1994a; Norman 1995; Thomson 1986). These conditions, however, do not apply to combatants. During armed conflict, soldiers may kill one another whether armed or unarmed, whether posing a grievous threat or idly standing by, and whether innocent or noninnocent. Even as soldiers threaten one another materially, they remain *innocent* aggressors. Most are coerced to fight. As they do, each is convinced of the justice of his cause. Material and moral noninnocence no longer characterize either party. Both aggressors and victims may legitimately kill one another during war and, at the same time, both lose their right to life as they face off.

The logic is almost counterintuitive. Ordinary aggressors lose their right to life because they pose material and noninnocent threats to others that less violent means cannot avert. Soldiers, however, lose their right to life once they assume a place in their nation's armed forces. It does not matter whether their nation is a victim or aggressor or their cause is just or unjust. Consider the German soldier who shoots at a defending Pole in September 1939. The Pole shoots back and misses. The German returns fire and kills the defender. Although history presents few unequivocal cases of blatant aggression, Germany's invasion of Poland is certainly one of them. Nevertheless, every Allied soldier knew that his German counterpart retained a right to self-defense even if his nation did not. But if a state is noninnocent, then its emissaries are equally culpable. If soldiers gain their right to self-defense when their state is victimized, they should lose it when their nation is an aggressor. But this does not seem to be the case. Aggressors and victims are equally vulnerable on the battlefield. The idea of moral innocence does not help us understand a soldier's right to kill any more than noninnocence explains away his right to life.

This is one of the peculiarities of armed conflict, and perhaps only an appeal to positive law solidifies a soldier's right to kill and, with it, the loss of his or her right to life. A state's right to wage war is a matter of customary and treaty law that complements a state's right to compel its citizens to fight and kill. As states evaluate the threats they face, they may call on their armed forces to implement military policy. Subject to international law, the world community recognizes the rights of sovereign states (and some quasi-state actors) to wage war in defense of vital interests and, at the same time, the right of each state to enact laws that strip some of its citizens of their right to life and accord them the right to kill. Each state, aggressor and defender alike, authorizes particular groups of individuals, namely its soldiers, to kill one another. We may be tempted to speak in terms of rights, of the right to self-defense and of the right to kill in self-defense, or in terms of moral and material noninnocence, but these only force the counterexamples described earlier. Nations go to war for a wide variety of reasons. Some are victims of bald aggression, while others face threats that only impinge on their honor. Nevertheless, each commands the authority to expend the lives of its soldiers while permitting them to kill others charged with a similar mission.

Noncombatants' Right to Life   International law makes a concerted effort to protect noncombatants from harm and affirm their right to life:

Protected persons [persons taking no active part in the hostilities, including members of armed forces who have laid down their arms and those placed *hors de combat*—literally "out of combat" and referring to wounded or captured combatants who can no longer fight due to sickness, wounds, detention, or any other cause] are entitled, in all circumstances, to respect for their persons, their honour, their family rights, their religious convictions and practices, and their manners and customs. They shall at all times be humanely treated, and shall be protected especially against all acts of violence or threats thereof. (Geneva Convention (IV), 1949d, Article 27)

The principle of noncombatant immunity is the cornerstone of international humanitarian law and shields noncombatants from harm during war. While its protection is sweeping, it is not, in principle, blanket or absolute. It is both inevitable and morally acceptable that noncombatants suffer harm during armed conflict. While civilians are immune from intentional harm, they may suffer as the unavoidable side effect of a necessary military operation. This is the doctrine of double effect. In other, far rarer cases, noncombatants may face intentional harm when a state faces an existential threat. This is the principle of supreme emergency.

When harm befalls noncombatants, belligerents are apt to appeal to the doctrine of double effect (DDE) and claim that they did not *mean* to harm innocents or that their deaths are a foreseen but unintended outcome of a legitimate act of war. Typically, the doctrine of double effect imposes several conditions:

1. The act itself must be morally good or at least indifferent.
2. The agent may not positively will the bad effect but may permit it.
3. The good effect must flow from the action at least as immediately as the bad effect. In other words, the good effect must be produced directly by the action, not by the bad effect. Otherwise the agent would be using a bad means to a good end, which is never allowed.
4. The good effect must be sufficiently desirable to compensate for the bad effect. (Connell 1967, 229)

While the DDE is an important principle of military ethics, it does not always work as many intend. By design, it permits harm that comes from pursuing a just cause or morally good act, and prohibits harm to noncombatants as a result of war crimes and other acts of war that intentionally and unnecessarily take their lives. Unfortunately, the DDE is rather elastic, easily encompassing nearly any unintended act of violence that a perpetrator declares necessary to prosecute a war.

Finding a legitimate expression for the DDE that properly discriminates between legitimate and illegitimate cases of harm to noncombatants requires a firm definition of intent. But this has proved elusive. What does it mean, for example, when a pilot who bombs a ball-bearing factory and kills thousands of civilians living nearby says that he did not *mean* to kill them? Are we concerned solely with the perpetrator's subjective state of mind? While this might be a reasonable interpretation of intentionality, it leads us to judge similar acts differently. Consider two pilots who bomb the same factory. The first aims at the factory and although he knows that some of his bombs will kill enemy civilians he truly does not intend to kill them. The second also aims at the factory but is pleased knowing his bombs will also kill enemy civilians. Does one act violate the DDE and the other not?

Cases such as these lead observers to ferret out alternative meanings of intentionality. One possibility imposes the test of failure: would a mission fail if the harmful effects were avoided? In each case above, the answer is no. Either mission could succeed if no civilians were killed. These acts, regardless of the death and destruction they bring to civilians, keep faith with the DDE. This is not true when a terror bomber requires noncombatant deaths to demoralize his enemy. The terror bomber cannot succeed without killing innocent civilians. Terror bombing intentionally causes harm and violates the DDE. Warren Quinn (1989) fleshes out the argument further. The critical question is whether "the victims are made to play a role in the service of the agent's goal that is not (or may not be) morally required of them and this aspect of direct agency adds its own negative moral force—a force over and above that provided by the fact of harming or failing to prevent harm" (p. 342). This moral fact is decisive for Quinn, who readily points out that a strategic bomber "perhaps . . . cannot honestly say that this [harmful] effect will be 'unintentional' in any standard sense, or that he 'does not mean' to kill them. But he can honestly deny that their involvement in the [bombing] is anything to his purpose" (p. 342; also see McMahan 1994a).

These arguments repudiate subjective intentionality and focus instead on the outcomes: Were civilian deaths part of the purpose one seeks to achieve? Was one's purpose morally defensible—that is, necessary to obtain a good end? Was the harm befalling noncombatants necessary, or were alternative means available to achieve the same goal at a lower cost? Answers to these questions determine the legitimacy of harming civilians during war. During armed conflict, the right to life—a central tenet of bioethics—weakens considerably as the result of the exigencies and vicissitudes of war.

The limitations war imposes on the right to life have important implications as we consider an important subsidiary of the right to life, namely, the right to receive medical care. Ordinarily, individuals enjoy the right to receive medical care as an extension of their right to life. While the few industrialized nations without universal health care may still dispute this, most nations and, indeed, the UN Declaration of Human Rights, recognize a person's basic right to health care. A combatant's right to life, however, is weak and this may jeopardize his or her right to speedy evacuation and medical care for wounds sustained in battle. Because soldiers have conditionally lost their right to life, one can credibly ask whether similar conditions constrain their right to receive medical treatment. This question is the subject of the following chapter. By the same token, the exigencies of war limit respect for a noncombatant's right to life and treatment during hostilities.

Noncombatant Immunity and Supreme Emergency Noncombatant immunity also suffers when nations face a supreme emergency—that is, a threat of such magnitude that it overrides the conventions of war and allows belligerents to intentionally harm noncombatants to bring an enemy to its knees (Walzer 1977, 251–268; Coates 1997, 260–264; Orend 2001). I will consider this problem again in chapter 8. Here, however, three points are important. First, existential threats remain obscure and difficult to define. Is the demise of the political community sufficient to trigger a supreme emergency or must a nation face genocide? The Nazis devastated Poland, killing and imprisoning many Poles. Is this sufficient to permit the Poles to attack German civilians indiscriminately, or must Germany threaten Poland with genocidal extermination? Second, there is little evidence to suggest that attacks on civilians do much to demoralize or cripple an enemy in any significant way. On the contrary, reprisals and terror attacks often have much the opposite effect (Quester 1990). Finally, existential threats, however defined, are in the eyes of the beholder. The British bombing campaign against Germany early in World War II, the American attack on Hiroshima, and many contemporary terrorists all repudiate noncombatant immunity in the name of supreme emergency. Yet, in retrospect, there is little to suggest that a nation's existence hung in the balance or, if it did, that egregious violations of noncombatant immunity had any significant strategic value. Should these conditions change, however, we would be compelled to ask whether medical professionals may set aside their professional duties and contribute their expertise to weapons development and other acts of war.

Autonomy and Dignity

Just as soldiering and war curtail a person's right to life, they also affect autonomy. Dignity and respect for autonomy, two distinct concepts, are central to bioethics and color nearly every dilemma perplexing health-care professionals. Dignity, the intrinsic value we attach to any human being, is a fundamental and overriding component of contemporary just-war theory and international humanitarian law. It animates the UN Declaration of Human Rights and the Geneva Conventions. It underlies respect for human personhood regardless of cognitive competence and protects individuals from humiliation, dishonor, ill-treatment, and servitude. In contrast, autonomy or self-determination reflects the cognitive capacity of human beings to legislate or determine their own ends and vision of the good life. As individuals contemplate these ends and the means necessary to realize them, they exercise the freedom to shape their own lives. Respect for autonomy cuts across deontological and utilitarian moral theories. For the former, it is a fundamental and defining element of Kantian ethics; for the latter, an essential component of human happiness. For both, respect for autonomy generates a firm basis for civil and political liberties that include political participation, representation, freedom of religion, assembly, and conscience, and equality before the law. Self-determination and respect for autonomy anchor these liberties and form the necessary components of human development.

Alongside the rights of the individual stand those of the community. A political community's right to autonomy or self-determination is a constant feature of international politics. Nation-states demand that others respect their autonomy, sovereignty, and territorial integrity. Emerging political communities make similar demands. Some settle for partial autonomy; others will wage war to gain greater rights. Some degree of autonomy is necessary to ensure aggregate welfare, provide security and stability, protect liberty, safeguard property, and promote economic prosperity. At the same time, the fully independent and autonomous state fulfills superaggregate interests, enabling a political community to realize its national ethos or "way of life" as it draws its linguistic, cultural, religious, and historical heritage into the state's political institutions. A well-developed national ethos serves two purposes. First, it offers a psychological anchor and source of pride for individuals—that is, a point of bearing for the development of their own identity. Second, a well-developed collective personality firmly grounded in the institutions of state allows a political community to pursue foreign and domestic policies that foster its own vision of human good and leave its mark, for better or for worse, on the world.

Autonomy in Bioethics

In bioethics, respect for autonomy spawns a number of derivative principles that guide medical practice. These include informed consent, respect for privacy, and confidentiality. Informed consent demands access to sufficient information to make an intelligent decision about one's own medical care under conditions free from coercion and undue influence. While these conditions are difficult to fully realize in practice—information is never sufficient, complete, or entirely certain, patients often lack competence, and even the most competent are never entirely free of pain, anxiety, dependence, or "undue" influence—medical practice has made tremendous strides in the last several decades to draw patients in as equal partners in the decision making process. Informed consent also entails informed refusal and the right to die as patients refuse medical treatment and life-saving care. Autonomy ensures privacy and confidentiality as it strengthens the doctor-patient relationship and alters the propriety of medical information. Patients gain greater access to their own medical records, while health-care professionals must guard sensitive patient information from those inside and outside the profession.

In and of themselves, these principles provoke little controversy today. While they may sometimes conflict with one another in the course of day-to-day practice, more serious problems arise when autonomy and its derivative principles conflict with the right to life and the state's duty to protect collective and individual life. The "right to die with dignity" is inherently problematic for the modern liberal state that must protect life, dignity, *and* autonomous decision making. No state can fulfill all three obligations simultaneously. If it grants free and autonomous decision making, the state cannot, at the same time, vigorously protect its citizens who choose to end their lives. Refusing care not only complicates a physician's duty to preserve life; it ultimately confounds the state's same duty. Liberal states resolved this dilemma slowly, gradually according near-sacrosanct status to respect for autonomy as competent and incompetent patients gained the right to refuse and withdraw life-sustaining treatment and, in some cases, demand physician-assisted death.

Although respect for autonomy enjoys widespread support, there is now a growing debate, indeed backlash, over and against excessive autonomy when patients unnecessarily risk their own lives. Often, this debate turns on the relative value of autonomy and life. While few nations allow doctors to treat competent patients by force (Gross 2005), physicians in many other nations are wondering whether the right to life, the duty to preserve life, and patient autonomy ought to be balanced more equally and in a way that might better serve a patient's needs (Veatch 1984; Childress 1990; Glick 1997).

Throughout this debate, respect for autonomy is juxtaposed with paternalism—that is, "self"-ruled versus "other"-ruled. Overlooked, however, is the fact that "self"-ruled also connotes "selfishly" ruled. Autonomous decision making generally promotes individual patient interests as distinct from those of the patient's family, ethnic group, or society at large. Patient needs are also at the center of medical paternalism. Autonomous patients decide by themselves about themselves. Paternalistic health-care professionals decide by themselves about their patients. Each decision maker looks after the welfare of the patient, and this emphasis is a staple of Western medical care.

However, the range of affected interests can easily change. A patient or doctor, for example, may wonder how the high cost of continued treatment affects the financial health of a child, spouse, or society. Normally, these concerns do not overly occupy patients or their doctors. They do occupy policymakers, however, who must wrestle with questions of macroallocation as legislators versed in utilitarianism aim to maximize aggregate utility. In some cases, macroallocation decisions may harm a particular patient's interests. Counting each individual equally, policymakers strive to satisfy the preferences of the largest number of individuals. For these calculations, the unit of analysis remains the anonymous, self-interested person. The unit of analysis changes dramatically, however, as one moves from individual or aggregate well-being to the superaggregate welfare that characterizes the state, its people, and its political community. From this perspective, the idea of autonomy as self-determination loses its force if by this we mean the self deciding by itself for itself. The individual is no longer of great concern to either autonomists or paternalists. Instead, each focuses its gaze on interests and reason of state. This transformation is especially pronounced during war.

Autonomy during Armed Conflict

Nations seldom wage war to protect the greatest number of citizens from harm. Rarely do some individuals give their lives so that many others may live. Instead, they die in the name of some national interest. The interest may be tangible, disputed territory for example, or such entirely abstract interests as honor and prestige. During war, individual interests vanish from calculations of costs and benefits as military leaders show little concern for aggregate utility. Soldier's lives are a means to a supremely important end. This end is not necessarily saving more lives.

The decisive shift in autonomy during war is not "who will rule?" but "whose interests will rule?" Military service, regardless of a nation's state of war, limits a person's autonomy, right to self-determination, and derivative civil liberties. Military personnel do not enjoy full autonomy. The state usurps this right out of consideration for the task military personnel must perform in the service of the common good. The nation and its army immerse themselves in a collective undertaking to further state or statelike interests. In this context, autonomy cannot mean personal rule of the self for the good of the self, for the good of the self is of little concern to the military. If anything, autonomy may mean rule of the self for the common, superaggregate good. Consider, for example, the autonomy of commanders-in-chief who, by definition, retain self-rule but rule by themselves for the benefit of the state, not for their own good. This is true of military commanders down the line. Successful military hierarchies know that flexible, autonomous, and creative commanders are the hallmark of great armies. In this way, any member of the hierarchy, from squad leader on up, is autonomous. While military planners higher up impose the ends of war, local commanders retain a considerable degree of freedom to decide the means necessary to achieve their objectives. But they do not decide in their own interests, nor do they necessarily weigh the welfare of those immediately under their command. Instead, they consider the common goal they are all fighting for.

Soldiers without command authority may also ask whether they are effectively fighting for the collective good they cherish. Lacking the information they need to answer the question, they often demur to those in command. As the locus of concern shifts from individual interests to reason of state, the knowledge necessary to maximize efficient outcomes is no longer the purview of the individual soldier but is invested with others. The assumption that those higher up command better information than those below drives every military hierarchy. But this is not always true, and sometimes soldiers may ask themselves whether they are fighting effectively or justly for collective interests. Refusing immoral orders because they violate the community's collective sense of justice is but one example of soldiers exercising their autonomy.

Observers sometimes note that a soldier's autonomy "dramatically decreases" as battle approaches (Howe and Martin 1991, 23). As the arguments in the preceding paragraph suggest, however, this may not be the case at all. Officers' autonomy may increase while ordinary soldiers assume the responsibility of gauging the morality of the war they fight. No soldier, whether enlisted or conscripted, sheds his or her moral responsibilities or decision-making capacity. Both may defer many decisions to others who command greater resources and information, understanding that the importance of individual interests—that is, of *their own* interests—diminishes in the face of collective welfare. Military service, therefore, limits autonomy in this way: self-rule is not always selfish, and the less selfish it becomes the less most individuals, particularly ordinary soldiers, have to say about it. At the end of the day, self-rule generally gives way to other-ruled. Because military service, particularly during war, limits autonomy, it necessarily curtails its derivative rights. These include both medical rights (informed consent, privacy, and confidentiality) and civil liberties (freedom of movement, assembly, and representation). But if war abridges autonomy and its derivative rights and liberties, armed conflict should have no effect on the protection that comes from human dignity.

Dignity: An Absolute Moral Right?

In its original etymology, *dignity* denotes worth and merit. *Human* dignity is the worth and merit we accord to human beings and to the preservation of their basic human qualities. Some of these qualities depend on sentience and include self-respect and independent thinking. Others depend only on the human form and include respect for bodily integrity and the modesty that sentient humans would demand regardless of their cognitive state. Dignity resonates with Kant's dictum to avoid treating others as means as one pursues one's own ends. Dignity also demands that states afford individuals the means to achieve self-respect and control of their own lives without fear or degradation. In the Kantian tradition, human worth and dignity are closely allied with autonomy. "Why do human beings have such an exalted value?" asks Daniel Statman (2001, 546). "Because," he writes, "they are rational beings capable of legislating universal laws and of freeing themselves from the determinism of the natural world. 'Autonomy,' says Kant, 'is then the basis for the dignity of a human being and of every rational creature.'" Undermining either robs individuals of their ability to freely self-legislate the ends of their own life (see Dillon 1995, 14–18; Spiegelberg 1970).

If dignity reflects the intrinsic value of humanness, it may also be absolute and inviolable. This is how Kant views it and how dignity is enshrined in the UN Declaration of Human Rights:

Recognition of the inherent dignity and of the equal and inalienable rights of all members of the human family is the foundation of freedom, justice and peace in the world. (Preamble)

All human beings are born free and equal in dignity and rights. They are endowed with reason and conscience and should act towards one another in a spirit of brotherhood. (Article 1)

In the eyes of the international community dignity is a prior, paramount human attribute that forms the fountainhead of a family of inalienable rights that include life, liberty, security, freedom from slavery, and recognition as a person before the law. As such, dignity is inviolable and its derivative rights nonderogable during public emergency, war, or the threat of war.

Elevating dignity to an absolute principle reduces moral decision making to the relatively simple act of identifying and condemning actions that violate human dignity. The international community resolves this issue unambiguously, and the first eighteen articles of the Declaration of Human Rights enumerate those inalienable rights that no nation may violate under any circumstances and irrespective of public emergency.

Paramount among these are the right to life, freedom from torture, slavery, servitude, and retroactive legislation, freedom of conscience, the right to recognition before the law, and the right not to be imprisoned for breach of contract. Any violation of these rights constitutes an inexcusable affront to human dignity (International Covenant on Civil and Political Rights, 1976, Article 4).

Nevertheless, the idea of absolute dignity, although appealing, may be unworkable in the moral atmosphere of medicine and war. Common experience shows us how even "inalienable" rights can conflict. I have already noted how self-respect and the state's duty to protect an individual's right to life clash when a person wishes to die with dignity. Aggressive interrogation to elicit information to prevent terror attacks poses a similar dilemma, because the right to life of some conflicts with the dignity of others. Which principle prevails in these cases? The answer is not always clear, nor do states resolve the issue in the same way.

It is clear, however, that states and individuals govern themselves by several principles of overriding significance and try, as best they can, to maximize all of them. When these principles conflict, intense dilemmas arise that require one to rank disparate norms. How a community ranks contesting norms will depend on the prevailing cultural milieu. Some democracies rank dignity and autonomy above life; others will place life at the top. There is nothing in liberal theory, per se, to determine how liberal states must rank basic rights and norms. Nevertheless, the very fact that these principles conflict undermines the absolutist position. Dignity directs us to avoid humiliating and degrading other human beings or committing any other act that deprives them of their autonomy as rational human beings. Normally, this prohibits taking innocent lives, torture, or ill-treatment. Nevertheless, we must ask whether the rights that the international community anchors in human dignity ever conflict or give way to other moral obligations.

Dignity and Self-Esteem

Competing principles characterize any moral dilemma, but is dignity one of several competing norms or a supreme principle that overrides all others when they conflict? To resolve this confusion it is useful to distinguish between dignity as a measure of the fundamental worth of any human being and dignity as self-esteem. In the former sense, which I will refer to hereafter simply as "dignity," dignity functions as an overarching moral principle that yields a number of subsidiary principles that we term "human rights," for they derive their authority from basic attributes of humanness rather than from contingent political arrangements. These derivative rights include the right to life, respect for autonomy, and self-esteem. To violate any or all of these rights is to deny a person his or her dignity. As derivative principles, however, they may occasionally conflict and none, therefore, is absolute. For this reason, some observers invoke Kant with caution, aware that his thinking may generate competing absolute moral injunctions (Beauchamp and Childress 1994, 60–61).

Dignity in the sense I will refer to as "self-esteem" underlies many of the provisions of humanitarian law. Self-esteem ranks high among Rawls's primary goods. It is a function of how one views oneself, that is, a sense of one's own value and confidence in one's own life plans, and of how others view oneself, that is, an indication of the respect individuals accord their fellow men and women as they pursue their vision of the good (Rawls 1971, 440). Without self-esteem, human endeavor is crippled. Degradation, humiliation, ill-treatment, and debasement, whether by physical, political, or psychological means, impair self-esteem and make it impossible for anyone to formulate much less realize the goals that will make them better people.

Nevertheless, self-esteem, however crucial for human growth and important among primary goods, is only one good among others that include liberty, opportunity, wealth, and income. Clearly, these can conflict, and when they do no single principle commands obvious authority.[4] Human dignity, on the other hand, is a statement about the absolute worth of human beings but is not an operational principle. In this sense, all of Rawls's primary goods together with human rights guaranteed by the international community contribute to human dignity. Yet dignity, as such, cannot resolve conflicts among is derivative principles. Self-esteem, respect for autonomy, the right to life, and the right to a decent life can all conflict. Affronts to self-esteem abound in war and suggest that respect for self-esteem may pose greater difficulties for contemporary just-war theory than for bioethics. This is largely true, although the concept of self-esteem in bioethics is not without its difficulties and ambiguities.

Dignity and Self-Esteem in Bioethics Self-esteem, as important a concept as it is, excites no great moral controversy nor is it the stuff of difficult bioethical dilemmas. Few would contest a physician's obligation to respect self-esteem and avoid humiliating a patient. Ordinarily, the principle of nonhumiliation extends to sentient and minimally self-reflective individuals; one cannot, as it were, humiliate an unconscious person or infant. But nonhumiliation is also part of a dynamic, two-sided human relationship that speaks to the idea of absolute dignity noted earlier. One covers the nakedness of an unconscious patient or cleans the dirt from his body out of respect for human dignity. Yet the patient himself never suffers humiliation nor may ever regain consciousness to know he once had. Instead, the failure to respect a person's basic human dignity shames and humiliates those around him. These observations push dignity beyond sentience to one of respect for personhood that depends solely on the mere fact that one bears the human form. It is self-esteem turned inside out: esteem for the self of another who may be incapable of self-recognition or understanding. Respect for self-esteem, in this sense, is oblivious to one's state of mind or behavior. It is an utterly basic human right that sometimes supercedes the significance we attach to other fundamental human rights. One can lose autonomy or the right to life under many common circumstances, but the situation is rare in which one may forfeit one's self-esteem. The same is true during armed conflict.

Dignity and Self-Esteem during Armed Conflict Self-esteem together with its subsidiary principles—nonhumiliation, nondegradation, and freedom from torture and servitude—form the basis of humanitarian law during armed conflict. If war sometimes sets aside the civil liberties that civilians enjoy during peace, human rights, insofar as they do not fatally conflict, remain inviolable. The overriding purpose of humanitarian law is to ensure that human rights do not go the way of civil liberties during armed conflict. Apart from the right to life, a person's rights qua human being protect one from humiliation, torture, and slavery, cruel and inhuman treatment, crushing poverty, ignorance, and political impotence. During war, there is a great temptation to inflict all this and more on one's enemy. The conventions of war hope to prevent these abuses from befalling combatant and noncombatant alike.

Humanitarian law and the laws of armed conflict articulate the principles that constrain the means of war. Early modern theorists took great pains to distinguish contemporary war from "primeval" forms of warfare that desired nothing less than annihilating an enemy, its people, and its resources. In contrast, post-Enlightenment warfare set for itself the simpler goal of disabling an enemy to the point of surrender while condemning hostilities beyond this point as unnecessary bloodletting and unwarranted suffering. Humanitarian law reflects this self-imposed restraint.

Nations impose restraints on themselves for several reasons. One lies in growing respect for humanitarian and natural rights emerging from the Enlightenment. While German military theorists of the nineteenth century were quick to counter with reason of state and the imperatives of war, the international community sided slowly with humanitarian law (Best 1980, 172–176). Respect for human dignity aside, the reasons for bolstering humanitarian law were eminently practical. As the modern nation-state consolidated its hold on armed violence and armed its citizens to kill, it was necessary to develop rules and guidelines to prevent domestic and international anarchy. Soldiers had to know who they could kill and who they could not, just as governments needed to know whom to honor and whom to hang (van Creveld 1991, 90). States had a vital interest in protecting their soldiers and citizens and so preferred disabling wars to those of annihilation. Finally, and unless wars and their battles were fought to the death, nations had to devise some way to surrender and end war. War convention does this by creating the terms of the fragile trust that allow one side to lay down its arms without fear of slaughter, and the other side to respect a flag of truce without fear of perfidy and betrayal. Without these conventions, war would be interminable.

International accords evolved slowly, but after World War II the Geneva Conventions (1949) formulated clear and concise rules governing the treatment of combatants and noncombatants during international armed conflict. On the battlefield, belligerents banned excessively cruel weapons that brought "unnecessary suffering and superfluous injury." Off the battlefield, humanitarian law extended sweeping protection to wounded and captured soldiers. Deprived of civil liberties and incarcerated for the duration of the war, prisoners of war gained the right to medical care, as well as freedom from torture, slavery, summary execution, and other forms of ill-treatment. In addition to the rights accorded imprisoned or wounded combatants, defeated and occupied civilians enjoyed freedom of conscience, respect for property and religious institutions, and freedom from reprisal. While occupying military forces might abridge noncombatants' civil rights—freedom of movement, expression, and assembly, for example—subject to the dictates of military necessity, they undertook to respect human rights including life, self-esteem, and freedom from torture and ill-treatment. Human rights underlie the protections offered all noncombatants: sick and wounded soldiers (the First and Second Geneva Conventions), prisoners of war (the Third Convention), and, in particular, civilians (the Fourth Convention).

Unlike concern for an individual's dignity, human rights conventions make no mention of *national* dignity, but national dignity may, like a nation's right to life, offer a justifiable ground for going to war. Article 51 of the UN charter recognizes only one justifiable cause for war: self-defense. Generally, self-defense signals a violation of territorial integrity or harm to some other vital national interest. But the definition is fluid. "Self-defense," for example, may justify anticipatory warfare, as a nation reacts to the threat of war rather than armed aggression. Self-defense may also hark back to earlier justifications for war, namely, to punish rogue nations who violate (or violated) the international order. Punishment may be rehabilitative, leading one nation to compel another to change its errant ways by force of arms. Or punishment may be retributive, aiming to right a past wrong by restoring territory or simply forcing miscreant nations to own up to past misdeeds. Affronts to national honor constantly intertwine with self-defense, suggesting that one may interpret a nation's "self" just as one does a person's "self."

Each "self" may suffer similar forms of humiliation or injustice and, in response, defend its "self" by armed violence. It is no accident that affronts to honor outstrips both self-defense and self-aggrandizement as a historical cause of war (Kagen 1995).

Absolute Human Rights?

Human rights are inviolable only insofar as they do not conflict with one another. While we often rank them equally, it is not difficult to imagine conflicts between different holders of competing rights. Ordinarily, any violation of self-esteem and its derivative principles prohibiting torture, humiliation, and degradation is unacceptable and morally wrong. But the right to self-esteem and freedom from physical abuse may collide with the right to life. Interrogational torture raises the difficult question whether violating the self-esteem of one individual is a greater affront to human dignity than permitting the deaths of others (chapter 7). While torture offers an extreme example, tension between life and the costs of maintaining it is at the heart of many dilemmas in bioethics and war, as we set goods that benefit some individuals against the inalienable correlates of human dignity we ascribe to any human being. Juggling these principles is difficult in its own right and exacerbated by the diversity of actors and interests present during armed conflict. Deontological concepts such as the right to life, autonomy, and self-esteem are central to any moral theory of war and medicine, but assessments of utility are often crucial. Sometimes only an appeal to utility that weighs the short- and long-term costs and benefits of pursuing one principle or another can resolve the dilemmas that arise when fundamental principles conflict.

Utility: Limiting Harm and Achieving Good

Whether defined by the value of human life or the integrity of the political community, both medicine and war strive to achieve good. How high a price are we then willing to pay? Must physicians strive to save life at any cost? Must nations prosecute war at all costs? While there might be some lives one will invest great resources to save or some wars nations cannot afford to lose at any price, the answer is generally no. The value of life is not absolute. It need not be saved at any cost.

The Nature of Utility Calculations

Whether facing a patient requiring particularly expensive care, allocating state resources for medicine and other goods, staging a battle, or going to war, one immediately calculates costs and benefits. There are several components to this process. Rational decision making requires an idea of the magnitude or relative value of the costs and benefits one faces, and an estimate of the probability one's action will succeed. Rational agents will also define the scope of those their actions should affect. The structure of reasoning is the same in medicine and war. Take, for example, a patient's decision to undergo surgery. The costs may include pain, a long recovery period, financial expenditures, and incapacitation or death, while the benefits may include a longer, pain-free life. These costs and benefits are not equally valued. Pain following surgery may be short-lived, while the specter of financial costs may overwhelm every other consideration. Incapacitation may be extensive or limited, short-term or long-term, so that one cost, limited and short-term incapacitation, for example, may pose acceptable risk, while another cost, such as extensive and long-term incapacitation, may bring one to refuse surgery. In this case, one must also have an idea of the probability that surgery will lead to one outcome or another. Death is an ever-present but considerable cost. One will only accept the risk of death if it is low or at least lower than the risk of death that comes from refusing medical care.

Probabilities work hand in glove with outcomes to determine rational decision making as a patient and her physicians weigh her best interest. In this example, surgery is certain to cause short-term discomfort (a minor cost), unlikely to bring death (a major cost), less than likely to incapacitate a patient (an intermediate cost), and more than likely to restore normal functioning (a major benefit). To make a rational decision one tallies the costs and benefits, assigns each a value, estimates probability, and compares the outcomes of different courses of action. Ordinarily, and this is true in the above example, the scope of these costs and benefits is confined to the patient herself and a function of her best interest whether measured by longevity or quality of life. Yet one may also expand the scope of decision making and consider the costs to other family members or society at large. These may be financial or emotional costs, and factoring them into calculations of expected utility creates a threefold decision-making process of defining the magnitude, probability, and scope of each cost and benefit. If surgery offers a sufficiently high probability that one will gain a valuable good, such as a long pain-free life, it becomes the rational choice. If, on the other hand, there is a good chance that both the patient and significant others will incur high costs, it may be rational to demur.

Similar calculations govern the distribution of scarce medical resources. Although life is precious, it is not the sole component of human happiness, so that it makes good moral sense to allocate scarce resources in a way that maximizes health care, education, employment, and other forms of welfare. Inevitably, this entails insufficient resources to save all lives at all costs. Instead, we focus our moral concern on procedural issues: "Are resources distributed fairly?" and "Are the affected groups represented in or party to the decision-making process?" (see Daniels and Sabin 1997). Medical expenditures will compete with other goods that people value. This demands that the competitive process be fair, accessible, and publicly accountable.

During war, we make decisions that are more complex. These first raise the costs and benefits of war. Costs may include death, pain and suffering, impaired civil liberties, and abridged human rights. Benefits include restoration of rights and liberties, long-term security, and the protection of life and property. Each of these costs and benefits varies in scope to include individuals (combatants, noncombatants, and injured soldiers) and collectives (states, nonstates, and international organizations). During war, states work assiduously to maximize incommensurable sets of interests. Ideally, political leaders and military planners strive to save the maximum number of civilian lives, salvage as many soldiers as possible for military service, and, at the same time, protect and pursue the interests of state. Since many goals are often impossible to accomplish simultaneously, politicians and the people they lead must determine their priorities. Utility calculations are difficult but essential, because planners must assess the costs and benefits of military operations relative to the goals they pursue. Wars, and the battles required to wage them, must be necessary—that is, they must bring about the good end that nations seek and do so at a reasonable cost. "Reasonable" costs are difficult to define, but holding them in line while securing supremely important benefits lies at the heart of the all-encompassing notion of military necessity that stands opposite to and often overrides many entrenched principles of bioethics.

The Principle of Military Necessity

Military necessity addresses both the ends and the means of war necessary to preserve the welfare of the state, its army, and its citizens. In neither case does necessity "know no law." On the contrary, it is an important moral principle in its own right as states choose wars for political and strategic reasons and as a means to protect their security, safeguard their autonomy, or uphold their dignity. Military necessity reflects a concern for the collective welfare of the political community that reaches beyond individual well-being and sometimes overrides the normative force of deontological moral principles central to bioethics.

Necessity often appears in municipal law to allow individuals to violate the law when they or others face a grievous, immediate, and otherwise unavoidable threat. Necessity is not a form of simple utility; it does not grant undisputed moral weight to any action that is simply cost-effective. Instead, it allows one to break the law in the face of a dire threat that cannot be otherwise averted. Invoking necessity justifies extreme measures, but only as a last resort. Military necessity works in much the same way. It allows nations to breach the peace for a morally justified goal, whether self-defense or the protection of a defenseless third party, when war is the only means available to safeguard these supremely important moral values.

The fundamental difference between ordinary necessity and military necessity comes to light when we ask ourselves, "What is at stake?" Ordinary necessity turns on a grievous threat to life or limb. Military necessity, however, is multifaceted; the idea of "reason of state," which guides military necessity, embraces the multiple and conflicting interests the state must protect. At one level, states must protect their citizens' lives, economic interests, civil liberties, happiness, and well-being. A state that no longer meets these expectations loses the trust of its citizens and forfeits its authority and legitimacy. War should impose the same obligation, leaving states to go to war for the sole reason of protecting the aggregate interests of their citizens. Unfortunately, this is not always the case. Sometimes states wage war with the hope of saving more lives than they sacrifice, but often impose hardship on all citizens to secure the integrity of something more than aggregate welfare. States fight to preserve honor, territorial integrity, culture, moral personhood, and the other organic attributes of statehood described earlier. War poses a constant danger of running roughshod over aggregate welfare. "Elevating the preservation of an abstraction—the state—above individual persons," writes Robert Holmes (1989, 112), "places no limits upon what may be done to achieve that objective."

Military necessity is a justificatory principle that operates at two levels. At one level, it legitimizes war and is part of the set of principles that comprise *jus ad bellum* and morally sanctioned war. This is *strategic* necessity, justifying war as part of the strategy a state chooses to secure its political interests. At another level, military necessity is *tactical*. It reaches to the means to wage war and justifies any measure that is efficient and allows a state to attain its military objectives. In this formulation, military necessity is unconstrained by any principle other than cost-effectiveness and the justice of a nation's objectives.

Does it now follow that the means of war are so unbridled that military necessity overrides most other significant moral principles, and leads, as Holmes believes, to unrelenting violence and destruction? While some suggest that military necessity admits of no built-in moral limits, it is not without cause that international instruments themselves restrict necessity to "the means necessary to subdue an enemy and which are not forbidden by international law"(Protocol I, 1977a, Article 35). This is a legalistic definition, but the moral parameters are inherent in the meaning of necessity. First, military necessity cannot, any more than ordinary necessity, rest on calculations of simple utility. It cannot justify war simply because it expeditiously achieves one's aims. Otherwise, war, or the threat of war, would always be the means of choice when the strong confront the weak. Second, only the threat of grievous harm justifies necessary war. In the international community, this translates into gross territorial infringement, egregious violations of human rights, and immediate threats to world peace. These are the causes of just war.

Military necessity, therefore, only justifies the means necessary to subdue—that is, disable and not annihilate—an enemy in pursuit of legitimate aims. Inherent in these aims are certain moral limits that seep into and infuse the means of war. Logically, these aims and means must mesh. It hardly makes sense, for example, to allow nations to defend themselves from territorial encroachment or protect others from human rights abuses, and then permit them to undertake means that permanently encroach on the territory of others or violate their human rights. The just means of war, *jus in bello*, demand that belligerents respect noncombatant immunity, honor human rights, and avoid indiscriminate harm. The ends may justify the means, but the ends are carefully circumscribed and, as such, also shape and restrain the means.

Constraining Military Necessity: The Principle of Proportionality

The legitimate aims of modern war engender humanitarian law while, at the same time, humanitarian law often bends itself to the exigencies of military necessity by allowing belligerents ample room to violate or, more precisely, override moral norms in certain circumstances. Supreme emergency, for example, will effectively gut humanitarian law when a nation or political community faces an existential threat. The doctrine of double effect sets aside a noncombatant's right to life under many circumstances of modern war. While each suggests that in a crunch military necessity supercedes the deontological principles of humanitarian law, necessity remains constrained by proportionality, a principle related to, but not identical with, utility and noncombatant immunity.

Proportionality limits *excessive* harm and draws on humanitarian concern for aggregate human life. An act violates the principle of utility when it produces more harm than it seeks to avoid, but it is disproportionate if securing an important goal incurs considerable human cost. "Excessive" cost is not synonymous with "unnecessary" cost. The cost one pays in noncombatant lives to secure a particular military objective may be necessary for a mission to succeed, yet may remain disproportionate if *too high*. Assessing proportionality is difficult because the benefits and costs of military action are not commensurable. The benefit is a military one, safeguarding national security, sinking a ship, or taking a strategic position, while the cost is measured by harm to noncombatants. As such, belligerents object to reprisals when *too many* civilians are killed; the doctrine of double effect will justify intentionally harming civilians only when *reasonable* numbers die. Applying this principle in practice, however, remains intensely problematic. The simplest way to determine excessive harm is to ask whether military planners have less costly, alternative means at their disposal to achieve the same goal. When this is not possible, planners may simply try to calculate civilian casualties and if this seems or feels too high a mission may be scrubbed. "Too high" is often a function of whatever the market—that is, domestic and international public opinion—will bear.

Bioethics, War, and Necessity

As nations go to war, military necessity defers to and at the same time curtails the force of humanitarian norms, noncombatant immunity, and proportionality. Military necessity presents an overwhelming challenge to bioethics unused to bowing before forces beyond its domain. In nearly all cases imaginable, bioethical norms should prevail in the conduct of medicine: physicians should respect confidentiality and patient autonomy, medical personnel should remain neutral, and patients should receive care solely subject to medical need. But during war, military necessity may override these duties. Strategic necessity—that is, the need to wage war in pursuit of legitimate national interests—firmly limits the medical rights that both combatants and noncombatant patients enjoy. Tactical necessity—the need to develop efficient means to wage war and achieve particular military objectives—will restrict access to medical care, will govern the distribution of scarce resources, and may compel physicians to lend their expertise to the development of weapons systems. This places military medical personnel in the awkward, if not untenable, position of causing avoidable harm, and while the principle of proportionality may prevent egregious harm, the harm may remain substantial nonetheless.

The necessities of war, therefore, reflect multiple interests. While a state's and its army's welfare are of first and foremost concern, neither is always an overriding force as one calculates the cost and benefits of waging war by various means. Military necessity functions within particular moral parameters that limit the ends and means of war. Nevertheless, military necessity retains a distinct if not superior status, if only because most individuals gladly weigh the interests of state above their own. Military necessity, therefore, joins the pantheon of other principles that guide medicine and war as first among equals, and forces the peculiar caregiving and noncaregiving dilemmas that characterize bioethics during armed conflict.

3
Medical Care for the Wounded

Caregiving dilemmas presuppose the *duty* of care, a presupposition so obvious that few would question it. Doctors have a professional duty to care for their patients. While one may debate a person's right to receive medical care from the state or from the workplace, no one would ask a nurse or physician "Why treat a sick person?" If one did, the answer would appear self-evident: One treats the sick because without care they will suffer or die. Death and suffering are prima facie evils and in the absence of compelling reasons to the contrary a physician has an obligation to treat a sick or injured person. A physician's duty to prevent suffering and death is professional. It is anchored, argue Pellegrino and Thomasma, in a "sacred trust" imposed on physicians by their choice of profession and by a concomitant promise to society to use medical knowledge for the good of patients.

A political right to medical care draws from the state's duty to safeguard its citizens' right to life and provides them the means to secure liberty. Beyond the minimal state, whose role is to provide basic security, more advanced liberal states should nurture what Mill ([1859] 1989) describes as the moral, practical, and intellectual development of its citizens. Surely this cannot take place in the absence of basic medical care. The sick make poor citizens. Nevertheless, while a state's duty to guarantee the right to life and provide adequate health care is of paramount importance, it is not absolute. While emphasizing a person's positive right to receive basic medical care, one must recognize that resources are limited and other entitlements—education, welfare, and defense—compete for the same resources medical care demands. This renders the state's position vis-à-vis health care different from the physician's.

Because the relationship between physician and patient is bilateral, it remains largely unaffected by conflicting rights and interests of third parties.

Military medicine, however, introduces a number of rights, duties, and interests that compete directly with those traditionally associated with the patient-doctor relationship. In the previous chapter I described how soldiers are not ordinary patients. Deprived of the right to life and many civil liberties that anchor medical care, it is not clear why and how soldiers gain a right to receive treatment when injured. After all, if a soldier is sent to die, why is it necessary to care for him or her when wounded? There is no obvious or compelling answer to this question. Nor can physicians simply fall back on their professional duty to care for the sick and injured, for during war they must struggle with the general dictates of military necessity. This may preclude them from providing the care they think necessary or from treating every patient that they can.

At the same time, any decision to provide medical care during wartime is not solely one for physicians in the field. Instead, it is primarily a decision for military commanders. This creates two classes of military medical decision makers. Dominique Larrey, Napoléon's medical director and chief surgeon, makes the point clearly when he comments on Napoléon's campaigns in Egypt and Poland (in 1799 and 1807). To offer optimum care, Larrey believed that military organizations should evacuate their wounded from frontline aid stations to larger hospitals in the rear "immediately after an engagement." But the decision is not only medical: "To these physiological arguments in favour of removing the wounded should be added others of a political nature. To the commander-in-chief alone it belonged to admit these, and to arrange such plans as would best serve the interests of the wounded, and support the spirits of the soldiers" (Larrey [1814] 1987, vol. 2, 147).

Underlying Larrey's remarks is the conviction that medical treatment is ultimately a military decision regardless of patients' right to medical care and irrespective of physicians' duty to their patients. Physicians may determine their patients' medical needs, but military commanders decide when and how to serve them consistent with military necessity and the prosecution of the war.

Evacuating and Treating the Wounded

As we ponder the question "Why treat the wounded?" it is useful to keep in mind that for much of recorded history, armies did not do all they could to care for their injured. It is one of the great ironies of military medicine that the advances war afforded to medicine did not readily benefit soldiers on the field. Medical care would not have advanced as it did in the nineteenth and twentieth centuries but for the need to treat increasingly severe wounds in wars that killed and injured soldiers in battle as never before. Yet, despite the great medical benefits that war sometime brought, soldiers were not often the recipients of this growing expertise. Quite the contrary; until the twentieth century there was a glaring gap between available medical technology and the ability to bring that technology to the battlefield in any significant way. The problem was largely organizational. Large, conventional armies lacked both the will and the way to efficiently evacuate soldiers from the battlefield and provide the necessary resources and personnel to staff a sufficient number of field stations and military hospitals.

Throughout history, wounded soldiers often fared worse than dead ones. Bestowed with honor and buried with ceremony, the dead lived on as exemplars for generations of young men. The wounded were not so fortunate. In most cases, they lay on the battlefield until the fighting ended. Engagements could be short, but days could pass before injured soldiers received treatment. Those with minor wounds returned to battle with minimal, if any, care while the seriously wounded often died before receiving treatment. Those who did not die received rudimentary care that often left them crippled, without pensions and reduced to begging. This picture had not changed much by the French Revolution. While the wealthy had access to experienced physicians, common soldiers made do with poorly trained and equipped barber surgeons.

Spurred by the carnage of Napoléonic warfare, Larrey was among the first to think seriously about evacuating the wounded during, rather than after, battle. With his invention of "flying ambulances"—light-weight carriages that could reach the front lines—as well as a dedicated corps of medical personnel to staff them and evacuate the wounded, Larrey's innovations would reshape military medicine (Larrey [1814]

1987, vol. 1, 77–83). Unfortunately, most European armies suffered mightily at the hands of Napoléon and ignored Larrey's innovations. Napoléon himself instituted Larrey's reforms for the benefit of the Imperial Guard, his elite corps, while neglecting the vast majority of his troops, who "were frequently abandoned through lack of transport on forced marches and retreats or were stuffed in buildings of every sort and left to die" (also see Richardson 1985). The situation did not improve by midcentury and the Crimean War (1859) earned the dubious distinction as one of the worst military medical disasters of all time. Twenty percent of the French force died of disease. The Turks had no medical personnel whatsoever. The British fielded nearly 100,000 troops and entered the war with "40 ambulance wagons, a pack mule and 10 litters for each regiment, no winter clothing, no shelter tents and a worthless corps of male nurses commandeered from the line" (Garrison [1922] 1970, 172).

During the American Civil War, Larrey's principles of evacuation garnered new interest as Jonathan Letterman, chief medical officer of the Army of the Potomac, improved Larrey's ambulance design, streamlined the organization and distribution of medical supplies, and introduced mobile field hospitals. Nevertheless, General Henry W. Halleck, the Union Army's general-in-chief in 1862, rejected a plan to establish a coordinated system of evacuation and treatment because he feared that "the presence of medical personnel on the battlefield would spread panic among soldiers who might view them as a harbinger of suffering and death" (Ginn 1977, 13). Even with Halleck's departure, Letterman's reforms came slowly.

Following the Civil War, Letterman's innovations gradually took hold in Europe, but the record of the major European powers in caring for the wounded remained spotty at best. Medicine had little to offer and what it did have, it did not always offer wounded soldiers. Physicians could treat saber and gunshot wounds and, if necessary, amputate limbs, only to stand by helplessly as infection carried off many of their patients. During the Franco-Prussian War (1870–1871), 65 percent of German amputees and 90 percent of French amputees died, a figure significantly *worse* than the 50 percent mortality rate among Union amputees during the Civil War half a decade earlier (Gabriel and Metz 1992, vol. 2, 220).

While medical care progressed in the intervening years, most notably in the field of antisepsis, few expended much effort to bring new technology to the battlefield. For most commanders, care for the wounded remained of secondary concern. While the British were careful to provide their civilian hospitals with adequate medical personnel and equipment during the Boer War (1899–1902), their military medical facilities languished, "incontestable proof," notes one historian, "of the insufficient provision made for the sick and wounded" (Pagaard 1986, 75).

Medical care improved significantly in the twentieth century. The Russo-Japanese War (1904–1905) became the first conflict where at least one side, in this case the Japanese, could claim that fewer men died of disease than from battlefield wounds. By the First World War death from both causes drew even. Still, medical care did not always command premium resources. The British medical corps, for example, entered World War I only to find themselves stripped of motorized transport to evacuate the wounded "on the grounds that the roads were already overburdened with more important supplies" (Gabriel and Metz 1992, vol. 2, 247). While medicine made considerable progress by World War II, particularly in the field of surgery, the German army, unlike the American, would consciously decide to minimize forward surgical care and neglect the seriously wounded.

The image of efficient care and prompt evacuation is relatively new, the result of medical care only large conventional armies can provide. The emphasis military medical history places on prominent postwar conflicts—Korea, Vietnam, the Middle East, the Falklands, and the Gulf Wars—reinforces this image. Here, indeed, the "Western" side to the conflict devoted vast resources to medical care. Nevertheless, we sometimes see how military commanders decide to forgo protection rather than accept a reduction in "mission capability." In Vietnam, flak jackets and helmets could significantly reduce head and chest injuries but were often left behind because they were too heavy or too hot to wear. (Neel 1991) Among indigenous troops the situation was far different. Guerrilla organizations—the People's Army of North Vietnam (PAVN) or Mao's Red Army, for example—could not provide anywhere near the level of medical care Western armies could offer, nor did they always provide the care they might have.

If, historically, treatment for the wounded is the exception rather than the rule, the question remains, "Why treat the wounded?" If political leaders could expend lives with large measures of impunity, why deplete scarce resources when these same lives no longer contribute to the war? Why be receptive to suffering if inured to death?

Why Treat the Wounded?

In the *Roman History*, Livy offers three reasons for treating the wounded: "military necessity," "patriotic duty," and the need to prevent "the demoralization of the fighting line by the misery of the wounded" (Garrison [1922] 1970, 52). The Byzantine emperor Leo VI echoed similar concerns in the tenth century: "Give all the care you possibly can to your wounded, for if you neglect them, you will make your soldiers timorous and cowardly before a battle, and, not only that, but your personnel, whom you might preserve and retain by proper consideration for their health and welfare, will be otherwise lost to you through your own negligence" (Garrison [1922] 1970, 80).

Military necessity, morale, and duty are compelling reasons for treating wounded soldiers. Military necessity is the most intuitively appealing: evacuation and care for the wounded preserve an army's fighting strength. Morale is another important benefit of medical care, without which soldiers are reluctant to fight. Duty emphasizes the state's obligation to care for those willing to die on its behalf.

While each of these arguments appears convincing, they do not withstand careful scrutiny. Though caring for wounded soldiers, in general, can salvage manpower, treating severely wounded soldiers does not significantly affect an army's fighting strength. Moreover, until the beginning of the twentieth century, far more soldiers died of disease than of any wounds inflicted during battle. Cost-effectiveness, therefore, lay in sanitation and hygiene, not in evacuation and medical care for the wounded. Military authorities failed to evacuate wounded soldiers simply because of the "unwillingness of armies to take military medicine seriously as a means of salvaging manpower" (Gabriel and Metz 1992, vol. 2, 216). The effect of medical care on morale is less than straightforward. Observers cannot agree whether medical care acts as a positive incentive, inducing soldiers to risk their lives, or whether lack of care is a negative incentive, unsettling healthy soldiers who fear going into battle without supporting care or who must bear the cries of those abandoned on the battlefield. Finally, the state's obligation to care for the wounded is fundamental, but it is not a patriotic duty—that is, a duty owed soldiers because of their willingness to fight. The duty of citizens to die for their country stands independently of the state's obligation to provide medical care to the wounded. The former is anchored in the nature of political obligation, while the latter is prepolitical and a function of basic human rights.

Medical Care and Military Necessity

Treating wounded soldiers in order to return significant numbers of salvageable soldiers to battle is not necessarily the most compelling reason to provide medical care. Prior to Larrey's and Letterman's reforms, military commanders realized that far from salvaging manpower, evacuating soldiers during battle actually reduced the number of men available to fight: "A Confederate report echoed the universal complaint of line commanders: 'If any from the ranks are drawn from the fight to carry off the wounded, they never return until the fight is over, and thus three are lost to the company instead of one wounded'" (Chisholm 1861, 92).

Without a properly organized and trained evacuation corps, only those presently fighting could remove wounded soldiers from the battlefield. While many were not averse to evacuation duty and only too happy to head for safer ground, this informal procedure wreaked havoc on manpower, particularly because several fit men were needed to evacuate a single wounded soldier and none was too quick to return to the fighting. Nor were the fruits of medical care overwhelmingly positive. The seriously wounded soldiers would, most likely, never fight again and the lightly wounded would, in most cases, recover without intensive care. Add to this the manpower required to remove soldiers during battle and the utilitarian argument for evacuation falls to the wayside. This was especially true throughout the nineteenth century, because military medicine had little to offer the seriously wounded beyond amputation.

The Benefits of Military Medicine

Resistance by field commanders to establishing evacuation and care as their first priority reflects their understanding that whatever the humanitarian benefits medical care brings, the military benefits are often marginal. Far greater benefit comes from sanitation, and there is no doubt that military medicine has made a tremendous contribution to preserving manpower by preventing infectious disease. Four to five times as many French and English died of disease in the Crimean War than died in battle. During the American Civil War, twice the 115,000 soldiers killed in action fell to disease (Garrison [1922] 1970, 172). By World War I, as noted, the numbers drew even; 51,259 Americans died in battle and 51,447 died from disease, primarily influenza. By World War II, Korea, and Vietnam, disease claimed very few combatants (Dupuy 1995, 140–141). These gains came from a better understanding of the sanitation and hygienic techniques necessary to reduce the spread of infectious disease such as influenza, whooping cough, and typhus as well as the development of vaccines against smallpox, yellow fever, typhoid, and paratyphoid at the end of the nineteenth and early twentieth centuries; the availability of tetanus antitoxin during World War I; and the discovery of sulfa drugs, penicillin, and other antibiotics during World War II (Garrison [1922] 1970, 107; Grissinger 1927, 345–347; Gabriel and Metz 1992, vol. 2, 215–268).

Few of these accomplishments, however, have anything to do with evacuating and treating wounded soldiers. In figures that have changed little in 150 years of American warfare, 20 percent of all casualties are killed in action (KIA), 65 percent suffer minor wounds and survive without extensive medical care, and the balance, 15 percent, suffer serious injury and benefit significantly from medical care. How much do they benefit? Working from the number of "hits" an army absorbs during battle, T. N. Dupuy (1995, 140–141) presents data that chart a steady rise in the number of soldiers who survive a hit during battle. Overall, 70 percent of the soldiers survived a battlefield hit in the Civil War, 73 percent in World War II, and 76 percent in Vietnam. Lest these gains seem modest, Dupuy emphasizes the dramatic increase in survival among the most critically injured. While 25 percent of the seriously wounded survived the Mexican War, 82 percent would survive Korea, largely the result of better evacuation techniques and better medicine.

Dupuy cites steadily increasing survival rates for the severely wounded as evidence that modern medicine can significantly improve attrition rates. He does not, however, distinguish between saving lives and returning soldiers to active duty. While the aim of medicine might be to save lives when possible, the goal of military medicine remains human salvage. Here, the gains remain modest. In the Civil War, for example, 2.2 million men fought for the North. Of these, 67,000 were killed in action, 43,000 died of their wounds, and while approximately 20,000 survived after sustaining serious injuries, many were amputees who could not return to duty.[1] By World War II the picture improved, but not to the extent one might expect given the tremendous advances in medical care of the preceding eighty years. Comparing World War II combat casualty care in the American army in 1944 and German army in 1941, Ronald Bellamy (1985, 407) describes the different approach of each medical corps: "The American organization was designed to save lives by emphasizing the treatment of the severely wounded as far forward as possible. . . . Contrariwise, the German organization was designed to maximize the return to duty by emphasizing the treatment of the lightly wounded. There were few surgeons [and] transfusions were rarely more than 500 ml."

To staff the facilities necessary to provide forward medical care, the American army devoted more than twice the personnel (8.7 percent of total strength) as its German counterpart (3.8 percent) to medical care. Nevertheless, each medical organization achieved similar results. For every 1,000 casualties, 215 American and 236 Germans died in action, a figure similar to the Civil War. Of those suffering serious wounds, 24 Americans and 81 Germans of every 1,000 casualties died. This should come as no surprise, because the German units "confined their surgery to men with wounds of such a nature that they would be able to return to their units and full duty within reasonably short periods of time after surgery." During intense fighting, soldiers suffering from abdominal and head wounds received no surgical care at all (Wiltse 1965, 603). Yet, despite the Americans' ability to save three times as many lives, the number of soldiers each medical organization was able to salvage and return to duty did not vary significantly. For every 1,000 casualties, the Americans returned 549 to duty while the Germans returned 399 to active duty and 262 to limited duty (the American figure is undifferentiated) (Bellamy 1985).

While these figures suggest that modern military medicine does much to salvage manpower, one must draw a distinction between moderately wounded soldiers—that is, those who will survive with minimal medical intervention—and the more severely wounded who require intensive, frontline surgical care. Dupuy's figures suggest that the vast majority of wounded are "walking" wounded who require minimal care. Discussing post–World War II casualties (Korea, Vietnam, and the Gulf War), Swan and Swan (1996) estimate that of all wounded, 65 percent are walking wounded who "should receive treatment but their wounds are sufficiently minor that they are survivable without treatment for the most part," 25 percent "require prompt surgical attention if they are to survive with the hope of a meaningful existence," and approximately 10 percent "are probably beyond salvage, even with maximal care." Mallory (1954, 58) suggests similar figures for the Korean War: 25 percent dead or mortally wounded, 10 percent severely wounded, and 65 percent requiring minimal attention "until they undergo definitive surgery." Koehler, Smith, and Bacaner (1994) put the percentage of severely wounded in Vietnam, the 1973 Arab-Israeli War, and the 1982 Israeli war in Lebanon at between 15 and 25 percent.

Treating the Severely Wounded

The hard moral question turns on the imperative to provide forward surgical care for those who will certainly die without it but will make no contribution to the war effort after they recover. The question about providing the care that most soldiers need to return to battle is not difficult. In Korea, for example, about half of the approximately 90,000 soldiers wounded required surgery. Half of these suffered wounds to the extremities and most, 80 percent, recovered to return to duty in some capacity (Reister 1973, 14). While those who did not return to duty either died or received a disability separation, most suffered severe abdominal, thoracic, or spinal-cord injuries—the very injuries the Germans did not

establish facilities to treat. For this reason, Bellamy "found no evidence
... that the increased salvage of [American] lives was associated with a
corresponding increase in the number of casualties who return to duty."
The severely injured simply did not return to fight. This was true in the
postwar period as well. Citing data from Vietnam and Israel, Koehler,
Smith, and Bacaner (1994) conclude that only 15 to 17 percent of
severely wounded American and Israeli soldiers requiring evacuation to
second-echelon care were returned to duty. Finally, one must consider
that the stamina of severely wounded soldiers returning to duty is often
fragile. Anthony Kellet (1990, 223) argues that "evidence of the Second
World War suggests a fairly strong relationship between wounding and
subsequent psychiatric breakdown after the soldier has returned to his
unit." Describing American losses in November 1944, Robert Rush
(2001, 323) emphasizes that "the highest percentage of casualties...
were among those soldiers returned to duty after being wounded."

These data reinforce, perhaps, what many military commanders have
intuitively known for a long time. Preventive care and hygiene go a very
long way toward preserving an army's fighting strength. Of those
wounded in battle, most require minimal medical care to survive and
return to duty. While improved medical care increases the chance that
the severely wounded will survive, most do not return to duty. Of those
that do, many are unable to fight as they did before. These data undermine arguments that ground medical care for the wounded, particularly
the severely wounded, in utility. The "walking wounded" require little
intensive care. Immediate evacuation and forward surgical care to benefit
the severely wounded do not bolster military manpower. Bellamy (1985,
410) concluded this much from his study of American and German care:

If conserving fighting strength and clearing casualties from the battlefield are
really the *only* reasons for combat casualty care, the German organization with
its lack of surgical capabilities should be considered a fine prototype. . . . In fact,
given the slow rate of return to duty of wounded casualties (probably less than
20% in the first month), it is easy to argue that there is no need for any surgical capability.

Why then evacuate and treat the severely wounded? The Americans
saved 57 more lives per 1,000 than the Germans. By the war's end this
meant the lives of more than 30,000 men.[2] But why save them if they

cannot return to duty? Bellamy (1985, 410) only hazards a guess: "Of course, there are other reasons for providing combat casualty care—reasons such as the morale of the soldier and the obligation of the nation to do all that is necessary to care for its defenders. Life saving surgery should be justified on these grounds, not because it conserves the fighting strength."

In a retrospective look at the Korean conflict, Mallory (1954, 58) also ponders this question, first invoking the right to life and then, perhaps realizing that he is skating on thin ice, raises utilitarian benefits for treating the wounded:

The medical effort expended on Group II [the severely wounded requiring continuous medical support and supervision] is justified primarily by the moral obligation to prevent loss of life. The salvage value of these casualties is limited for direct military purposes, but of considerable importance to the gross national output; especially when we contemplate the heavy financial obligation assumed by the Government in the event of mortality.

While one doubts that the cost of caring for a seriously wounded veteran is less than the government's obligation upon a soldier's death, others were also quick to draw on utilitarian arguments. In an era when medical care could return few to duty, Dunant ([1862] 1986, 122, n. 1) bolstered his humanitarian appeal with utility, pointing out how quicker care would avoid unnecessary amputation and reduce the number of cripples as well as the pensions that governments pay the disabled. Similarly, others hoped that speedy evacuation would root out stragglers who feign injury and malinger among the wounded (Ginn 1977, 15). Nevertheless, the utilitarian grounds for treating the seriously wounded remain relatively weak. For this reason, observers appeal to additional benefits, most notably morale. Medical care raises morale—that is, it does not so much affect the military usefulness of the injured soldier as much as it affects the fighting fitness of the healthy and makes them more willing to risk their lives during war.

Medical Care and Morale

While many commentators note the relationship between medicine and morale on the battlefield, they do not necessarily focus on the evacuation and treatment of the wounded. From ancient times until the twentieth century, disease could decimate and demoralize an army far more quickly than wounds inflicted in battle could. Livy (*Roman History*, XXV, 26), for example, describes a plague during the siege of Syracuse in 212 BC as a "calamity affecting both sides." As increasing numbers of soldiers succumbed, "their feelings became so brutalized . . . that they not only did not follow their dead with tears and decent lamentations but they did not even carry them out and bury them. . . . Some, preferring to die by the sword, even rushed alone upon the outposts of the enemy" (Garrison [1922] 1970, 53). This scene of deteriorating discipline must have been repeated countless times throughout history, so that proper sanitation and hygiene could have an overwhelming impact on the morale of troops if they could prevent or contain epidemics of infectious disease.

It should also be remembered that for a long time military medicine did not often have much to offer wounded soldiers. Did the prospect of the following care so enthusiastically described by Larrey ([1814] 1987, vol. 2, 43–44) in his memoirs inspire or demoralize French soldiers? "I was obliged to take off both thighs of a soldier. Besides the sphacelus in his extremities, produced by the total disorganization of the parts, his face, hand and breast were burnt. Notwithstanding the loss of these limbs, and the enormous burns with which he was covered, this man survived, and was completely cured. . . . Another lost both his arms, and yet was perfectly cured." Larrey was enthusiastic, of course, because he saved men's lives and restored them to relative health. But did his patients agree that they were "perfectly cured," or would they rather die? Does death affect morale any worse than the likelihood of living as a double amputee in an age where prostheses (especially for double-leg amputees) were hardly developed, veterans' pensions were meager at best, and many disabled veterans were reduced to begging (Garrison [1922] 1970, 122, 128)?

Improving Military Morale

What, then, is the relationship between military medicine and morale? Morale is a positive frame of mind necessary to undertake a dangerous or difficult task that helps offset the costs one faces. The ultimate cost of military service is death and that cost, together with a person's unwillingness to incur it, is a function of risk or the probability that one will die in battle. One way, then, to raise morale is to reduce risk. Competent leadership or body armor, for example, may do this. Alternatively, or in addition, one may offset costs with increased benefits. Some benefits are simply material. Plentiful food, good pay, warm clothes, and the prospect of a college education will raise morale to the extent that some, members of a volunteer army for example, are prepared to risk their lives. Negative incentives, the threat of punishment for desertion, may also underlie the motivation to risk one's life. Other soldiers may require more valuable goods that sometimes come after death: posthumous honors or the fulfillment of some ideological or religious goal, for instance. Other benefits may be social, so that soldiers may risk their lives if there is a good chance they will earn the approbation and support of their family or comrades-in-arms. Camaraderie may be the single greatest factor motivating soldiers to fight, not so much in the name of ideology, but to support and defend their comrades-in-arms: "In the heat of battle, it ceases to be an idea for which we fight, or a flag. Rather we fight for the man on our left and we fight for the man on our right" (*Four Feathers*, 2002). Or, as Stephen Crane puts it in *The Red Badge of Courage* ([1895] 2003, 37), "There was a consciousness always of the presence of his comrades about him. He felt the subtle battle brotherhood more potent than the cause for which they were fighting. It was a mysterious fraternity born of the smoke and danger of death."

These simple citations reaffirm the findings of large-scale studies of combat motivation among American troops in World War II. While ideology was an important component of "precombat" motivation—that is, the willingness to go to war—"primary-group" cohesion accounts for soldiers' readiness to risk their lives during combat (Chodoff 1983). They find security as part of a small, cohesive, interdependent, and trusted group whose members will do their utmost not to let one another down. They risk their lives in combat to protect the lives of their comrades and to preserve self-respect in the eyes of their fellow soldiers (Lazersfeld 1949; Stouffer et al. 1949, 130–149). Guarding one another's back may also be the surest route to survival in life-threatening situations. None of these motives, moreover, operates in a vacuum but only in the context of a well-structured, formal, and often coercive organization that nurtures leadership, enforces discipline, rewards merit, and trains and delivers soldiers into combat zones in the context of a highly organized social structure (Williams 1989, 155–174).

Nevertheless, these factors do not tell the entire story about morale. In a detailed study of an attritional eighteen-day battle in the Hürtgen Forest in November 1944, Rush (2001) writes how heavy casualties decimated American units within days. While replacements replenished depleted units, soldiers no longer knew one another, and primary group cohesion evaporated. By any standard account, the units should have stopped fighting after three days. Yet they did not stop and, instead, fought with great tenacity and staggering casualties until defeating the defending Germans. Rush accounts for this by citing positive and negative incentives. The positive incentives lie in organizational, not primary-group, cohesion. The military remained organized and efficient, and continued to provide replacement troops, supplies, and services to troops throughout the battle. This same organizational cohesion collapsed on the German side and seriously eroded morale. Negative incentives were coercive: first sergeants moved behind the company to ensure that soldiers moved forward. Those who did not fight faced punishment and sanctions. Morale was so low in the German Army that only the threat of execution kept many soldiers at the line.

Morale and the Role of Medical Care

Medical care fits into this complex structure of incentives at the level of organizational cohesion. An effective military, one that commands the allegiance of its members and one that soldiers will die for, must provide services and support. Describing the factors that made morale among American soldiers fighting in Vietnam the highest he had seen in three wars, General William C. Westmoreland, commander of American forces in Vietnam, cites: " 'Creature comforts', post exchanges, recreational facilities, rest and recuperation . . . open channels of complaint and information, participation in civic action programs, the rotation systems and the expectation of swift evacuation and excellent medical treatment" (Kellet 1982, 247). It is difficult, however, to measure the effects of medicine alone. Lack of medical care in a conventional army signals the collapse of organizational cohesion in general. An army that does not provide medical care is also not providing mail, food, supplies, and replacement troops. These factors combine to decimate morale.

Nevertheless, medical care alone can affect morale in two ways. First, battlefield medical care comforts the wounded even when it cannot save many lives. The willingness to evacuate soldiers and tend to the severely wounded as they die marks the care and fraternity one feels toward soldiers in the field. Failure to provide care engenders a sense of abandonment. This aspect of medical care, rather than acute care to save the critically injured, preoccupied Henry Dunant at Solferino in 1859. Second, as medical care has improved, it has reduced the risks soldiers face. However, medical care may not reduce the risk of death as much as it minimizes the risk of pain and suffering. These are two, distinct consequences. While medical care has reduced mortality among severely wounded soldiers, it has provided many more with relief from pain and suffering. This is true of medical care in general. Assuming that soldiers fear unattended pain and suffering at least as much as they fear death and injury itself, this is no trivial benefit. Nineteenth-century calls to care for the wounded appealed to the former; medicine could do little for the latter. Without adequate medical care and, just as importantly, without the willingness of other soldiers to evacuate the wounded, soldiers face abandonment, pain and suffering, injury and death, and organizational disintegration. How much and what kind of care is necessary to avoid these outcomes?

One may speculate, for example, that German soldiers benefiting from the medical system Bellamy describes above, a system that eschewed life-saving surgical care in favor of more efficient care for moderately or lightly wounded soldiers, were no less (or no more) eager to fight than their American counterparts. German care was adequate because it fulfilled two functions. First, it treated the wounded as efficiently as possible commensurate with available resources, and second, it alleviated, or should have tried to alleviate, the pain and suffering of those severely wounded by providing comfort care. It included "definitive care for the lightly wounded (wound incision and cleaning rather than formal wound excision), simple life supporting surgery when technically possible and further preparation for the evacuation of the seriously wounded"

(Bellamy 1985, 406). Seriously wounded soldiers might not receive anything beyond stabilizing and comfort care until evacuated to surgical facilities as far as 100 kilometers to the rear, a process that heavy fighting might delay for many hours and during which many soldiers would die. The American medical organizations reduced the mortality of seriously injured soldiers by providing advance surgery closer to the front lines. However, because each medical organization offered a reasonable prospect that it could alleviate pain and suffering and provide the care necessary so most injured men would recover, there is no reason to think that soldiers' morale was affected one way or another by the kind of medical care available.

Anecdotal evidence from guerrilla armies also suggests that minimal medical care is sufficient to maintain morale. Medical care in the People's Army of North Vietnam (PAVN), for example, highlights the substantial gap between medical expertise and the means available to practice modern medicine, a picture probably characteristic of many modern guerrilla armies. On the one hand, surgeons were highly trained, while, on the other, they faced a chronic lack of basic supplies such as bandages, anesthetics, IV lines, and surgical equipment. Battlefield conditions constantly forced doctors to evacuate their staff and patients or to work in tunnels and rooms dug underground to escape American bombers. Conditions there were abysmal, electrical supply sporadic, and ventilation poor. Supplies were often improvised from material on hand. Downed American planes were stripped of every item that might be medically useful: metal hardware to set bones or make braces, plastic insulation for IV lines, flare tubes for stethoscopes, and parachute cloth for surgical thread and bandages. Medical staff used coconut shells for IV bottles, and bamboo shoots for emergency tracheotomies. But there was no substitute for anesthesia, and not since the early nineteenth century does one encounter such harrowing tales of unanesthetized cranial and abdominal surgery and amputation (Dai 2004, 380).

Lacking not only medical supplies, the North Vietnamese Army was also without facilities for timely evacuation during battle. The luxury available to large conventional armies since Larrey's time allowing them to dedicate troops to evacuate the wounded during battle was nonexistent. The wounded could expect evacuation only once the fighting ended.

Carried literally on the backs of their comrades, the wounded found their way to aid stations several kilometers to the rear and received perfunctory care before evacuation to larger hospitals. Often without motorized transport, litter bearers transported the injured by bicycle or raft, or bore the wounded by hand for days or weeks on end. During this time, the seriously injured died, while otherwise treatable wounds often suffered gangrene and forced amputation (Zumwalt, n.d.)

Did the level of medical care available to North Vietnamese soldiers affect morale? This is difficult to say. Soldiers were reasonably assured they would not be abandoned on the field and that they would receive whatever care was available. They probably also knew that they would die of major wounds and suffer amputation for severe wounds to the extremities. Ideology might have carried many through in spite of the prospect of less-than-optimum care:

There was little alternative to the hardship [North Vietnamese military surgeon] Dr. Le Cao Dai's patients endured. Limited medical supplies, combined with a constant influx of wounded whose lives teetered on the brink of life or death, did not afford Dai the luxury of delaying treatment for a more ideal time. And while medical conditions were nightmarish, it was, said Dai, a price we paid for victory. (Zumwalt, n.d.)

Dai's last line is telling. Not only does it describe the ideological fervor that imbued many, it also speaks to the relationship between military necessity and medical care. On the one hand, medical care and the supplies necessary to provide it were limited by circumstance, because American bombing destroyed many supply trains in transit, and by policy—that is, by a conscious decision by policymakers to allocate certain resources to medical care in the first place. On the other hand, medical care, however, abysmal, was sufficient to maintain the fighting force and uphold morale among soldiers. The Vietnamese case also highlights the relationship between medical care and organizational integrity. For conventional armies, comprehensive medical care is an integral part of the armed forces' capacity to fight. Failure to provide this care is a sign of widespread organizational disintegration, as will happen, for example, when an army is close to defeat. In guerrilla armies, on the other hand, poor medical care does not necessarily impinge on the army's organizational capacity to wage war as it continues to provide competent leadership, supplies, and personnel.

Medical care affects morale in this indirect way. Material and ideological incentives often motivate soldiers to risk death. Soldiers also know that the risk of death is ever-present and never entirely absent. Unattended pain and suffering, on the other hand, are considerably more corrosive. The cries of men left dying on the battlefield must damage morale more than the deaths of the fallen themselves. For this reason, acute care for the moderately wounded together with stabilizing and comfort care that reasonably reduces the risk of unattended pain and suffering among the most severely wounded, although not necessarily dedicated to saving their lives or reducing the chances these soldiers will die, will go a long way to prevent demoralization. For reasons of morale and for further reasons I will explore below, the duty to provide adequate medical care to salvage those lightly or moderately wounded and comfort the severely injured takes precedence over saving some soldiers' lives when aggressive medical care demands considerable resources. In military organizations that lack the resources of the well-developed armies of industrialized nations, medical personnel can only offer minimal care similar to the care PAVN provided its soldiers. In these cases, minimal care is adequate and sufficient to offset the negative effects of no care at all. Moreover, the effect of medical care on morale is limited, so that more than adequate care probably does not affect morale positively. That is, it is doubtful that very advanced medical care instills any sort of superior fighting spirit. On the contrary, once adequate care is available, ideology is certainly a powerful enough incentive to overcome the threat of death while superb care, despite Westmoreland's claim to the contrary, will not sustain morale once an army has lost its will to fight.

In general, then, medical care has the greatest effect on morale when it is lacking entirely, when evacuation is absent or inefficient, when hospitals are cesspools of neglect and infection, and when soldiers are abandoned in their final hours. This raises the risk of death, instills a fear of unattended pain and suffering, and underscores neglect and abandonment. While none of this typifies modern armies today, it was close to the norm through the end of the nineteenth century. Yet this does not demand more than adequate medical care to meet the needs of the moderately and lightly wounded and alleviate the pain and suffering of those wounded severely. Morale does not offer grounds for extensive life-saving surgical capabilities nor sufficient reason to save the 30,000 wounded men the Germans let die. One may have to search for these grounds elsewhere.

Utilitarian justifications for evacuating and treating severely wounded soldiers, whether for reasons of salvaging soldiers for battle or increasing morale, fall short in several respects. In many cases, commanding officers were well aware that using existing resources to evacuate and treat the severely wounded was often inefficient. Nor was medical care necessary to keep morale among the troops high. Soldiers both desire and deserve medical care, but this tells us little about what kind of medical care is necessary to preserve morale. Adequate care combined with material and ideological incentives could maintain sufficient morale without having to provide forward surgical units. For this reason, perhaps, utilitarian justifications of intensive battlefield medical care are not pressed with much enthusiasm. Instead, nonconsequentialist justifications calling on obligation and humanitarian duty might be more convincing.

Medical Care and Political Obligation

"Is there any Government that would hesitate to give its patronage to a group [of voluntary orderlies and nurses] endeavoring . . . to preserve the lives of useful citizens, for assuredly the soldier who receives a bullet in defense of his country deserves all that country's solicitude" (Dunant [1862] 1986, 126–127).

There is strong intuitive appeal to the argument that the state is obligated to care for soldiers who risk their lives on its behalf. This claim suggests mutual obligation: the state, through its national and/or military health-care system, "has a moral obligation to provide medical care for those whom society sends into battle" (Dolev 1996, 785). If medical care was not readily available in the past, it was only because the state did not understand its obligation to those who shoulder the responsibility of military service. Presumably, this would change as the modern state took note of its duty to protect its citizens gone to war. And, indeed, Gabriel and Metz (1992, vol. 2, 62, 88) link the growth of military care for the wounded with emerging notions of citizenship that followed the French Revolution:

The idea of citizen obligation to the state based on general reciprocal obligations was established early. It was the established principle of citizenship that called into existence a state's obligation to care for the citizen-soldier gone to war to protect the community. . . . As soldiers were increasingly asked to serve in wars on grounds of national identity and loyalty, it was inevitable that governments would come to recognize some responsibility for treating and caring for the sick and wounded as a reciprocal obligation of military service.

This view is inaccurate. While there are recorded instances of soldiers, principally mercenaries, whose contracts for services stipulate the provision of medical care and disability, the modern state was never quick to come to the aid of its wounded citizen-soldiers. Moreover, the political duty of common citizens to fight, suffer injury, and possibly die for their state does not entail an obligation on the state's part to provide medical care. The obligation to die for the state emerges from the duties that citizenship imposes on the individual. The state's obligation to provide medical care for the severely wounded stems from its humanitarian obligations to relieve pain and suffering. This duty obligates the state, whether one is a civilian or a soldier. The latter have no special claim to medical care simply because they risk their lives during war. This argument proceeds in two parts, first examining a citizen's obligation to die for the state and then the state's obligation to relieve pain and suffering. Each stands independently of the other. There is no implicit or explicit bargain, nor any reciprocal obligation, to provide medical care in return for military service.

The Citizen's Obligation to Die or Suffer Injury for the State

The obligation of citizens to die for their country does not sit well with the rationale of individualism and egoism that justifies the modern state. After rejecting the divinely ordained authority of the medieval and early modern state, theorists were left with a quandary: How, in light of the natural and unlimited freedom of human beings, could the state gain coercive authority? The answer from the standpoint of Hobbes, Locke, and other thinkers lies in contract and agreement. Under certain conditions individuals would agree to restrict their own freedom and allow the state, in the form of a sovereign assembly or monarch, to regulate their lives for the express purpose of safeguarding the security of each and every citizen. Men and women exchanged a measure of freedom for a measure of security.

Contractual Obligations to Die for the State   For the most part contractarian obligations entail political participation, obedience to the law, and payment of taxes. But does it mean dying for the state? Hobbes, for example, equivocates. On the one hand, the prospect of death, as Walzer (1970) notes, signifies the failure of the state. One contracts with the state for personal, not collective, security. Having to die for the state repudiates the legitimacy of the state, thereby leaving individuals free to break the bonds of contract and disassociate themselves from the state's coercive power. On the other hand, Hobbes ([1651] 1996, chapter 21, p. 152) refuses to release citizens from military duty when the security of the state is at stake: "When the defense of the commonwealth requires at once the help of all that are able to bear arms, everyone is obliged; because otherwise the institution of the commonwealth, which they have not the purpose or the courage to preserve, was in vain."

This passage has rankled scholars, for it greatly muddies Hobbes's view of obligatory military service. While Deborah Baumgold (1983) favors a presumptive obligation to die for one's state with few exceptions, Walzer concludes that Hobbes's commitment to the inalienable right of self-preservation overrides obligatory military service. The very need for military service, in Walzer's opinion, undermines the social contract, and Hobbes, in spite of his protests to the contrary, cannot get very far trying to obligate citizens to die for their state. Others believe that Hobbes was sensitive to this weakness and therefore generally excluded citizens from military service and relied, instead, on a paid army of professionals bound to the state by an ordinary contract (Dolman 1995).

These interpretations leave ordinary citizens generally, if not entirely, free from the obligations normally associated with democratic citizenship, leading one to ask whether liberal states can ever obligate any citizen to go to war. Walzer (1970, 89), in fact, says they cannot. "Indeed," he writes, "the great advantage of liberal society may simply be this: that no one can be asked to die for public reasons on behalf of the state." And, while private reasons may suffice to drive citizens to risk their lives in defense of hearth and home, a state can hardly wage war if its only recourse is to invoke self-interest. Instead, the state must appeal to collective welfare.

Utilitarian Grounds to Die for the State   If contract theory is stymied by its attempts to justify a citizen's duty to die for the state, utilitarianism may fare somewhat better. The liberal, utilitarian state does not rest on an agreement of contracting members but on the state's successful defense of collective happiness and well-being. This requires the state to provide security, a function it assigns to the police and military. Charged with safeguarding civil liberties and the overriding duty to protect aggregate interests, the state may obligate citizens to military service and, indeed, send some of them to their death.

Utilitarianism is often accused of failing to take individuals qua individuals seriously—that is, it may theoretically subjugate a few for the benefits of the many. The flip side of this argument, however, is that unlike contractarianism, where each person stands before the state and can judge the entire state by how the state's action affects the welfare of a single individual, utilitarianism does not allow this move. The state is not obligated to protect the singular interests of atomized individuals but to safeguard aggregate welfare, so that the moral basis of utilitarianism certainly allows the liberal state to sacrifice some individuals for the interests of others. Moreover, certain inefficient outcomes of rationality that may prompt some to free-ride rather than contribute to a collective good demand that the state forcibly conscript young men and women into military service and severely punish those who desist.

Yet, utilitarianism does not create an overwhelming case for obligating citizens to die for their country. Utilitarianism compels citizens to serve when aggregate interests are at stake, on the assumption that the deaths of some will save the lives of many. This may occur as a state faces existential dangers or the threat of genocide. Hugo Bedau, for example, demands that citizens risk their lives in the service of the state when war poses an immediate threat to its citizens. In contrast to the obligation to serve in the Vietnam War, Bedau (1971) argues that Israelis facing Arab armies in 1967 shouldered the obligation to take up arms in defense of their nation because the lives of their compatriots were at stake. Obligations of this type are unilateral; the state neither promises nor is obliged to offer anything in return. Most often, however, wars are not fought to save a nation from destruction but, as in Vietnam, for interests that have little to do with the aggregate welfare of its citizens. In these circumstances, utilitarianism says little about the obligation to die for the state.

Superaggregate Interests and the Duty to Die for the State   Only by moving beyond personal and aggregate interests may one enlarge the scope of obligation to embrace the wars most nations fight: wars of honor, ideology, and territorial aggrandizement. These wars do not protect self-interest or the interests of the greatest number but speak to the common, indivisible good that characterizes Rousseau's vision of the General Will described earlier. Cognizant of the collective good, citizens of the enlightened state do not realize their potential by pursuing narrow self-interest but by gradually leaving self-interest behind and identifying with the greater interests of society and the state. "They die willingly for the sake of the state," writes Walzer (1970, 92), "not because the state protects their lives—which would be as Hegel argued, absurd—but because the state is their common life." By the French Revolution, the state commanded the allegiance of its citizenry to the extent that great waves of citizens, the *levée en masse*, rose up spontaneously in its defense. For these French citizens, individual interests were incoherent outside the framework of the nation-state, a view markedly different from that of Locke or Hobbes, who were only too happy to release individuals from their commitment to the state and return them to their natural freedom should the state collapse.

The French tradition of collective consciousness, the General Will, and the privileged interests of the state resonated on the Continent. Through Herder, Hegel, and later thinkers, the state serves as an essential actor in an evolutionary process necessarily fraught with war, revolution, and conflict, but one expected to bring a greater measure of freedom or progress than humankind previously experienced. The duty to serve the goal of an ever-expanding notion of freedom obligated citizens to risk their lives during war. Investing the state or common way of life with a higher purpose subordinates private to public interests. The emerging superpersonality, whether identified with the nation-state, a people, a grand metaphysical idea, or more recently, with pan-national religious movements, exerts a powerful influence on citizens and individual members of the community, calling on them to abjure personal interests and give their lives in defense of higher ideals. Great sacrifices are expected to protect a particular way of life and idea of the good so that a people, nation, or religion may leave its mark on the world. Whether war serves individual or aggregate welfare is immaterial.

Dying for the State and Medical Care

While contract theory, utilitarianism, and collectivist theories of the state all obligate their citizens to serve their country (or people or religion) to one degree or another, this obligation, as weak or as strong as it may be, says little about medical care or special entitlements due those who are wounded or who die fighting. The obligation to die or suffer injury for one's nation is, at best, a unilateral obligation. Walzer has demonstrated how traditional contract theory cannot easily generate this obligation at all. Utilitarianism charges the state with protecting aggregate welfare and may therefore allow the state to coerce some into military service. The state's duty to offer conscripts medical care, however, is not part of a reciprocal agreement or bargain. Military service does not create a special entitlement; individuals cannot condition their military service on the provision of medical care. There is nothing in the moral obligation to die or risk injury in the service of the state that grants soldiers privileged access to medical resources.

A state provides medical care commensurate with its resources, but on the basis of the same obligation it fulfills when it raises an army, namely, to protect the welfare of as many citizens as possible. A state conscripting soldiers must therefore provide medical care insofar as this care serves the aim of safeguarding aggregate interests—that is, care that turns on returning wounded soldiers to battle. Once severely wounded and unable to return to duty, a soldier's welfare is no longer of *special* concern. That is, soldiers have no unique entitlement to receive medical care simply because they risked their lives. The same utilitarian logic that obligates individuals to die for their country may militate against medical care, directing the state to abandon the wounded when they no longer serve the common good. Similar arguments govern medical care for those answering the call of the General Will. The state does not make war to protect aggregate interests but fights to protect a supremely important collective good. Such a state is bound to commit its resources to obtain that good. One might even find states of this nature behaving considerably more recklessly than utilitarian governed states, committing vast resources to obtain some abstract good that offers no immediate benefit to any large number of private individuals. Their imperative to provide medical care is also dictated by return to duty and salvage.

A Rawlsian Contract?   One might wonder, at this point, whether a more elaborate and complex contract of the kind Rawls has in mind is sufficient to create mutual obligations, so that the duty to die for the state generates a reciprocal obligation to dedicate care to the severely wounded. In a hypothetical Rawlsian contract it is reasonable to suppose that citizens would blindly agree to risk their lives for their state, assuming that the burdens were distributed equitably and the ends and means of war were just. This would apply to citizens of either the Hobbesian or Rousseauian mold. A individualist who sees nothing but instrumental value to the state might reason that the probability of having to die for the state is very low while, at the same time, the probability of saving one's life and property if others are prepared to fight is very high. Rational, self-interested agents might then agree to a system of fair military service. Moreover, knowing the inclination of rational individuals to avoid harm's way, these same agents might also allow the state to take coercive measures to conscript soldiers. Once the veil is removed, those facing death in war could not, without violating the cognitive consistency characteristic of rational beings, then opt out. Additionally, the Rawlsian citizen may be sufficiently versed in human psychology to endow the state with intrinsic worth beyond its role of protecting the life of each and every citizen. The state may serve as a vehicle for national culture or language, or more generally "a way of life" that one wishes to perpetuate. Or, the state may provide nonmaterial goods—identity, fellow feeling, solidarity, and support—without which an individual might not be able to live. As such, the contracting citizen may realize that life without a state is worse than death. In this case, too, a binding agreement to participate in an equitable conscription plan is not out of the question.

   In such an arrangement individuals may consider medical care as a condition of risking their lives. However, I do not think that this particular provision will stand alone; rather it will stand relative to military necessity and reason of state. Rawlsian citizens might formulate the following rule: *Distribute scarce medical resources during war to best aid the war effort but, at the same time, provide a safety net of adequate medical care for all.* They may then consider priority medical care for critically wounded soldiers. What might be the basis for this decision? First, contracting agents may consider the vagaries of human psychology and conclude that soldiers fight better, and, therefore, better protect the welfare of everyone else, if assured that cutting-edge medical care is always available. We have seen, however, that this claim is empirically weak. Aggressive medical care for the severely wounded does not enhance an army's manpower or significantly contribute to its morale. Alternatively, contracting agents may consider the gratitude they owe soldiers who risk their lives. A nation may indeed owe its soldiers a debt of gratitude, but however deserving soldiers are of appreciation, there is no obvious reason that they should be rewarded with scarce medical resources—a fundamental primary good.[3] On the contrary, to grant priority to soldiers based only on the fact they risked their lives threatens to invoke a morally arbitrary and stilted criterion that devotes medical resources to the welfare of young males at the expense of others—children, the disabled, the elderly, and most women—who cannot fulfill their civic duties in the same way. The state does not owe soldiers exceptional treatment beyond that which can be justified by expediency. There is no bargain or claim right that grants combatants special entitlements. Absent a compelling utilitarian argument, medical resources remain to be distributed based on medical need whether the patient is a combatant or noncombatant.

Medical Care and the Liberal State   The theoretical difficulty inherent in the liberal state's ability to find good grounds for medical care that cannot be justified by expediency is reflected in the history of military medicine. Until World War I, the liberal, European states had a deplorable record for military medicine. Medical care in the British navy, for example, was probably the worst in Europe. Impressment was the favored method of conscription, flogging was rampant, and wounded sailors were often thrown overboard (Gabriel and Metz 1992, vol. 2,

118). This is hardly the picture of reciprocal obligations between ordinary citizens and the emerging liberal state. Napoléon's attitude toward medical care was, at best, ambivalent. On one hand he had great regard for the wounded, often ordering officers to give up their horses to carry the wounded. On the other, he "seems to have shared the traditional view that soldiers drawn from the lower social orders simply did not count for much." While Larrey had a free hand to develop evacuation and supply strategies for Napoléon's Imperial Guard, the rest of his army often left the wounded languishing on the battlefield for days on end (Richardson 1985). During the Crimean War, staggering losses did not move the British to provide anything more than abysmal care for their wounded. The mortality rate at the British military hospital in Scutari was 44 percent but would drop to 2 percent by the war's end, owing to Florence Nightingale and the dedication of a few other well-trained nurses (Gabriel and Metz 1992, vol. 2, 170). This was no great feat of medical technology; it only reflected the desire to treat the wounded like human beings. Neglect best sums up the attitude of most European armies toward their wounded. It is noteworthy that the best record of military medical care prior to World War I belongs to Japan, hardly the paragon of the enlightened, liberal state.

So where are the fruits of this heady talk of bargains and reciprocal obligations between the emerging state and its citizens? During the nineteenth century, medical care had little to offer most of the wounded, and those whose lives it might save were often militarily useless amputees. As a consequence, few armies devoted significant resources to medical care. The situation improved for many soldiers as medicine offered the prospect of returning significant numbers of what were previously considered "seriously wounded" to duty. However, the imperative to care for the remaining seriously wounded remains unjustified by calculations of expected utility. Nor is the obligation to provide extensive medical care to the severely wounded, one we can readily derive from a citizen's willingness or duty to die for the state. Contract and utility underlie this duty but do not entail the duty to aid the wounded unless it serves reason of state. But reason of state cannot justify medical care for the severely wounded if they do not return to duty.

At best, we might look for the duty to provide medical care to the severely wounded in the state's prima facie duties to prevent pain and suffering. These are not reciprocal obligations generated by an individual's contribution to the state. Rather, the state owes medical care to each individual on the basis of each person's basic human rights. For this reason, perhaps, it was the outcry from civilians moved by humanitarian concerns that led to immediate, albeit often ad hoc, improvements in medical care. Dunant ([1862] 1986, 124–125), it will be remembered, did not trouble himself with a plea to military authorities to provide better care for the wounded but appealed instead to "the humane and philanthropically inclined." These appeals do not rest on the state's unmet reciprocal obligations due soldier qua soldiers, but on the state's duty to protect soldiers qua human beings from harm.

The State's Obligation to Relieve Pain and Suffering

During armed conflict soldiers are wounded, some horrifically. Surely they would like to live, but the state does not owe them their life unequivocally. Individuals lose their right to life when they take up arms; the state is only obligated to prevent *unnecessary* death. The right to life is conditional and subordinate to military necessity; as long as most wars continue, military planners will expend human life with relative impunity. Once wounded, soldiers have no claim-right to priority care unless they can return to duty. Those that remain seriously wounded and without a reasonable chance to return to duty have no special status. Soldiers who cannot return to duty can only appeal to the state's duty to prevent harm, the same appeal any individual can make. The relationship between a soldier and the state offers no ground for offering combatants prior access to medical care.

Both contractarian and utilitarian theories impose on the state the obligation to protect its citizens from harm. Whether citizens exchange freedom for security or entrust the state to maximize aggregate welfare, they generally expect the state to do its utmost to prevent harm from befalling them. Among the forms that harm takes, most noteworthy are death, and pain and suffering. If, during war, states do not have an unequivocal duty to protect and preserve the lives of certain classes of

individuals, namely their soldiers, states are not relieved of their humanitarian duty to prevent unnecessary pain and suffering. To the extent
that death as well as pain and suffering are an inexorable part of war,
this duty will labor under the limits imposed by military necessity.
But military necessity, as noted in the previous chapter, can only
justify *necessary* and proportionate harm; it cannot, except on the pain
of self-contradiction, condone unnecessary suffering. Assuming access
to moderate medical resources, the duty to prevent pain and suffering
and provide the wounded with minimally adequate care, remains
absolute.

Humanitarian duties are not, as is sometimes assumed, a supererogatory or philanthropic impulse to help those less fortunate (as Dunant
suggests). On the contrary, humanitarian obligations are prepolitical,
unilateral, and nonreciprocal, derive from an individual's basic human
and not political rights, and antedate any political arrangement, contract,
or bargain. As such, they apply equally to all persons. Every individual
commands the right to freedom from unnecessary pain and suffering
irrespective of the contingencies of war. The care necessary to alleviate
unnecessary pain and suffering represents a baseline of *minimally adequate* medical care that should command a sufficient share of resources
to meet the needs of wounded combatants, civilians, and prisoners
of war—that is, those who cannot claim priority care or additional
resources based on their future contribution to the war effort. Allocations beyond this point are subject to rational deliberation among policymakers, who may decide to allocate additional resources to medical
care. But minimally adequate care remains the basic right of every sick
or injured person. What does this mean for the wounded soldier?

Adequate Care for the Wounded   By World War II, cutting-edge
medicine included blood-preservation techniques, burn treatment, and
antibiotics such as penicillin and sulfa drugs. For the most part, these
innovations made their way directly to the battlefield, often at the
expense of the general public. Nor did the Allies spare expense as they
deployed significantly larger numbers of medical personnel to care for
their wounded than did the Germans. The American policy of providing
prompt evacuation of the wounded together with technologically

advanced, forward surgical facilities continued through Korea, Vietnam, and the Gulf Wars. Israeli and British military medical care is similarly sophisticated (Danon, Nili, and Dolev 1984; Israeloff 1985; Rozin, Klausner, and Dolev 1988).

Although the kind of advanced surgical care that the United States, Israel, or Britain extends to its soldiers is now the norm in Western armies, it is not morally obligatory to provide such care for all the wounded. Military necessity governs medical care and grants priority to those capable of returning to duty. For those unable to return to duty, humanitarian duty—not utility, morale, or reciprocal obligation—sustains a wounded soldier's right to receive medical care. Beyond those wounded whose recovery aids the war effort, medicine must treat the remaining classes of wounded noncombatants (severely wounded soldiers and injured civilians) by criteria that apply equally to all. As such, every army must consider its resources and ask what kind of medical care it should provide its soldiers.

Consider the conclusion of a team of American medical officers commissioned to study German military medicine at the end of World War II:

> To the German Army, surgically understaffed and underequipped, and seemingly with a lower moral conception of the medical mission than our own, a seriously wounded man who could not fight again, even if his life were saved, was not worth bothering with, or expending precious time and supplies upon. But if, by means of preventive medicine, even one man could be spared an infectious disease which would incapacitate him for only three days, then preventive medicine was the field upon which the harshly realistic Wehrmacht would concentrate its efforts. (Wiltse 1965, 611–612)

In light of the preceding arguments, however, there is nothing to infer that a policy of expending scarce resources to save the lives of severely wounded soldiers is morally superior to one that does not. On the contrary, a policy limiting medical care may be justified on both utilitarian ("realistic") and nonconsequentialist grounds if it returns a maximum number of soldiers to duty and fulfills the state's humanitarian duty to prevent unnecessary pain and suffering by offering palliative care to the severely wounded.

Palliative care, normally the purview of patients suffering from fatal diseases, is the minimal medical care that a military organization must provide to the severely wounded to meet its humanitarian obligation. Palliative care does not endeavor to cure ill patients or extend their lives, but to preserve their dignity and self-respect, and relieve pain and suffering before they die. Palliative care is not normally an issue of any significance in military medicine, for every effort is made to save soldiers' lives regardless of cost. If a state commands sufficient resources to provide sophisticated care for all their sick and injured, *and* seriously wounded soldiers are treated on a par with any other similarly injured person, then there is no moral impediment to providing acute care to any injured person. However, most countries, even the wealthiest, do not have sufficient resources to provide advanced medical care to every citizen in need. States, therefore, use many methods to ration resources. This is their right insofar as these methods are reasonably fair. Without going into a detailed discussion of which methods are fair, let me simply suggest that they cannot be fair if they grant priority to seriously wounded soldiers. After caring for its lightly and moderately wounded soldiers—that is, those who will return to duty—the state turns its attention to all the seriously injured, both civilians and soldiers, as a single class. At this point, the remaining resources should be available to all those in need on the basis of a universally acceptable and equally applied criterion of distributive justice. Generally this is medical need, commensurate with pain and suffering and, perhaps, with the quality of a patient's remaining life years or similar criteria (Callahan 1988; Daniels 1988). Unfortunately, this lesson is frequently lost, and nonmilitary medical needs are often given short shrift to the detriment of the basic human rights all should enjoy.

Inadequate Medical Care for the Wounded If a surfeit of resources sometimes leads to the overtreatment of seriously wounded soldiers at the expense of similarly wounded civilians, there is a woeful tendency to simply ignore the seriously wounded when resources are not plentiful. Here, too, human rights suffer, not those of civilians per se but of the wounded in general. In two accounts, Norman Bethune, the Canadian medical advisor to Mao's Eighth Route Army in the late 1930s, graphically describes the state of military medical care available to guerrilla fighters in China:

The beds weren't really beds and the hospitals weren't really hospitals. . . . The staff did what they could, but there were no adequately trained personnel among them. There were no anesthetics . . . no regular operating rooms, none of the regular instruments required for surgery. Bandages were washed after use, hung out to dry, and then used again. There was only homemade thread for stitching up wounds. Medical supplies were mostly pills of local manufacture and dubious value. Probes were made of wire. For tweezers and pincers pieces of iron were used. There were no training facilities for doctors or medical attendants of any kind. (Allen and Gordon 1971, 193)

And

There are 175 wounded here, scattered among the houses. This is what is meant by a "hospital" here. It would break your heart to see them—lying on brick k'angs with only a little straw beneath them. Some have no coverlets—none have blankets. The wounded are crawling with lice. They have only one uniform, and that they have on. It is filthy with the accumulated dirt of nine months' fighting. Their bandages have been washed so often they are nothing but dirty rags. Three men, one with the loss of both feet through frost-bite gangrene, have no clothes at all to wear. There is only a coverlet for them. Their food is boiled millet— that's all. All are anemic and underfed. Most of them are slowly dying of sepsis and starvation. Many have tuberculosis. (Allen and Gordon 1971, 199)

It is important to see the difference between these two accounts. The first describes lack of medical expertise and equipment. "Think of it:" wrote Bethune, "200,000 troops here, 2,500 wounded always in hospital, over 1,000 battles fought in the past year. And to handle all this, no medical supplies, only five graduate doctors, 50 Chinese untrained 'doctors,' and one foreigner!" (Allen and Gordon 1971, 290). The need was so great that it is impossible to meaningfully raise questions of ethical priorities. Justice, as Hume reminds us, requires *moderate* scarcity without which there is either enough for everyone, or so little that desert and need are meaningless criteria for distributing resources. During Mao's guerrilla war, medical resources were in such short supply that Bethune simply did the best he could with whatever he had. By bringing his operating theater as close to the front as possible and organizing crews of stretcher bearers to evacuate the wounded as soon as possible, he simply tried to stretch his meager resources as efficiently as possible.

The second account, on the other hand, has little to do with medical expertise and a great deal to do with neglect. It calls to mind the state of many a wounded on European battlefields during the nineteenth century. Why were the wounded left in such a state unless military commanders and civilians alike felt there was no need to expend any resources whatsoever on their behalf? This attitude, no doubt, is fueled by lack of available medical expertise, without which it may well have been futile to treat the wounded. But this does not explain lice, filth, inadequate clothing, and substandard food. Humanitarian care remains an imperative regardless of the state and availability of medical care, a point driven home by Dunant, Nightingale, and others but, again, lost on some military commanders.

Excessive Care for the Wounded   Once return to active duty is doubtful, a soldier's claim to medical treatment turns on the same criteria that dictate medical treatment for any individual. Lest one argue that medical personnel can only make this determination on an ad hoc basis subject to the condition of a particular patient at a particular time, let me suggest a more general statistical approach. Soldiers suffering from certain wounds will have a particular probability of returning to duty. Once this probability is low, then the patient loses his or her priority to receive medical care and joins the pool of all similarly injured individuals. Thus, rather than deny the general public access to penicillin as the United States did in the middle of World War II, authorities should first distribute the drug on the strength of military necessity and then by reason of medical need for all affected patients. But this was not the case. The lion's share of penicillin made its way to the military without discriminating between classes of wounded soldiers (chapter 5). The same rule holds true for the distribution of neurosurgeons or vascular surgeons, for example. The U.S. army was proud of its ability to provide technologically advanced medical care in Vietnam:

An outstanding feature of medical service in Vietnam was the quality and extent of care given in the battle area. Any type of medical or surgical specialist was available in the combat zone. For example, by the spring of 1968, there were 10 neurosurgeons at five Army hospitals, supervised by a board-certified neurosurgeon. Sophisticated operations were handled as a matter of routine. (Neel 1991, 57)[4]

But what claim do severely wounded soldiers have to these resources if they are in short supply? This question is particularly poignant, for at least one-third of head injuries were the result of soldiers' failure or unwillingness to wear helmets (Neel 1991, 55). Do they have a stronger claim to this expertise than the folks back home? I do not see how. Beyond medical need, a criterion that should put them on the same footing as anyone else, there are no good grounds for flooding a war zone with excessive numbers of specialists. Any other policy is inherently unjust, as is a policy of granting greater disability benefits to veterans than to those noncombatants suffering similar injuries from disease or accident (Gal 2001, 225–244).

The Limits of Military Medical Care

In the final analysis, it is not utility or the obligation of the state to care for those who risk their lives on its behalf that anchors the obligation to provide medical care. Instead, simple humanitarian duty renders the state responsible for caring for wounded soldiers. While nations strip some of their citizens of their right to life, place them in harm's way, and empower them to kill during war, the state cannot strip citizens of their right to be free of unattended pain and suffering. And this remains the sole, overriding purpose of military medical care for the severely wounded. Palliative care meets the conditions of utility, state obligation, and humanity. An efficient use of resources, palliative care reinforces morale and distributes scarce resources to those most likely to return to battle rather than recover from serious injury. Palliative care allows the state to meet the obligation imposed by human rights. Palliative care under these conditions also squares with a physician's minimal obligation to provide beneficent care. Should a military organization command sufficient resources to move beyond this point in any significant way, physicians will use these resources to better the condition of their patients. However, they must also realize that there are others with legitimate claims against these resources that the military may fail to take into account. These may be civilians or other medically needy individuals.

Thirty thousand lives are not trivial. Without forward surgical care, the number of American soldiers dying from wounds during World War II might have easily increased by 50 percent, from 60,000 to 90,000 men. Yet it is entirely possible that a comparable, if not greater, number of

American civilians died from similar forms of trauma because surgical personnel and medical supplies, like penicillin, were dispatched for the benefit of the military. Moreover, like any disaster, war does not allow the most efficient use of medical resources. It is the nature of military medicine to see short periods of intense activity followed by longer periods of little to do. One wonders, for example, whether some of the ten neurosurgeons in Vietnam in 1968 might have saved more lives, many more lives, had they remained at home.

For many, asking this question might be unsettling. Combat soldiers, particularly the seriously wounded, demand the best medical care a nation can muster in order to maintain a nation's fighting force, strengthen morale, and meet the state's obligation to care for its defenders. These arguments surface repeatedly and remain difficult to dislodge. On close examination, however, they are not altogether compelling. They suggest unequal treatment where none is due, and harm the rights of those who deserve state protection. Addressing the question of care for the wounded demands that we draw as clear a distinction as possible between moderately wounded soldiers who will return to duty and severely wounded soldiers who will not, and between sufficient care for the moderately wounded to restore them to combat readiness and palliative care for the severely wounded to relieve their pain and suffering. This suggests a baseline for minimal military medical care. When less care is available, and a nation can no longer protect the minimal human rights of its citizens, it loses its reason of state and may consider surrender. When resources are abundant and a nation easily meets its minimal requirements, it will then consider how to distribute the balance of its resources fairly and without discriminating in favor of severely wounded soldiers. The right to medical care is an abiding problem for military medical ethics precisely because of the tendency to grant inordinate weight to the welfare of all soldiers during war. The other patient rights that soldiers enjoy are similarly problematic, not because we grant them too much weight but because we run the risk of granting them too little.

4

Patient Rights for Soldiers

Soldiers are not ordinary patients. Their special status as combatants whose life, liberty, and dignity are limited by choice or circumstance attenuates habitual concern for their welfare and autonomy. Soldiers are not fully autonomous individuals nor, unless freely enlisting, have they elected to restrict their liberty. Positive law allows nations to conscript young men and women and place their lives in jeopardy in the service of the state irrespective of their wishes. Without autonomy in its most expansive form, its derivative patient rights—informed consent, confidentiality, and the right to die—weaken. The right to refuse treatment is near nonexistent because, in many cases, soldiers must accept medical care (Moskop 1998).[1] Confidentiality—the duty of medical personnel to refrain from disclosing privileged information—is feeble, and medical workers may sometimes find themselves obligated to denounce their patients, particularly enemy soldiers, to the authorities. Finally, the right to die, one of the most enduring byproducts of patient autonomy today, is entirely transformed during war. Rarely do soldiers ever ask to die, but faced with overwhelming pain and suffering, or injuries that may impede a mission and affect the safety of others, they, or others, may ask to end their lives. This is not the right to die in a hospital by withholding or withdrawing life-sustaining treatment, but an act akin to active euthanasia on the battlefield.

What rights, then, do soldier-patients enjoy? As autonomy dissipates, informed consent, confidentiality, and the right to die shrivel and shrink. Medical care assumes a distinctly paternalistic flavor, not simple paternalism—doctors manipulating their patients' choices for the patients' own good—but paternalism writ large, as doctors and military commanders direct patient care for the good of others. Self-rule, as I suggested in chapter 2, gives way to other-ruled, while selfish interests yield to collective concerns and superaggregate welfare. Reason of state overwhelms autonomy and the patient rights soldiers and sailors can claim.

Informed Consent during Armed Conflict

Informed consent is a measure of respect for autonomy and entails an obligatory decision-making process. Respect for autonomy requires health-care professionals to provide a patient with the information necessary to make a responsible decision—that is, one that will best restore their health or quality of life. Because informed consent entails *giving* consent, it is impossible to meet its conditions solely by furnishing information. It is not possible to partially preserve informed consent by providing patients with pertinent medical data while denying them the right to refuse care, as some proponents of mandatory inoculation in the military have suggested (see the following section). The act of informing alone has no bearing on the principle of informed consent. Information is helpful to any patient who wishes to monitor side effects and is a basic axiom of beneficent care.

Informed consent is neither a necessary nor a sufficient condition of good medical care; its purpose is to preserve respect for autonomy, not ensure quality treatment. Often these go hand in hand. When autonomy is respected, patients are better informed and will comply with treatment and recover more quickly. But this says nothing about consent. Paternalistic physicians can also provide abundant information because they expect that informed patients have a better chance of recovery than patients kept in the dark. Consent may also go awry and undermine medical care, as when patients decide to forgo life-saving treatment. Generally, there are few conflicts between physicians and their patients; often both agree on the same course of treatment. Conflicts only arise when patients make the wrong decision and choose to ignore sound medical advice. When they do, the options are not very palatable. Either the patients must suffer the consequences of their own stupidity or be treated by force (Gross 2005). Consent adds little to good medical care simply because it serves the principle of autonomy, a different master entirely.

The right to informed consent, like autonomy, diminishes with military service. Allowing soldiers to refuse medical treatment undermines discipline, increases risk to others, reduces manpower, and may abet malingering as untreated soldiers sicken and are withdrawn from combat. These are probably good arguments but they remain hypothetical. Oddly enough, the few cases of soldiers refusing treatment that punctuate the literature make quite the opposite impression: wounded soldiers gallantly refusing treatment to rally their troops are the stuff of military lore.

More than this, however, are the logical difficulties of a sustained right of informed consent in the military. Informed consent is intimately linked to respect for autonomy. Restrictions on the latter constrain the former. As collective interests overwhelm individual welfare, the information at one's fingertips recedes and decision making passes to others. Individuals can only exercise self-rule over a domain of interests they know; what they do not know they must cede to others. Ordinarily one knows, or can know, one's own state of health. But individual welfare is not the focus of military medical care. While medical personnel work to provide good medical care, they are obligated to provide the care necessary to maintain soldiers as a fighting *force*—that is, a corporate personality. I have already noted in the previous chapter how this does not necessarily include aggressive care for soldiers who cannot return to duty. Soldiers do not receive medical care to guarantee their health as individuals but to preserve the health of a larger organism, a common good quite distinct from the interests of the soldier as patient. Only those commanding sufficient resources to evaluate collective interests can exercise informed consent. This is not the common soldier as patient but generally those in command.

All this leaves informed consent as an artifact of peacetime civilian medicine with but marginal importance for soldiers during war. Ordinarily, this creates few problems and troops accept medical care without question as part of their duty to serve as good soldiers. Difficulties arise, however, with unproven or relatively dangerous forms of medical treatment. Reviewing the U.S. army's protocol for protecting soldiers against novel biological and chemical agents, some observers criticize the military for its failure to obtain informed consent. The debate raises two issues. First, it highlights the limits of informed consent in the military. Second, it draws attention to the element of risk: very high risk, particularly that accompanying investigational drugs, demands informed consent. The argument is compelling, but one must be careful to avoid confusing medical risk with military risk. Only when the latter, not the former, is very high is it sometimes necessary to secure a soldier's consent.

Treating Soldiers with Investigational Drugs

In recent years, the specter of unconventional warfare prompted military officials to develop defenses against chemical and biological weapons. Apart from protective gear, defensive measures include drugs and vaccines against an array of toxins and pathogens that rogue states or terror organizations may utilize. In most cases, potentially useful vaccines and antidotes undergo rigid testing and approval before the military uses them to treat its troops. But it is the nature of war to introduce novel weapons at unexpected times, so that the arsenal of medical defense is rarely up to date.

Improvising medical care to meet rapidly changing battle conditions, however, may run afoul of conventional research guidelines that demand rigorous testing before introducing new drugs for human use. As the American army developed defenses against chemical and biological weapons, several measures prompted sustained debate in the bioethics and medical community. During the 1990 Gulf War, the U.S. Department of Defense (DoD) requested special waivers to treat American troops with pyridostigmine bromide (PB) and botulinum toxoid (BT) to protect them against nerve agents and botulism without obtaining informed consent from each serviceperson. The U.S. Food and Drug Administration (FDA) had yet to approve either compound. As such, they were "investigational drugs" that required informed consent before use. The DoD asked the FDA to waive the informed-consent requirement, citing a reasonable chance that Iraq would deploy biological and/or chemical weapons and claiming that the chemical compounds, although investigational, offered the best available protection against the Iraqi threat. Moreover, it was "not feasible" in the DoD's opinion to obtain informed consent from U.S. servicepersons. The FDA agreed and issued an interim ruling that included the following provisions:

1. At the request of the DoD to use an investigational drug, the FDA commissioner could waive informed consent when it was "not feasible" to obtain it and when no other treatment is available.
2. The DoD request must be limited to a military situation that involves "combat or the immediate threat of combat."
3. The request must facilitate a military mission and preserve the health of servicepersons so that allowing informed consent and permitting some servicepersons to refuse treatment endangers national security and adversely affects the best interests of military personnel.
4. An institutional review board must approve the request. (Rettig 1999)

The final, 1999, ruling differs from the previous ruling in one respect: only the president of the United States, rather than the commissioner of the FDA, may approve the army's request to waive the informed-consent requirement for using an investigational drug (U.S. Food and Drug Administration, 1999).

Informed consent flared again in 1998 when the U.S. Secretary of Defense ordered the inoculation of all U.S. service personnel against anthrax, one of the deadliest pathogens in anyone's arsenal. In contrast to PB and BT, both investigational drugs, the vaccine for anthrax enjoyed long-standing approval from the FDA. This allowed the DoD to argue that the anthrax vaccine is a standard, therapeutic treatment that military personnel could not refuse. Critics argued that the FDA approved a vaccine against subcutaneous anthrax, not the inhalation anthrax that soldiers might encounter in battle. The DoD, therefore, required a presidential waiver to vaccinate soldiers without their consent. In either case, once the DoD decided to treat American soldiers without their consent, either because prior FDA approval made consent unnecessary or because the president waived the requirement, a dissenting soldier's only option was to resign from the service if he or she wished to refuse treatment (Annas 1998; Katz 2000–2001; Cummings 2002; FitzPatrick and Zwangziger 2003).

The ensuing debate is a harbinger of an emerging bioethical dilemma that many nations may face as they prepare for chemical and biological warfare. On the one hand, respect for patient autonomy demands consent to medical treatment. While most competent patients retain this right under any and all conditions, soldiers do not. As military personnel, they must accept medical treatment. On the other hand, war is a longtime testing ground for medical research and experimentation that lead to advances that benefit soldiers and civilians alike. Confronting novel wounds and injuries, medical science improvises and experiments to prevent injury and return wounded soldiers to active duty. When this does not permit informed consent, military necessity challenges an entrenched principle of peacetime bioethics.

The Inherent Limits of Informed Consent

Observers agree that military authorities may treat their troops with standard therapeutic drugs without their consent, either because service personnel freely waive their right to informed consent and/or because the free exercise of informed consent may endanger military discipline, increase casualties in the field, or encourage malingering (Howe and Martin 1991). This argument, as already noted, is incomplete. Conscripts do not freely waive their right to informed consent in the way enlisted personnel do. Nevertheless, it would be wrong to think that conscripts constitute a fundamentally different class of military personnel. Moreover, the harmful consequences of obtaining informed consent are largely hypothetical. Were they certain, the effects of seeking informed consent might be just the opposite that some suppose. Fear of the same consequences that make standard therapeutic care compulsory might also make investigational drugs mandatory if failure to consent erodes discipline or increases casualties.

Some of these worse fears are realized when soldiers are asked to assent to inoculation. Prior to the Boer War, the British army successfully field-tested a vaccine against typhoid, a disease that ravished armies. In spite of the vaccine's success, the British army authorized inoculation on a voluntary basis only. The response was not enthusiastic. Citing the short-lived but sometimes severe reaction some soldiers experienced following inoculation, together with the entirely groundless fear that vaccination would imperil their virility, 95 percent of British soldiers refused treatment (Pagaard 1986). Astonishingly, American soldiers rejecting anthrax vaccines one hundred years later would refuse for the very same, unfounded reason (Miller 2002). The results for Britain were disastrous: while 6,000 soldiers fell in battle, 14,000 troops died of typhoid during the war (Gabriel and Metz 1992, vol. 2, 222).

The failure of voluntary consent highlights the inherent limits and complexity of informed consent in the military. Ordinarily, medicine knows the risks of informed consent, namely, that patients sometimes make the wrong decision based on spurious information. This is forgivable because the supreme importance of maintaining respect for autonomy outweighs the cost of one misinformed or stupid decision. This is certainly a compelling argument, but unavailable to anchor informed consent in the military. Respect for autonomy is not nearly as important among soldiers as among civilians. More importantly, the outcome of faulty decision making reaches beyond the individual patient. An ordinary patient who refuses a vaccine in the face of a deadly threat suffers, at worse, his own death. Ordinarily, this is an acceptable outcome provided the patient is competent and well informed. In other settings, however, it is unacceptable, not because a person dies but because he decimates a fighting force. This is true as long as the mortality rate from disease is higher than the risk of inoculation. The tragedy of the British experience during the Boer War is not the death of 14,000 men per se, but the decimation of the British army that cost them dearly in their fight against the Boers.

Not only is informed consent problematic because soldiers may weigh spurious information, but often because they tend to weigh the right information wrongly. In many cases, investigational drugs are, in fact, sufficiently risky to convince any self-interested person to refuse treatment. Yet this decision, however rational and well informed it may be, may easily harm collective endeavors. This is the essence of any collective-action problem that plagues institutions like the military and a difficulty that only coercion can generally overcome (Hardin 1982). Agents of the state or military hierarchy who command sufficient information about the nature of the collective good and the means necessary to obtain it, will override informed consent and coerce individuals to accept treatment. Military medical ethics only *permits* informed consent, and thereby reverses the burden of proof generally incumbent on medical personnel. During war those seeking informed consent must explain how it does not impair the functioning of military operations and why they simply do not command their troops to follow an order. Quite often, this explanation lies in the risk they face.

Informed Consent and Military and Medical Risk

Explicit in the FDA's ruling is a cost-benefit analysis that weighs informed consent and military necessity. The president can waive informed consent after determining that "conditioning use of the investigational new drug on the voluntary participation of each member could significantly risk the safety and health of any individual member who would decline its use, the safety of other military personnel, and the accomplishment of the military mission."

How can someone make this decision? Are the parameters of risk the same for "the safety and health of any individual member" and "the accomplishment of the military mission"? This proviso touches on a deeper question: Is military *medical* risk any different from military risk in general? That is, to what extent is it permissible to risk soldiers' lives, either by inoculating them with an unproven drug or by sending them off into battle with unknown odds of survival in order to complete a necessary mission? Consider the following case. Army A considers a target vital and is willing to commit the troops necessary to take the objective, knowing casualties (killed and wounded) will approach 50 percent. Thus in the Hürtgen Forest, typical of the ferocious offensive battles the Allies waged against Germany at the end of 1944, the 22nd Infantry Division lost 2,805 soldiers or 48 percent of its men to capture one village and 6,000 yards of forest in a battle that lasted eighteen days (Rush 2001, 280, 82). Then or now, few have questioned whether the risk was acceptable. Replacements simply took the place of killed or wounded soldiers until the division accomplished its objective.

Now consider a scenario in which the Germans had incapacitating chemical weapons to hold back the Americans rather than dense forests, foul weather, and entrenched defenses. Consider further that this weapon would seriously incapacitate, but not kill, every exposed soldier. The antidote was untested but was expected to bring death or impairment to nearly 50 percent of those who received it. The risk of dying from exposure to poison gas, on the other hand, was relatively low, say 3 percent, just as it was in World War I (Dupuy 1995, 141). By any calculation of medical risk, inoculation was foolhardy and carried a risk that a single rational patient would refuse. Because opting out, however, would destroy any semblance of a fighting force, coercion remained the only solution. The only remaining question is the following: What level of risk may military commanders impose on their soldiers?

FDA directives instruct the president to weigh "the extent and strength of evidence of the safety and effectiveness of the investigational new drug in relation to the *medical* risk" (emphasis added). The FDA fails to consider, however, that in a situation similar to the one just described, an investigational drug might be consistent with acceptable *military* risk. Because medical and military risks are incommensurable, one must fall by the wayside. Investing the president, who happens to be commander-in-chief of the armed forces, with the authority to waive informed consent makes this a straightforward decision. The president's duty answers to reason of state, allowing him or her to order the army to vaccinate soldiers commensurate with acceptable military risk. This risk may be significantly higher than the risk ordinarily associated with acceptable medical treatment. As in the Hürtgen Forest, some military goals can push the risk of death or injury to extremely high levels. Nevertheless, we can ask whether there is an upper limit: how high can risk go before consent becomes obligatory? Rarely do military commanders solicit consent from their soldiers. Yet, consent is sometimes mandatory when soldiers are called on to risk their lives. Supererogatory, heroic actions offer an instructive parallel to the problem of informed medical consent in wartime.

Informed Consent and Extreme Military Risk

The President may award, and present in the name of Congress, a medal of honor of appropriate design, with ribbons and appurtenances, to a person who while a member of the Army, distinguished himself conspicuously by gallantry and intrepidity at the risk of his life *above and beyond the call of duty.* (USC 2000, Title 10, §3741; emphasis added)

Soldiers risk their lives all the time and are never asked to consent. Why do we then find it necessary to sometimes ask for volunteers and then award them medals when they are killed or wounded? The idea of supererogatory action in the military, illustrated by soldiers who sacrifice themselves for their fellow soldiers or volunteer for suicide missions, is a peculiar notion. What makes an act heroic and beyond the call of duty? Soldiers have a duty to risk their lives in the service of the state and to subordinate their own interests to the collective good they all seek. What then, makes them heroes? Why must they volunteer for some missions and not others, and how do answers to these questions enrich our understanding of informed medical consent?

Consider two related cases. In the first, a soldier falls on a grenade to save five of his fellow soldiers. By most accounts, this behavior is supererogatory and the soldier receives a medal for an action above and beyond the call of duty. In the second, a squad must run a diversionary attack to draw fire that will undoubtedly kill them all. The company commander asks for volunteers. They are all killed and each receives a commendation similar to the one awarded to the solider who fell on a grenade.

Why are these actions supererogatory and why do they require consent? One condition of supererogatory actions is undoubtedly high risk. But how high? Soldiers often face life-threatening situations, yet the outcomes are far from certain. The casualty rate relative to the number of soldiers mobilized is generally low. Of the 4.3 million soldiers mobilized for the Vietnam War, 127,000 were injured (3 percent), a figure that has declined steadily since the Civil War.[2] Among combat soldiers engaged in battle, however, casualty rates may easily exceed 50 percent (Dupuy 1995, 138). Yet these risks do not merit special commendation, nor are the soldiers who endure them taking supererogatory action. It seems that overwhelming, near *certain* risk of death is the criterion one searches for.

Yet certain risk is insufficient. Nor do soldiers commanded to face certain death necessarily merit commendation. Consider whether a commanding officer might order soldiers to fall on a grenade or, more extreme still, push them to their death to save others. We would repel in horror at such an act of murder. We cannot kill our own soldiers, if by that we mean not to simply risk their lives, but willfully cause their deaths. The line is fine but not merely semantic. Soldiers lose their right to life vis-à-vis the enemy. The enemy can kill them but their own commanders cannot, and those who order their soldiers to die become directly responsible for their death. To avoid the charge of murder, the enemy bears responsibility as the proximate cause of soldiers' deaths. Their own officers merely place them in harm's way. Compelling soldiers to act in the face of certain death, however, is to murder them. For this reason, they must consent and, as it were, sacrifice themselves. For this, they deserve a medal.

Yet not all acts of duress under conditions of extreme risk constitute murder. Troops reluctant to fight are often coaxed out of their foxhole or trench at the point of a gun. They are pushed forward, sometimes to certain death or injury. Yet no one awards them a medal. If anything, we condemn their fearfulness. This case affords one more intuition differentiating heroic from ordinary action, namely, the idea of fairness. In a situation where all face similar slim odds of survival, extreme risk does not characterize supererogatory behavior. Part of this problem is relativism: exceptional behavior must be extraordinary. If everyone faces the same odds, no one is a hero. More than this, however, is the intuition of fairness. Soldiers can accept risk and danger, provided all face the same threat equally and no one is excused for frivolous reasons (Williams 1989). An action becomes supererogatory when the risk it entails is both overwhelming and impossible to distribute equally so that some must assume an unequal burden. Once a person or persons are singled out for disproportionate risk, they must give their consent.

Consent hinges on indivisible extreme risk that cannot be distributed fairly among soldiers. To order soldiers to give their lives under these conditions and without consent is to murder them. These criteria apply directly to the problem of informed medical consent. The use of investigational drugs—that is, unproven drugs that provide a therapeutic benefit and maintain the fitness of a fighting force—does *not* meet the conditions requiring informed consent. Although their risks might be very high, investigational drugs do not demand consent if the risk is militarily necessary and is distributed fairly. Testing experimental drugs to enhance general human knowledge rather than provide a direct therapeutic benefit, however, presents a different sort of problem, particularly during war. Would FDA guidelines permit experimentation, or even force participation, if an experiment is necessary and a subject's refusal would "endanger national security and adversely affect the best interests of military personnel"? The fairness condition precludes this: experiments distribute risk unfairly and, therefore, demand informed consent. Nevertheless, the necessity condition should prompt another look at consent and experimentation.

Informed Consent and Experimentation   Informed consent is the centerpiece of modern medical research. Since World War II, research protocols have changed dramatically to protect patients and, in particular, vulnerable patients—soldiers, occupied civilians, and prisoners of war—from wanton medical experimentation. The Nuremberg Code regulates medical research in the wake of Nazi atrocities and stipulates unequivocally that "the voluntary consent of the human [experimental] subject is absolutely essential" (Nuremberg Code, 1947). Experimental research strives for "fruitful results for the good of society, unprocurable by other methods or means of study" and is distinct from therapeutic treatment that ministers to a particular patient or class of patients. "Research," in the opinion of the influential *Belmont Report* (National Commission for the Protection of Human Subjects of Biomedical and Behavioral Research, 1979, 3) is "an activity designed to test a hypothesis, permit conclusions to be drawn and thereby to develop or contribute to generalizable knowledge."

Most commentators, therefore, agree that the high risk of experimental research, in either a military or a civilian setting, requires informed consent. Of course, the risk need not be particularly high. Any procedure that threatens the health and well-being of a healthy person requires his or her consent. But we have already seen that risk alone is insufficient to require informed consent during war and that FDA guidelines are insufficient to regulate research that might be militarily necessary. If extreme risk is not a constraining factor, then certainly lesser risks should not stand in the way of necessary research.

Military necessity guides legitimate medical research during war, a point sometimes overlooked by focusing solely on the abuses of medical experimentation. Moreover, it is the nature of military medicine to experiment, if by this one means securing "fruitful results for the good of society, unprocurable by other methods or means of study." Consider, for example, the history of penicillin development. In 1942 and 1943, desperately ill civilians could receive penicillin only if this would aid the war effort—that is, provide knowledge useful to the military. While there was never an informed-consent protocol as we know it today, one assumes that physicians discussed the costs and benefits of treatment with their patients. This was not true for soldiers on the battlefield. Researchers knew little about using penicillin under battlefield conditions and had no way of finding out without trying it on wounded soldiers. These studies were clearly experimental. Howard Florey brought penicillin to North Africa in mid-1943 precisely so he could test it on soldiers, observe its efficacy, and modify practice accordingly:

It should be clearly understood that the object was not primarily to ascertain whether penicillin was capable of dealing with gram-positive organisms in septic conditions; this we consider had been amply shown in England already. The main problem was to learn to employ the small quantities of penicillin likely to be available for service use to the best advantage. The work, then, had been designed to give an answer to the question, "Can penicillin be used effectively in the field at all?" and "If so, how much is required and at what place in the Army organization can it be used to best advantage?" (Bickel 1972, 198–199)

This description emphasizes the experimental nature of the work of Florey and his colleagues. Yet no one ever thought to obtain informed consent.[3] One might argue, of course, that values and attitudes have changed since then, particularly since the international community reasserted humanitarian law in the postwar period. Nevertheless, the question remains whether today, in the atmosphere of modern bioethical norms, it is ethical to test drugs on soldiers without their consent in the way penicillin was tested during World War II. I do not think that we can resolve this question by simply citing the *Belmont Report*, guidelines that regulate experimentation in peacetime but do not take into account the exigencies of research during war.

One immediate response invokes the therapeutic value of penicillin treatment. After all, these were wounded soldiers; researchers are treating them first and experimenting second. But this avenue is not entirely helpful. The Advisory Committee on Human Radiation Experiments does not recognize any morally significant difference between sick and healthy research subjects and requires informed consent form both (Moreno and Lederer 1995). More importantly, one could convincingly argue that ill subjects, particularly soldiers, require *greater* protection from exploitation than those who are healthy. This demands greater concern for informed consent, not less. But soldiers do not enjoy full autonomy. It is permissible to use them as means, to treat them for their good *and* the good of others. For these reasons, perhaps experiments that are both therapeutic *and* experimental can dispense with informed consent. This harks back to emergent need as one possible exception to informed consent. Maybe these cases are simply more prevalent during war.

Were this the case, the question of informed consent would be easy to resolve with the following guideline: *It is imperative to respect informed consent when experimenting on military personnel. However, informed consent may be waived in an emergency at the discretion of the attending physician.* This is an extension of the "not-feasible" rule that regulates investigational drugs. During war, it is often necessary to experiment with new treatments to treat novel wounds and, at the same time, infeasible to obtain informed consent under battlefield conditions. Therefore, physicians may waive informed consent at their discretion.

This guideline, however, immediately generates a far-reaching and excessively broad definition of *emergency* that not only includes immediate danger to the subject-patient but threats to other significant interests as well. These latter interests could easily embrace the welfare of other injured soldiers, together with the well-being of healthy soldiers whose health must be preserved to fulfill their military roles. As a result, nearly any wartime situation is an emergency that demands that military personnel test new treatments as quickly as possible. Unfortunately, this guts the principle of informed consent one is trying to protect. How then does one prevent healthy soldiers from falling victim to medical experimentation when the only criterion of a necessary medical experiment is military necessity?

The criteria for demanding consent for medical experimentation parallel those driving the consent requirement for supererogatory action. Experimentation, in general, is simply another form of action above and beyond the call of duty. Risk is often high and not apportioned fairly. Human experimentation, like supererogatory action, should be a measure of last resort necessary to achieve an important military aim unobtainable by other means. Many medical experiments, unlike investigational drugs, violate the condition of risk and fairness and, therefore, *require* informed consent. But this leaves two other classes of experimentation to consider: unnecessary experiments or experiments whose goals researchers can achieve by other means, and controlled experiments similar to those that tested penicillin and sulfa drugs on wounded soldiers. The former are impermissible regardless of consent and the latter may not require consent at all.

Controlled experiments under battlefield conditions do not require consent. One obvious reason is feasibility. Generally, it is simply impossible to obtain consent. But this not sufficient to permit experimentation. Instead, one must evaluate the distribution of risk. Considering the question of treating the wounded with penicillin or sulfa drugs during World War II, it is clear that neither treatment protocol carried an obviously greater risk of death or morbidity. That is, neither treatment posed extreme risk, a necessary condition for demanding informed consent. Moreover, what risk there was fell equally among the wounded soldiers affected. None could claim deferential or inferior status. Finally, military need was compelling: penicillin would prove to be one of the most effective "weapons" of the Second World War. These circumstances differ markedly from those surrounding experiments testing the effects of LSD, radiation poisoning, or chemical and biological agents of the sort the U.S. military conducted on soldiers without informed consent since the end of World War II (Moreno 2001). These experiments singled out soldiers for exceptional risk in experiments whose benefits often elude us today. When risks are distributed unfairly, the burden of obtaining informed consent shifts back to the military. No consent, however, can justify an unnecessary experiment. "Necessity" is elusive. During the normal run of war, generals and presidents determine what is necessary. Medical experimentation, however, requires a more subtle, interdisciplinary mechanism. Time is often of the essence during war but most often, it does not bear down on medical researchers in the way it excites military commanders. Institutional review boards, already required by the FDA, are certainly the order of the day.

Informed consent is a marginal right of military personnel and crops up only when military medical personnel contemplate the need for experimentation. Experimentation is long the hallmark of great military medicine. Since ancient times and certainly since Ambrose Paré (1968, 138), the renowned sixteenth-century military surgeon, military surgeons have experimented on wounded soldiers to test new therapies and on healthy soldiers to formulate new defenses. The history of military medicine is often one of medical experimentation on wounded soldiers in an effort to save their lives, reduce suffering, and return them to duty. While the Nazis abused military medicine in a way previously thought unimaginable, it would be a mistake to let Nazi abuses rather than the long history of medical achievement guide our thinking. Consent does have its place in military medical ethics but, more often than not, it is the exception rather than the rule. The principle of confidentiality—long a staple of bioethics—is similarly constrained by the exigencies of war.

Confidentiality

Pearl Buck (1986) tells the poignant story of a Japanese doctor who finds a wounded American serviceman stranded in enemy territory. As he treats the man's wounds, the physician struggles with his medical duty to cure him and his civic duty to turn him over to the authorities. In the end, he nurses his patient back to health and releases him rather than divulge his identity and condemn him to the horrors of a Japanese POW camp. Readers cannot help but admire his humanity and applaud his actions.

Buck's story brings the problem of confidentiality into sharp relief, because the imperative to remain neutral and respect a patient's confidentiality creates difficulties for medical personnel who may have a duty to divulge militarily relevant information and/or denounce their patients to the authorities. The horns of the dilemma emerge as humanitarian law first commented on the subject:

No person engaged in medical activities shall be compelled to give to anyone . . . any information concerning the wounded and sick who are, or who have been, under his care, if such information would, in his opinion, prove harmful to the patients concerned or to their families. Regulations for the compulsory notification of communicable diseases shall, however, be respected. (Protocol I, 1977a, Article 16)

The fact that medical personnel may not be "compelled" by the authorities to violate confidentiality does not mean that they have no moral obligation to do so. Realizing that confidentiality may easily conflict with military necessity, the 1977 Protocols to the Geneva Conventions call on medical personnel to exercise independent judgment as they weigh their conflicting obligations: "It is up to each authority to reach a judgment on what attitude it intends to take with regard to military requirements and with regard to its humanitarian obligations" (Protocol II, 1977, Article 10, Paragraph 4701).

Military requirements may demand that physicians divulge information important for the war effort and/or remand their patients to military authorities so they cannot return to active duty. Humanitarian obligations, in this opinion, emphasize confidentiality and the obligation "not to divulge any information that might be harmful to [a physician's] patient or the latter's relatives" (Protocol II, 1977, Article 10, Paragraph 4696). In some ways, this dilemma is reminiscent of those that plague confidentiality during peacetime, particularly in psychiatric settings, because it demands that health-care professionals weigh the good of their patients against the welfare of morally significant third parties. In other ways, however, the problem is radically different, for wartime poses particular dangers not experienced in peacetime. Before I address these dangers, however, it is important to understand the place of confidentiality in biomedical ethics.

The Importance of Maintaining Confidentiality

Confidentiality represents a fiduciary responsibility on the part of a physician to respect patient privacy and refrain from divulging information to third parties who do not contribute to the patient's medical care. On the one hand, confidentiality is a derivative principle of autonomy. Unless a patient's condition threatens others, medical information remains a patient's property, the sole purview of patient and doctor. Medical information, however interesting and useful to others, does not fall into the public domain simply because it is medical. Nor can attending physicians appropriate it at their discretion. On the other hand, confidentiality enjoyed a hallowed place in medicine long before patient autonomy became an overriding norm of bioethics. Without trust, doctors cannot treat their patients effectively, and they cannot maintain trust without keeping secrets, particularly those that come to light during medical treatment. As a result, confidentiality is a mainstay of medicine, protected by law and medical ethics.

The common exceptions to confidentiality cite imminent dangers to third parties that dangerous criminals or mentally unstable patients may pose. When a diligent emergency-room physician noticed a distinctive tattoo on the arm of Richard Speck, the infamous mass murderer of student nurses in Chicago in 1966, he earned justifiable praise for denouncing Speck to the police. But Speck's doctor had only a fleeting clinical relationship with his patient. More importantly, the police sought Speck for heinous crimes. The situation is far different when a physician treats a patient who *may* commit a crime. This very question occupied the California courts in 1969. When a patient divulged his intent to kill and later murdered his girlfriend, the court famously ruled "the protective privilege ends where the public peril begins" (*Tarasoff*, 1976). Confidentiality is not inviolate but falls before the welfare of other individuals.

While clinicians support the intuitive principle behind the ruling, they sometimes find it difficult to apply in practice. While no one wishes to harm a third party, the dilemma of violating confidentiality turns on assessing the magnitude and probability of the harm a patient poses. Is a patient after murder or intimidation? Is there a reasonable risk he will carry out his threat, however dangerous, or are his words largely empty? These questions are exceedingly difficult to answer when posed about a *potential* criminal and definitive answers can be very difficult to come by. As a result, respect for confidentiality is the rule rather than the exception of modern medicine, necessary to maintain the trust a patient and physician require to ensure quality medical care. Only severe and certain threats to the welfare of third parties are sufficient to justify a breach of confidentiality. Similar threats limit the right of confidentiality during war.

Confidentiality in War: The Peacetime Analogy

During war, enemy soldiers often receive medical treatment. Sometimes these prisoners may divulge important military information. More likely, however, the Protocols envisioned insurgents or guerrillas who find themselves in a doctor's care without anyone immediately realizing they are enemy soldiers. Here a physician must then consider, as did the Japanese doctor in Pearl Buck's story, whether to denounce their patients to the authorities. Like their civilians counterparts, military medical personnel must evaluate the likelihood of serious harm a patient and the public will suffer should they denounce a patient or conceal his presence.

In contrast to a strong obligation to break confidentiality when third parties are threatened with grave and imminent harm, the Protocols side with the weaker argument, namely, that under certain conditions medical personnel are *permitted* rather than *obligated* to violate confidentiality. The choice between military necessity (i.e., the duty to aid the war effort) and biomedical ethics (i.e., the duty to protect confidentiality and, with it, a patient's welfare) is left unresolved. This led the International Committee of the Red Cross (ICRC) to permit physicians to decide for themselves whether to violate or maintain confidentiality. While one cannot be compelled to denounce patients, a physician "retains the freedom to denounce a patient on the basis that he may legitimately wish to prevent the patient pursuing activities which he considers to be dangerous for other human beings, just as, in peacetime, he may wish to prevent a criminal from continuing his criminal activities" (Protocol I, 1977b, Article 16, Paragraph 676).

The peacetime analogy is unsatisfactory: enemy soldiers are not criminals. Criminals are noninnocent material threats, while a captured or wounded soldier is just the opposite: morally innocent and no longer a material threat (chapter 2). Criminals commit or are likely to commit a crime that threatens another individual. Soldiers, on the other hand, are not criminals unless they grievously violate humanitarian law and commit war crimes. If anything, soldiers more closely resemble mentally ill and potentially violent patients who constitute a danger to the community. The decision to turn these patients over to the authorities rests on the probability that they pose grave and imminent harm to others (Beauchamp and Childress 1994, 418–429; Michalowski 2001). Because, in these circumstances, the costs of maintaining confidentiality pale beside the benefits of violating it, doctors have a moral and usually a legal duty to breach confidentiality. Similar reasoning should *obligate* combat physicians to denounce patients who, if released, are always a threat. The obligation is that much stronger when one considers important differences between soldiers and unstable, potentially violent patients.

First, it is exceptionally difficult to estimate the threat a patient poses during war. Unless a patient is entirely incapacitated, in which case neither repatriation nor incarceration presents any moral difficulty if adequate medical care is provided, there is no way to know whether soldiers will return to their threatening status. They will certainly try, however. Unlike potentially violent patients, soldiers are mentally stable and focus intense effort on returning to duty. While one cannot know the exact nature of the threat particular soldiers will pose, one can assume with reasonable certainty that they will join those whose job it is to kill one's own. Combatants always present a reasonable chance of grave harm, so that the potential for harm is sufficient to outweigh the dangers of violating confidentiality.

Second, one must ask whether soldiers, friendly or enemy, possess any significant right to confidentiality whatsoever. If not, the dilemma disappears. Soldiers lose their right to life regardless of the threat or danger they pose to others. Cooks are as vulnerable as commandos. Similarly, it stands to reason that the estimate of harm freed soldier-patients may do is quite irrelevant to any assessment of their right to confidentiality. Privacy and confidentiality are derivative rights, and therefore combatants' claims to these lesser rights might be as tenuous as their claim to the full autonomy from which the rights derive. This holds true whether soldiers are one's own or the enemy's.

A Friendly Soldier's Right to Confidentiality   Confidentiality derives much of its force from autonomy, and Sissela Bok (1989), for example, links the two closely. Confidentiality is essential so patients can exercise "individual autonomy over personal information." "Without some control over secrecy and openness about themselves, . . . their thoughts and plans, their actions, and in part their property," she writes, "people could neither maintain privacy nor guard against danger" (p. 120). Here, we might ask, what dangers are important to guard against during war?

There is no doubt, for example, that among ordinary patients confidentiality forestalls harm to self-esteem, job security, or social status that may result if personal information or private thoughts are suddenly made public. During war and among one's own soldiers, the scope of the private sphere decreases and that of the public expands as collective welfare takes precedence over an individual's private good. Thus, a wide range of private information is relevant during war that is not particularly interesting in other settings. This includes a person's emotional stability, propensity for aggression or unsocial behavior, or difficulty with authority—anything, in fact, that could upset the discipline and cohesiveness necessary to maintain effective fighting capabilities. This does not mean that all private information is fair game, but it does mean that more information that is private is important for nonmedical reasons than one finds in a nonmilitary, peacetime setting. It also means that the concept of harm pushes beyond that which befalls the individual patient. Harm to a patient is juxtaposed against harm to others. While this, as noted earlier, is also true in nonmilitary settings, the range of potential harms to others is greater in the military and particularly during war. Among civilians, one is concerned with the occasional patient who threatens others. During war, however, every soldier may potentially harm (just as he may aid) collective well-being. The danger only grows when a patient is an enemy soldier. All this leaves confidentiality during war hanging rather precariously unless we can consider other arguments to salvage wartime confidentiality.

Apart from respect for autonomy, Bok considers three alternative justifications for a person's right to confidentiality. First, she suggests, human relationships would irreparably founder without confidentiality and respect for personal secrets. Second, a doctor's "pledge of silence creates an obligation beyond the respect due to persons and to existing relationships" (p. 120). Finally, sick or injured individuals will avoid medical care without an assurance that a physician will respect confidentiality.

These are quite different arguments and carry far less force in military medicine than they do in ordinary medical practice. Consider the last one first. It remains unclear whether patients will avoid care knowing caregivers may violate confidentiality (Bok and Kottow 1986; Berlin,

Malin, and Dean 1991; Beauchamp and Childress 1994, 423). Regardless of what may happen in a nonmilitary setting, fear of disclosure will not disrupt military medical care simply because soldiers generally lack the option of seeking medical care elsewhere should they take issue with rules that compromise their confidentiality. More importantly, soldiers have no right to refuse medical care and may face compulsory treatment regardless of concerns that doctors will violate their confidentiality. This may ensure acute care but might certainly affect psychiatric care, which soldiers may avoid, fearing violations of confidentiality. The data, however, are lacking.

The question of whether a doctor's "pledge of silence" creates an obligation begs the question. Why should a doctor make a pledge of silence to begin with? Possible answers draw us back to previous discussions. Physicians honor confidentiality out of respect for autonomy and a desire to protect patients from harms of varying degrees. But if autonomy is limited and preventing harm to others offsets harm to a patient, then a military physician does not always have solid grounds to tender a pledge of silence. Finally, consider the delicate weave of human relationships that violations of secrecy might undermine, as Bok's first justification suggests. Undoubtedly, this is possible, but much depends on which set of human relationships one has in mind. Confidentiality, for example, is essential to preserve the small-group cohesiveness so vital for military morale. Dilemmas arise when officers ask soldiers to inform on their friends. Violating confidentiality may undermine discipline and solidarity, consequences that merit careful consideration before breaching trust. In a larger sense, a nation's entire war effort depends on confidentiality and the ability to keep secrets. Yet the effects of violating medical confidentiality are not so clear. On the one hand, limited confidentiality may not affect the quality of medical care that armies provide in what is already a paternalistic and coercive setting. On the other hand, flagrant violations of confidentiality may undermine trust in the organization as a whole. Medical personnel may only divulge pertinent information; irrelevant information remains protected by confidentiality. Nevertheless, the grounds for respecting confidentiality among one's own troops are often weak and, under these circumstances, it is all the more difficult to justify the duty to respect confidentiality among one's enemies.

An Enemy Soldier's Right to Confidentiality   Whether enemy soldiers captured in battle or presenting for treatment have any greater or lesser claim to confidentiality than one's own soldiers remains an interesting question. Neither category of soldiers seems to have an inherent and unrestricted right to their personal information insofar as this affects the common good. Moreover, enemy soldiers have no place in one's military organization or society at large, so that it is difficult to invoke the threats to organizational or social integrity that sometimes protect confidentiality. Violating enemy soldiers' confidentiality will affect neither group solidarity nor the web of human relations that bind society. It will hardly keep them from seeking medical care, for their only recourse is to die. Moreover, they have already made the choice to seek care knowing they may be denounced. The only reason to respect the confidentiality of wounded enemy soldiers is, ironically enough, that, once wounded, they are no longer soldiers but find themselves in the same position as any other patient. Paradoxically, as noncombatants and now "ordinary" patients, enemy soldiers may enjoy a stronger right to confidentiality that one's own soldiers in spite of the threat they pose as enemies. This dilemma drove the framers of the Protocols in two mutually exclusive directions. It, therefore, deserves closer attention.

Apart from the harmful consequences of protecting the confidentiality of enemy soldiers, it is important to understand that unlike one's own soldiers, they have no inherent right to medical care. If enemy soldiers have forfeited their right to life, why do they have any right to medical treatment at all? Why not simply let them die of their wounds on the battlefield? The answer is that wounded soldiers are no longer soldiers. They are *hors de combat*, no longer part of the threat facing one's nation. Once *hors de combat*, captured and wounded enemy soldiers recover their right to life, their right to confidentiality, and their right to receive the same medical care as other noncombatants. Nevertheless, enemy prisoners' right to receive life-saving medical care demands that they remain noncombatants for the duration of the war. Many early conventions were clear, perhaps chivalrously so, on this point: "[Wounded enemy soldiers] who, after their recovery, are recognized as being unfit for further service, shall be repatriated, [while] the others (that is, recovered enemy soldiers) may likewise be sent back, on condition that they shall not again, for the duration of hostilities, take up arms" (Geneva Convention, 1864, Article 6). Enemy soldiers, therefore, must not return to duty. Otherwise, they forfeit their right to life-saving care. Paradoxically, enemy soldiers regain their right to life as they lie dying but lose it once they have recovered.

Enemy soldiers are not entitled to medical care, nor are physicians required to treat them simply because they are sick or wounded. Medical care for wounded enemy soldiers is only justified when these soldiers are no longer a threat. Physicians can only nurse patients back to health knowing that they will sit out the remainder of the war. Acting otherwise flies in the face of their duty to aid the war effort and undertake those means necessary to subdue an enemy. Wartime enemy patients differ from peacetime patients at least in this regard. As a result, physicians are not neutral. A dominant argument running through the Protocols and their commentaries implies that physicians owe allegiance to no one but their patients. But this cannot be right. They surely owe allegiance to the side they are fighting with. They are *required* to denounce their patients; doing otherwise undermines the basis for medical care to enemy soldiers, who only enjoy medical care as long as they are not a threat. Only the specter of gross abuse, torture, or ill-treatment—not general and ill-defined "harms"—is sufficient to exempt medical personnel from the obligation to denounce enemy patients. For this reason alone, Pearl Buck's Japanese physician could not denounce his patient. Two observations, however, are important.

First, military physicians who consider violating confidentiality, like those contemplating the limits of informed consent, find themselves in much the opposite situation of their peacetime colleagues. For civilian physicians the burden of proof falls on those who violate confidentiality. During war, the burden of proof falls on those who *do not* violate patient confidentiality and protect their patients because they fear they will suffer grievous abuse and mistreatment. Second, physicians have no special moral responsibility when it comes to denouncing or sheltering an enemy soldier. Any person has a prima facie obligation to help others. In most cases, this means denouncing enemy soldiers, while in rare cases it demands sheltering them if human rights are at substantial risk. The right to confidentiality in this case is not only nonabsolute; it is also relatively weak when military necessity is at stake.

Battlefield Euthanasia and the Right to Die

Turin, 1537: Being in the City, I entered a stable thinking to lodge my own and my man's horse, where I found four dead soldiers, and three which were leaning against a wall, their faces wholly disfigured, and neither saw nor heard, nor spoke; and their clothes did yet flame with the gunpowder that had burnt them. Beholding them with pity, there happened to come an old soldier, who asked me if there were any possible means to cure them, I told him no: he presently approached them, and gently cut their throats without choler. Seeing this great cruelty, I told him he was a wicked man, he answered me that he prayed to God, that whensoever he should be in such a case, that he might find someone who would do as much to him, to the end he might not miserably languish. (Paré 1968, 21–22)

Palestine, 1799: When the army reached Jaffa, Napoleon, worried that the Turks would catch his army, consulted with Dr. René-Nicolas Desgenettes. According to Desgenettes, Napoleon said, "If I were in your place, I should put an end to the sufferings of our plague patients and, at the same time, to the danger they represent for us, by giving them opium." Desgenettes, however, disagreed, relating to Bonaparte that his duty was to preserve life. Bonaparte stated that his duty was to preserve the army. Napoleon said, "I shall not try to overcome your scruples, but I believe I shall find people who will appreciate my intentions more than you do." (Peterson 1995, 153; also Feinberg 1998)

Eventually, Napoléon found someone who did and, by some accounts, poisoned fifty French soldiers sick with the bubonic plague that ravished his army.

These are two very different stories that test our intuitions in different ways. The first, by Ambrose Paré, evokes a measure of sympathy for the killer and his victims. Paré says no more, but one is left with the distinct impression that while Paré as a doctor would not euthanize soldiers, he was happy someone else did. Unlike Napoléon, the killer had no further interest than to relieve the suffering of the wounded.

Napoléon, on the other hand, had a myriad of interests on his mind apart from the best interests of sick men. He was concerned, first and foremost, with getting his forces out of Palestine before the Turks overtook him. His retreat was chaotic and there were no facilities for transporting ill soldiers. Others feared that the Turks would torture any living patients, either to extract information or to avenge Napoléon's ruthless treatment of Turkish prisoners of war. Napoléon's dilemma was a classic one: what to do with wounded soldiers one cannot care for and one cannot abandon? Are there ever any instances when it may be permissible to let them die or kill them?

The Right to Die: Looking beyond the Patient-Soldier

Competent patients maintain the right to refuse any treatment including life-sustaining care. Most nations safeguard a patient's autonomy by guaranteeing informed consent and considering coercive treatment an actionable battery. Because informed consent is meaningless without the concomitant option of informed refusal, patients command this right as well. Soldiers, on the other hand, have no such right. They may not refuse standard medical care, nor may they refuse treatment commensurate with acceptable military risk. However, the care soldiers receive and their duty to accept treatment assumes that medical care will effectively restore their health and return them to duty. Soldiers who are seriously or terminally ill, so that there is no chance they will return to duty, no longer labor under the restrictions that constrain an ordinary soldier's choice. They revert to noncombatant status and regain the moral rights all patients enjoy, including the right to refuse treatment. For this reason, for example, there are no grounds to deny severely wounded soldiers the right to refuse an amputation. Whether they accept or reject surgery, they will not return to duty and, therefore, remain unsalvageable as soldiers. They should enjoy the same right as any patients facing a similar situation, a right that military organizations rarely recognize.

Unable to return to duty, critically wounded soldiers revert to nonmilitary medical status. This happens in the case Paré describes. The old soldier who decides to kill his wounded comrades first asks Paré whether he can do anything to help them. Paré might have replied that while he cannot cure them, he can make them comfortable until they die. But he does not. He responds that there is nothing he can do. Only then does the old soldier kill them. Yet Paré remains horrified; he calls the killer "a wicked man" but does not say why. Is he responding to the ethics of the Hippocratic oath, to canon law, or to the law of the land? Any one of these would be sufficient to prohibit euthanasia, and it would make little difference to Paré had the stricken soldiers consented to their deaths in some way. Yet "consent" is the old soldier's response. He does not invoke the consent of the wounded, for they cannot speak, but he does draw on the hypothetical consent of an ordinary, rational, and reasonable individual in similar circumstances, an interpretation of autonomy that modern jurisprudence and bioethics utilize for imputing informed consent (President's Commission for the study of Ethical Problems in Medicine and Biomedical and Behavioral Research, 1983, 132–136). When patients are incapable of expressing a wish to die, doctors and judges may rely on a substituted judgment to withhold or withdraw life support (Jonson 1998, 266–270; Mason and McCall Smith 1999, 413–448). Unaware of the intricacies of modern bioethics, Paré nevertheless seems persuaded by this argument and lets the matter drop.

While our sympathies may lie with the old soldier, a sweeping policy allowing soldiers the right to die on the battlefield, much less assist them, might be problematic. What conditions must they meet to gain this right, what sort of consent is necessary, and what means may they or others take to fulfill their wishes? I have already noted that a soldier's right to refuse treatment is virtually nonexistent when relatively healthy, but aligns with those of any other patient when severely or terminally ill. Soldiers as patients unable to return to duty may then exercise their right to die by either withholding or withdrawing treatment. If local law also allows physician-assisted suicide, then there is no reason to exclude these patients from exercising this right either. Whether withholding or withdrawing life-sustaining care from consenting patients, a physician's assistance is instrumental as soldier-patients exercise their right to die. The harder cases, of course, are those soldiers who have not professed a wish to die or, as in Paré's case, demand more "active" means to bring about their deaths. Paré's case, however, is not a problem of military medical ethics. While it presents the difficult dilemma of euthanasia and brings us to reflect on a soldier's right to die, military necessity is not at stake, nor does reason of state offer any compelling reason to end the life of the wounded soldiers. Before considering Paré's case further, let me therefore first turn to Napoléon's dilemma.

Military Necessity and the Right to Kill Wounded Soldiers

The intriguing problem remains Napoléon's: medical personnel must see to the welfare of their patients, while military personnel must see to the welfare of the army. What happens when these priorities conflict? Did Napoléon have a right or perhaps even a duty to kill critically ill soldiers who were slowing his retreat and endangering his army? If any argument will be coherent, it will be some version of the "last-resort" claim and will go something like this: *If wounded personnel significantly slow a retreat or otherwise thwart some other important military mission because there is no reasonable possibility of taking them along and caring for them, and if it is reasonably certain that abandoning them will deliver them to a more tragic fate, then it is permissible to kill them prior to retreating or undertaking the mission at hand.*

Like most questions decided on the basis of competing utilities, this one stands or falls on the likelihood and magnitude of the harm it poses to various parties. Assume for a moment that the first part of this hypothetical situation is true and there are instances when an army cannot bring along its wounded without slowing down the others. This may occur during a retreat or as a small patrol is trapped behind enemy lines (Stouffer et al. 1949, 144) The army, or patrol, then faces several options: to bring their wounded along and risk capture, to leave them behind hoping they will be found and cared for, or to kill them. The severity of the soldiers' injuries compounds the problem. Although suffering from the plague, Napoléon's soldiers, unlike those described by Paré, could benefit from care. Despite the high mortality rate, Larrey describes how he cared for plague victims. Nevertheless, Napoléon's plague-infected soldiers faced a mortality rate of over 90 percent (Larrey [1814] 1987, vol. 1, 182–206).

Prior to his difficulties in Palestine, Napoléon had not killed any of his own soldiers. So why did he start now? Why not just leave the soldiers where they lay until the Turks arrived? Surely this was better than abandoning them along the road, as they did with others during the hard march back to Egypt. With transport scarce, soldiers ill with the plague fell unattended by the wayside. Fearful of contagion, few offered assistance, leading some infected soldiers to inflict themselves with "ordinary" wounds in the hope their comrades would care for them. Yet even under these conditions, abandoning soldiers and letting them die seems far less severe than killing them. So why not simply abandon the wounded, perhaps heavily sedated, rather than kill them? Either they would die anyway or the Turks would care for them.

Letting patients die of their underlying disease rather than hastening their death by means unrelated to the treatment of their disease (such as lethal injection) is generally the line most draw between permissible forms of "passive" euthanasia and the more "active" forms that many construe as killing. The former include withholding and withdrawing life-sustaining treatment and, in some U.S. states, assisted suicide, while the latter comprise lethal injection at the hands of others. Active euthanasia, in contrast to its passive forms, requires a competent patient's informed consent in those nations that permit the practice. Critically ill patients are allowed to die when pain, suffering, and sometimes financial costs overwhelm the benefits of continuing to live. Ordinarily, patients make these decisions when competent. For never-competent patients or those who failed to execute explicit instructions when they were competent, most authorities permit substituted judgments based on the preferences of reasonable persons in similar situations (President's Commission for the Study of Ethical Problems in Medicine and Biomedical and Behavioral Research, 1983).

The calculus for allowing wounded soldiers to die is the same, but the scope of costs and benefits broadens. The decision to abandon wounded soldiers weighs the cost of taking them along, the probability they will reach medical treatment in time to receive care, and the risk their evacuation imposes on others. These costs and benefits are compared to the value of individual soldiers' lives, most often an expendable commodity during war, and the likelihood they will be found and well treated by the enemy. Decent treatment at the hands of an enemy, once a foregone conclusion, is an increasingly endangered practice, because substate parties in many current conflicts no longer respect the rights of wounded or captured combatants. The crucial consideration, however, turns on the harm soldiers will bring to others if they are *not* allowed to die. Obviously, this concern does not affect the decision of ordinary patients. When ordinary patients are not allowed to die, their welfare alone suffers. When wounded soldiers are not allowed to die—for example, if others insist on carrying them along—they may bring considerable harm to others. If we allow ordinary patients to die when the benefits exceed the cost, then it is permissible to allow wounded soldiers to die in similar circumstances, taking into account general welfare and the costs to others. Ordinary patients, however, must consent to their deaths. They decide by themselves for themselves when they demand the right to die. Only their interests count. If they refuse, it is because the benefit of dying does not outweigh that of living. One cannot imagine letting a patient die who did not want to. The fate of wounded soldiers, on the other hand, is decided by oneself and others for the benefit of others. Patient autonomy is weak among soldiers. Nor are critically wounded soldiers singled out for exceptionally risky treatment; they face significant risk of death whether abandoned or carried along. This differs from a situation that might require one soldier to remain behind to cover those retreating. His or her act is supererogatory and requires personal consent. Absent meaningful autonomy and the need for consent, critically ill patients may find themselves without recourse if abandoned to military necessity.

Apart from calling on the distinction between killing and letting die and appealing to utility, abandoning the wounded may also invoke the doctrine of double effect (DDE). As noted in chapter 2, the DDE is primarily a military doctrine allowing one to harm the innocent when that harm is necessary, unavoidable, and unintentional. *Unintentional* means "incidental": harm befalling innocents can in no way facilitate a mission's success. The DDE also allows us to draw a tighter distinction between killing and letting die. Ordinarily, the difference turns on prohibited acts of commission and permissible or forgivable acts of omission, between causing a death and allowing it to happen. But the distinction is not hard and fast. One might envision instances of passive acquiescence to death tantamount to murder—for example, when a person stands idly by while a hated spouse or despised business associate drowns. Failure to prevent an avoidable death while, at the same time, reaping its benefits highlights an intentional act and strips the bystander of innocence. The moral distinction between killing and letting die turns on these factors: the manner of death, intentions, *and* benefits to others (Norman 1995, 77–82).

Acts of omission combine with lack of intention to justify abandoning seriously wounded soldiers when the alternative poses a grave threat to others. Wounded soldiers are abandoned so that a mission may succeed; they are not abandoned to die. Their death, although inevitable, adds nothing to the mission's success. In extreme situations, utility and the DDE may come together and leave commanders the option of abandoning a wounded soldier. Too little is actually known of the historical circumstances surrounding Napoléon's decision to leave his ill soldiers behind, but Napoléon, like the five-man patrol caught in enemy territory in a contemporary war, may justifiably abandon the wounded, perhaps to let them die, if carrying them along jeopardizes a mission or endangers the lives of other soldiers.

None of the foregoing arguments—the distinction between killing and letting die, utility, and the double effect—say anything, however, about killing the wounded. In fact, they lend considerable weight to prohibiting the practice. While soldiers have lost their right to life vis-à-vis the enemy, they retain it vis-à-vis their own officers. Commanders may place their soldiers in harm's way but they may not kill them. Exposed to the risk of certain death, soldiers must often give their consent. Nor does the DDE help. Permitting unintentional harm under carefully controlled conditions, the DDE forbids intentional harm. At best, one may invoke utility on the assumption that sufficiently harmful consequences may overwhelm the prohibition against willful murder.

Only the prospect of "a fate worse than death" is sometimes sufficient to intentionally end another's life. By some accounts, Napoléon feared the Turks would torture and mutilate his soldiers. Had the British rather than the Turks pursued the French, Napoléon might happily have left his wounded where they lay and let the British care for them. Fearful, however, that the Turks might recall the execution of 3,000 Turkish prisoners of war in Jaffa, Napoléon had reason to fear that his men might not fare well at Turkish hands. But is this vague fear sufficient grounds to kill them? As things turned out, the Turks did not harm the survivors but delivered them to the British navy. Napoléon, in retrospect, had no cause to kill his soldiers, and this fact alone shows how difficult assessing utility can be. Whether this is always true is difficult to determine. In a painful account 150 years later, a World War II medic agonized over his role in the mercy killing of "fatally wounded" soldiers as the British retreated from the China-Burma front. "He had entered the war 'to save lives, not to take them,'" recounts his interviewer, "but he knew only too well the cruel and terrible fate of mortally wounded men falling into Japanese hands" (Smith 1999, 252). Unlike Napoléon, who worried about the welfare of his entire army, the medic here has only one interest at heart: his patients' welfare. Were these patients to face certain torture, a medical worker might, as Swann argues, successfully defend the decision to euthanize them (Swann 1985; Beam 2003). Barring these circumstances, it is exceedingly difficult to establish grounds that would allow commanders to kill their soldiers when they might just as easily have abandoned them. In spite of our sympathy for Paré's old soldier and, perhaps, for Napoléon's dilemma as well, killing wounded soldiers remains a wicked act.

It is, I think, sufficient to leave it at that. It is interesting to speculate, however, how modern medicine might have handled Paré's soldiers, assuming that it could not effectively treat their wounds. Palliative care and rigorous pain management would most likely be the order of the day. But, if pain breaks through and remains unmanageable, we show little tolerance for active euthanasia. We simply live with these cases as infrequent although tragic outcomes of a way of life that abhors murder and fears the consequences should it ever threaten to become commonplace. We sympathize with Paré's old soldier just as we may with a woman who smothers her desperately ill husband. And, while we may excuse their behavior, we have no way to formulate any principles to guide the practice of killing wounded soldiers. An officer killing his own wounded men to prevent significant harm from befalling either the wounded or the healthy, must enter the dock and defend himself; there are no guidelines to justify his action ex ante. Instead, he must invoke the "necessity defense" (chapter 7) and attempt to convince others he acted to prevent immediate, grievous, and otherwise unavoidable harm to others. Few and far between, these hard cases would make bad law.

One final case remains to complete this discussion. Consider the situation of critically ill soldiers who cannot tolerate evacuation and fear the consequences of abandonment or capture. May they ask others to kill them? Our intuitions lead in two directions. Killing on request is still murder. People who assent are no different from anyone else who kills wounded soldiers. In this case, they only add informed consent to the other justifications they will bring to the bar as they defend themselves. Whether their peers will excuse their behavior depends on how they evaluate utility, intentionality, the wounded soldiers' state of mind, alternative avenues of action, and other pertinent facts. On the other hand, we would probably judge the situation differently if the wounded soldiers simply asked others for the *means* to kill themselves. We balk at moral condemnation, because we can never know whether the wounded soldiers would turn the weapon on themselves or die defending their position. Still, the larger problem of helping others commit suicide remains. Resolving this issue depends much on the way particular societies judge assisted suicide. Concerned about the slippery slope, nations that permit assisted suicide establish strict guidelines and regulatory mechanisms to evaluate competence, consent, and need. Clearly, these factors would be difficult, if not impossible, to evaluate during war. Without any means to obtain prior authorization for assisted suicide, only the same ex post justificatory process required of homicide remains. Those helping others commit suicide will have to defend themselves. Unfortunately, there are no smoking guns. No one, neither judges nor perpetrators, would ever know whether abandoned, wounded soldiers died of their wounds, killed themselves, or were killed in battle. The circumstances necessary to determine, let alone evaluate, assisted suicide are nonexistent.

Dying, Letting Die, and Killing

This section moved rapidly from the right to die and the right to let die to the right to kill. Paré's case delivers several lessons. First, it draws our attention to the right to die that severely wounded patients enjoy when they will not return to service. Salvageable soldiers may not refuse any treatment that will restore them to combat. Permanently incapacitated soldiers, on the other hand, revert to civilian-patient status and may choose to end their lives by refusing or withholding treatment. Paré's story also makes us wary of active euthanasia, as he recoils when the old soldier kills severely wounded soldiers. While this case highlights the heinousness of homicide, it may leave room for isolated cases of excusable homicide that can only be judged ex post and on their merits.

Napoléon's order to poison his plague-infected soldiers sharpens the distinction between abandoning wounded soldiers and killing them, as we consider his alternative courses of action. Abandoning a wounded soldier is permissible if it is necessary and it is the only means available to safeguard supremely important military objectives and/or the welfare of other soldiers. Napoléon, however, pushes the envelope when he asks whether he may kill his critically ill soldiers. His chief medical officer refuses, citing his duty to protect life. Napoléon counters, citing his duty to protect the army. But the facts do not bear him out. He might leave his wounded to die, but not kill them. His ex post defense would have failed. This may not be true in every case, but one has to hope that the exceptions to homicide will be sufficiently rare that the rule against killing one's own soldiers remains paramount.

Patient Rights in War and Peace

Each category of patient rights—informed consent, confidentiality, and the right to die—highlights the different claims battlefield actors make to medical care. During war, the individual interests of soldier-patients are subordinate to the collective welfare. Their claim to medical care is entirely a function of their contribution to war. One treats soldiers, with either standard or investigational drugs, to maintain the integrity of a collective fighting force, not to care for particular patients. The dilemma of confidentiality emphasizes the close connection between enemy soldiers' right to medical care and the threat they pose. Physicians may provide care only insofar as their patients no longer constitute a material threat. Care depends on the assurance that enemy patients cannot return to their threatening status once they recover. Physicians must, therefore, consider denouncing their patients precisely so they can treat them. Finally, the vagaries of soldiers' right to die show how combatants' right to medical care depends on their salvage value. Salvageable soldiers command the right to medical care but lose the right to die. Unsalvageable soldiers lose their right to priority medical care but gain the right to die when they can no longer fight.

These dilemmas also highlight a noticeable shift in the burden of proof during war. In peacetime, those *violating* patient rights must justify their action; during war, those *upholding* patient rights generally bear the burden of proof. Considering investigational drugs, this may not be immediately obvious, because FDA regulations stipulate that informed consent is a rule that only the president can waive when obtaining consent is not feasible, contrary to a servicemember's interest, or not in the interests of national security. The reality, however, is quite the opposite. The military prevailed by arguing that obtaining informed consent, ordinarily a good thing, is just not feasible during war. Since the option to refuse will usually debilitate a fighting force as key troops choose to opt out, the burden shifts to those who must prove that it will not. Only then will authorities require informed consent. Absent mitigating circumstances, confidentiality, like informed consent, is the exception rather than the rule. What can these circumstances be if enemy soldiers, by definition, are always threats? One possible answer comes from Pearl Buck. Faced with the prospect that patients will be ill-treated, or face certain death or abuse, physicians may find sufficient cause to maintain confidentiality. The right to die, by its very nature, also shifts the burden of proof. Military medical personnel will always deny patients the right to die unless they are no longer fit for duty.

Finally, each of these cases draws attention to the fact that the principles at stake—consent, confidentiality, and the right to die—appear during war in a nonmedical setting and in ways that are not always controversial. In rare cases, soldiers are sometimes asked to volunteer for or give informed consent to certain missions. Why is this so? The answer turns on both risk and fairness. High risk alone is insufficient to demand consent. Combat soldiers face high risk all the time, and devastating casualty rates are not unusual in many situations. To require consent, however, this risk must be distributed unevenly and fall on the heads of relatively few individuals. So it is with medical informed consent. Risk alone, even the high risk of an investigational drug, is insufficient to require informed consent from soldiers if medical risk is no higher than military risk and distributed fairly among all troops. Experimentation, on the other hand, demands a subject's consent because the risk is not distributed equally or fairly. Confidentiality, too, plays an important part in the war convention, because captured soldiers need not divulge certain information. Confidentiality is respected because captured soldiers are innocent (that is, they are not criminals) and nonthreatening. The same principles apply when we consider violating the confidentiality of enemy soldiers who require medical care, respecting confidentiality when they are nonthreatening, and violating it when they are. Finally, the right to die surfaces, albeit rarely, when wounded soldiers are left behind, or ask to be left behind, enemy lines to die rather than risk jeopardizing a mission by being carried along. The issue turns on military necessity and the duty to maintain the fitness of one's unit, if in their wounded state, the wounded can no longer contribute to, and may even jeopardize, a mission's success. The same reasoning governs the disposition of soldiers who wish to refuse medical treatment and die. They regain their right to die when no longer militarily useful.

Clearly, we have come a long way from peacetime bioethics. Patient rights during armed conflict differ radically from those guiding medical care in times of peace. During war, respect for autonomy and utility rework themselves. Utility broadens to encompass the well-being of others and preservation of the collective good. Autonomy and its subsidiary principles—informed consent, confidentiality, and the right to die—contract, making room for external agents to make decisions on the behalf of others. As utility and autonomy wax and wane, many patient rights pass from the hands of soldier-patients to the hands of those charged with the collective welfare, with the expectation that costs to some individuals are offset by benefits to others. This is the logic behind triage and the subject of the following chapter.

5

Wartime Triage

Triage means nothing but sorting or culling. Referring once to the sorting of common goods, today it signifies the sorting of casualties into groups before delivering medical care. Attributed to Dominique Larrey, although undoubtedly practiced in an ad hoc manner whenever physicians had to deal with numerous casualties, triage procedures ordinarily divide the injured into three groups: those who will die regardless of care, those who will live regardless of care or require only minimal care, and those who will die without care. The dilemma of triage is not in the sorting but in the ranking: how should authorities allocate scarce medical resources among these three groups? That is, which group should be treated first?

The international provisions governing the distribution of medical resources during wartime are a bundle of contradictions. Based, in principle, on the neutrality of medical personnel and their duty to provide medical care to those in need regardless of national affiliation, humanitarian law seriously questions whether military necessity can ever dictate how to distribute these resources. The First and Second Geneva Conventions state: "Only urgent medical reasons will authorize priority in the order of treatment to be administered" (Geneva Conventions I, II, 1949, Article 12, Paragraph 3). Commenting on this directive, the 1977 Protocols declare: "This is a reminder to the personnel taking care of the wounded that they shall ignore the nationality or uniform of the person they are taking care of. The only reason for treating one patient before another shall be because his wounds require more urgent care, independently of any non-medical considerations" (Protocol I, 1977b, Article 10, paragraph 453).

At first glance, this reminder is eminently sound. It reiterates a twofold distribution principle of medical need and nondiscrimination that is grounded in fairness, respect for dignity, and the priority of patient well-being. At second glance, it is intensely problematic, ignoring the first rule of triage that guides belligerents during war: to return the greatest possible number of soldiers to combat and expend existing resources upon the "maximum number of salvageable soldiers" (U.S. Department of Defense, 1988, 3:12). In contrast to principles guiding the Geneva Conventions, the rule of salvage embraces a different twofold principle of distribution. First, utility overrides medical need when distributing scarce resources. Second, utilitarian triage emphatically favors the welfare of one's own soldiers over that of both one's enemy and one's own civilians. Therefore, if the principles laid out in the Protocols are correct, then the principle of distribution that animates triage during wartime is wrong.

The Moral Dilemmas of Triage

For better or for worse, Henry Beecher set the stage in 1971 for all subsequent discussions of ethics and triage with his now-famous account of penicillin triage:

When the wonders of penicillin were new, but recognized, and the supply heartbreakingly meager, a small shipment finally arrived in North Africa during World War II. The hospital beds were overflowing with wounded men. Many had been wounded in battles; many had also been wounded in brothels. Which group would get the penicillin? By all that is just, it would go to the heroes who had risked their lives, who were still in jeopardy and some of whom were dying. They did not receive it, nor should they have; it was given to those infected in brothels. Before indignation takes over, let us examine the situation. First there were desperate shortages of manpower at the front. Second those with broken bodies and broken bones would not be swiftly restored to the battle line even with penicillin, whereas those with venereal disease, on being treated with penicillin, would in a matter of days free the beds they were occupying and return to the front. (Beecher 1971, 209–210; also Howie 1979)

Beecher stokes our indignation by describing a situation that pits the bald utility of war against all that is just. The reality, however, may have been none of this. The wonders of penicillin were new, but not entirely recognized. While the Allies were field-testing penicillin for battle injuries, they approved its use to treat gonorrhea in September 1943 but remained unconvinced until July 1944 that penicillin could prevent surgical infection better than sulfa drugs (Office of the Surgeon General, 1944; Bickel 1972, 200–207). By then, supplies had increased dramatically, so that any question of how to distribute penicillin among troops was largely moot.

The British, on the other hand, were keen to use penicillin in surgery when the drug was scarce and wondered how to distribute it among their troops. Military commanders wanted it to treat thousands of troops sick with gonorrhea but by one account, Howard Florey and Hugh Cairns, the scientists who developed penicillin during World War II, felt it was unacceptable that penicillin should be given to "scallywags with self-inflicted wounds rather than genuine battle casualties." The decision then fell to General L.T. Poole, Director of Pathology in the War Office, who decided (after reportedly conferring with Winston Churchill) that the medical corps should use penicillin for the "best military advantage" and this meant restoring gonorrhea-incapacitated soldiers to their units (McFarlane 1998).

Even this story, told by one of Florey's biographers and so similar to Beecher's, is not entirely accurate. Florey objected to using penicillin for treating gonorrhea precisely because it was effective. Having demonstrated its ability to cure gonorrhea, Florey and his staff wanted to learn how to use penicillin to prevent gas gangrene, care for burns, and treat head, chest, and abdominal wounds under battlefield conditions (chapter 4). Poole, therefore, did not need to choose between successfully treating those injured in battle and those infected in brothels but between continuing to conduct clinical trials and using penicillin for an effective, proven purpose. This already blunts the acute moral dilemma that Beecher describes. Poole chose to discontinue clinical trials until supplies increased and, in the meantime, to use penicillin for an effective purpose.

Nevertheless, many worried about the political fallout and the reactions of the families of wounded men if the authorities had decided to treat soldiers suffering from venereal disease before attempting to treat the wounded with a new, experimental drug. This provides the story of penicillin triage with a novel twist as we see how antagonistic moral attitudes associated with venereal disease and prostitution can affect decision making and prevent the search for alternative solutions, namely, regulating prostitution to control sexually transmitted diseases, which could ease the dilemma scarce resources pose. Ignoring the so-called political ramifications, Poole authorized his staff to use penicillin to treat gonorrhea among British troops in Algiers (Hinds 1976, 29–51). While this may have been, as many thought, the "right" decision, the decision-making process was not right, for it ignored the moral imperative to weigh alternatives when resources are scarce and lives are at stake.

Although the story of penicillin triage may not have been the high drama Beecher supposed it to be, I will use it to introduce three distinct ethical problems of triage. First, penicillin triage raises the general question of whether salvage value or medical need should govern the distribution of scarce resources during wartime. Both are criteria for triage during war. Among soldiers, medical need did not always guide the allocation of resources and among others, it rarely did. POWs did not benefit from penicillin and only a fraction of existing supplies made its way to Allied civilians (Wilson 1976, 204; Adams 1991).

Penicillin triage also provides a starting point for two other subjects overlooked in triage discussions. For most observers penicillin triage presented the difficult dilemma of allocating a scarce drug during war. At the same time, however, it also posed the problem of distributing a unique medical resource, namely, scientific knowledge. While the British discovered penicillin prior to the war, the Americans developed the deep fermentation technique necessary for mass production. Britain and the United States shrouded production details in secrecy and censored scientific information heavily. Yet one must seriously ask whether the international community, including the Germans and the Japanese who were never able to develop penicillin during the war, should have had access to life-saving medical knowledge. No one but Allied researchers knew its secrets, and while this seems intuitively sound policy, it is difficult to justify if humanitarian law has any validity whatsoever. As it was, penicillin research commanded resources second only to the atomic bomb and remained a closely guarded secret until the end of the war. Penicillin, however, was not a bomb but medical treatment. Was there not some humanitarian obligation to provide the secrets of its production to the enemy, in the same way there is an obligation to provide medical care to the enemy when wounded?

Penicillin triage also focuses our attention on the imperative to solve the tragic dilemma that Beecher describes by searching for alternatives beyond having to choose between saving the critically wounded from surgical infection or curing gonorrhea and returning stricken soldiers to duty. When venereal disease beset American and British troops, Poole's dilemma assumes that there were no alternative avenues to reducing venereal disease short of redirecting the supply of penicillin. But the scourge of venereal disease plagued armies long before the advent of penicillin, and military organizations found that they could reduce the incidence of sexually transmitted disease by establishing and supervising brothels for their troops. These are never as effective as antibiotics, but if penicillin remained in short supply and the military could reduce the incidence of venereal disease by closely regulating prostitution, then is there not a moral obligation to do so? While English and American officials steadfastly refused to consider the idea, and the United States went so far as to legislate against brothels serving military troops, both the Germans and the French supervised prostitution for the benefit of their soldiers. Thus, a curious moral dilemma emerges. Which is the ethically superior doctrine: regulated prostitution or penicillin triage? More generally: when do extreme bioethical dilemmas compel policymakers to search for alternate solutions, however unpalatable? J. Howie (1979) describes the political uproar politicians would face from penicillin triage. Apparently this was nothing compared to the hue and cry they could expect from legalized prostitution. Yet how can one fail to resolve a life-threatening bioethical dilemma in a way that preserves at least some of the lives of those threatened?

Triage, Medical Need, and Military Utility

A cursory look at the instruments governing triage appears to reveal a situation that is hopelessly confused. The Geneva Conventions advocate medical need, while NATO's operational directives emphasize distributing medical care solely based on military salvage. Both medical need and salvage are objective criteria for care that entirely replace subjectively oriented criteria such as "quality of life" that characterize peacetime bioethics. "Medical need" reflects the care necessary to save patients' lives and restore their health to a generally well-recognized standard of care. This criterion is sometimes referred to as an "egalitarian principle," for it distributes medical care without regard for patients' rank or affiliation. Combatants, noncombatants, enemies, and friends all receive needs-based treatment equally.

"Salvage" is a criterion of medical care unique to war and looks well beyond the interests of an individual patient. During war, medical personnel do not treat individual soldiers qua discrete patients but as components of a fighting *force*: a living, collective entity. To maintain this force medical personnel bear the obligation to salvage soldiers—that is, return as many to duty as quickly as possible. The principle of salvage favors combatants over noncombatants, the less wounded over the severely wounded, and friend over foe. Salvage, like medical need, speaks to a specific and *objective* measure of quality of life distinct from a patient's *subjective* evaluation of his or her quality life that guides ordinary medical care. Salvage and medical need are entirely consistent with the abridged autonomy characteristic of combatants. Salvageable soldiers may not invoke subjective quality of life to refuse treatment, however painful or onerous, if it will return them to military duty. Those beyond salvage, on the other hand, may not appeal to any special right to secure medical care when resources are scarce. Once critically wounded, combatants unlikely to return to duty revert to noncombatant status and lose their privileged claim to scarce medical resources.

Criteria based on medical need and salvage fundamentally conflict with one another, and it is always tempting to blend conflicting principles rather than choose between them. In his study of triage, for example, Gerald Winslow suggests that the parties to Rawls's original position would choose an egalitarian principle of distribution that would treat the wounded according to medical need while, at the same time, making allowances for very severely wounded and those with special skills. Severely injured individuals, whose care would consume inordinate time and resources, move to the back of the queue while those with special skills and who are "immediately useful"—medical or military personnel—move to the front (Winslow 1982, 152). Winslow's model is largely needs-based, with what he considers minor adjustments for calculations of utility that serve the common good.

Citing Larrey rather than Rawls, Robert Baker and Martin Strosberg reach a similar conclusion. Recalling Larrey's contribution to battlefield care during the Napoleonic Wars, Baker and Strosberg (1992) chide commentators for overlooking Larrey's revolutionary, egalitarian medical philosophy as he and his medical team sought out the most critically wounded for immediate care rather than providing treatment in the haphazard order the injured arrived in from the battlefield. They, like Winslow, anchor an egalitarian principle of distribution in the rational decision making of objective and rational agents. Soldiers, they argue, expect casualties. Not knowing, however, who will number among the injured, rational soldiers will choose a principle that will guarantee the injured the greatest chances of survival. That is, they will choose an egalitarian principle that will treat the most severely wounded first, without distinction of rank and irrespective of utility. Baker and Strosberg do not consider adjustments, but the same rational agent would—as Winslow suggests—probably push the extremely injured to the back of the queue and those who can save more lives once treated, to the front.

Unfortunately, these analyses, intuitively appealing as they may be, raise more problems than they solve. Winslow, for example, never quite explains how to translate his suggestions into coherent and, more importantly, fair policy. Once allowing for "immediate usefulness," the burden of medical care shifts back to salvaging soldiers rather than treating based on medical need. Who and how does one decide on the criterion of "immediately useful"? Rank is the obvious measure, but it just as obviously flouts egalitarianism and probably efficiency as well. Melding utility and need is arbitrary at best and, perhaps for this reason, Baker and Strosberg decline to reintroduce utilitarian criteria. However, their historical analysis is incomplete. In spite of their admiration for the "staunchly egalitarian" character of the French army, Napoléon, as noted in the previous chapter, did not extend Larrey's reform beyond his Imperial Guard, and most of his soldiers received far less than exemplary care. Napoléon simply refused to allocate medical resources to soldiers who were easier to replace than to treat. Similarly, Baker and Strosberg overlook the significance of utility as they review guidelines for distributing penicillin to American civilians in World War II. Arguing that medical need generally governed the distribution of penicillin, they conclude "no attempt was made to weigh allocations in favor of those most capable of contributing to the ongoing war effort" (Baker and Strosberg 1992, 118). In fact, the situation was much the opposite. While authorities certainly made room for desperate cases, the entire story of penicillin triage (below) is one of utility and salvage as the lion's share of production went to the military and to civilians whose medical conditions and subsequent treatment could provide knowledge essential to the war effort. Focusing solely on *civilian* distribution presents a skewed picture. Neither example Baker and Strosberg bring—medical care in Napoléon's army or the distribution of penicillin among civilians in World War II—suggests that egalitarianism traditionally overrides utility. Nevertheless, the tension posed by two disparate distributive criteria continues to vex triage decision making. Rather than try to choose between salvage and medical need or utilize them tandem, it is simpler to use them separately in situations for which each is best suited.

Conventional and Mass-Casualty Triage
In a conflict as recent as the Falklands War, British medical personnel distinguished between *conventional* triage and *mass-casualty* triage. The former distributes medical care based on need, while the latter appeals solely to salvage and utility. Conventional triage first cares for those requiring immediate resuscitation and/or immediate surgery, then those who require resuscitation and early surgery, and then those who require no resuscitation and who may delay surgery. Conventional triage operates under a straightforward egalitarian principle based on medical need. Mass-casualty triage, however, reverses the order when "an overwhelming number of seriously injured or otherwise incapacitated individuals, within a limited area or multiple areas and a brief period of time, are placed upon locally available medical facilities quite unable to supply normal medical care for them." Under these conditions, patients who require "some form of surgery to save life and limb, short operating time and have good quality survival" take precedence over those with

"serious and often multiple injuries" who need difficult and time-consuming treatment (Ryan 1984, 195–6; Marsh 1983; Ryan, Sibson, and Howell 1990).

During conventional triage, medical supplies are ample so that if these supplies are properly managed, medical personnel can successfully treat all of the wounded. Mismanage casualties, however, and time will kill the most severely wounded even when supplies and personnel are plentiful. The guiding principle is to save as many lives as possible; when resources are adequate this translates into first treating those whose injuries are most severe. This is the rationale behind conventional triage and the one Larrey ([1814] 1987, vol. 2, 142) describes when he writes that "I attended to the Imperial Guard, but according to a rule which I established, dressing those first who were most grievously wounded without regard to rank or distinction." Putting aside the fact that apart from the privileged status of Napoléon's Imperial Guard, access to medical care in the Army of the Republic was neither adequate nor egalitarian, Larrey describes here, as elsewhere, a state of conventional triage. By treating the most severely ill first, he hoped to treat all in good time despite pitiful working conditions, long nights of amputations, and horrendous wounds and suffering. Moreover, given the limitations of late-eighteenth-century military medicine and typical recourse to amputation, he probably thought little of salvaging, as opposed to simply saving, most wounded soldiers. His return-to-duty rate certainly could not have been better than that of medical personnel during the American Civil War, described in chapter 3. Soldiers returning to battle generally required little care, while those requiring Larrey's constant attention finished their military career either dead, disabled, or discharged.

The prospect of salvaging soldiers is a product of twentieth-century medicine and then, even here, the prospects are not always bright. But the dilemma of mass-casualty triage only arises when medical resources, and particularly time, are in short supply. There is no time to treat everyone regardless of how efficiently one sorts the casualties. Conventional triage turns solely on rationally managing resources on the assumption that proper management will deliver adequate care to everyone who needs it. During mass-casualty triage, this assumption disappears; it is no longer possible to save everyone. Attention turns to saving the greatest number. Ordinarily, these are also the least severely wounded, who will return to battle quicker than others do. But this need not be the case. Consider the following perspective on triage drawn from the Korean War:

Triage rests on the premise that the greatest good must be accomplished for the greatest number under varying conditions of warfare. . . . Life takes precedence over limb, function over anatomical defects. We must always repair the defect which is most serious first. Thus when we were studying arterial injuries we found a sharp increase in the amputation rate after a lag period of 8 hours. Nevertheless, when a casualty is admitted with a perforated bowel and a perforated popliteal artery, the bowel injury must be repaired first as severe shock may interrupt the operation prior to completion and life must be protected over limb. (Howard 1954, 105)[1]

Lacking sufficient time and/or personnel to give the best care to both patients, medical personnel face a situation analogous to mass-casualty triage. Assume two soldiers enter the surgical unit simultaneously (case 1). Treating the less seriously injured solider first and letting the second perhaps die, returns one soldier to duty. Treating the more seriously wounded first and amputating the limb of the second, saves both, but neither returns to duty. If the purpose of mass-casualty triage is to save the greatest number of lives, doctors must save both. If the purpose is to salvage soldiers, they must allow one to die.

This scenario suggests that saving the maximum number of lives—that is, simple utility—and salvage are, in some cases, two disparate principles. Neither criterion is identical to medical need, which targets the worst off. Imagine that a third causality enters the surgical unit suffering from severe, multiple wounds and requiring the attention of the entire staff (case 2). The principle of medical need demands that that soldier receive treatment before the others. Given the extensive care this patient requires, the moderately wounded patient might die and the lightly wounded might lose an arm. This is the worst possible outcome.

In contrast to conventional triage, mass-casualty triage cannot treat the worst-off causalities first. Instead, it must exploit its resources to save the greatest number. The question remains, "saving the greatest number of whom?" Simple utility suggests saving as many lives as possible; salvage turns on saving as many lives as are fit for duty. In many cases, the outcomes of using either principle are identical since doctors will save more lives by focusing on those who do not require inordinate care. These will also be the same soldiers most likely to return to duty. But as case 1 demonstrates, this need not be true. If the outcomes of simple utility and salvage diverge, one must choose.

Two points are salient as medical personnel consider their options. First, a rational agent could choose either simple utility or salvage, assuming that the least wounded are generally the most salvageable. Should the outcomes differ, one might generally favor salvage on the assumption that most agents would place the welfare of the fighting force above the welfare of the most individuals during war. Moreover, those beyond salvage lose their unqualified right to medical care, thereby leaving only those who are salvageable with priority access to resources. The rest, those unsalvageable, then join the pool of all other sick and injured patients who compete for the balance of resources. Second, the case suggests that while a rational agent might reasonably choose simple utility or salvage, that agent would not choose a criterion that treats the wounded exclusively on the basis of medical need when facing the conditions of scarcity that characterize mass-casualty triage. This is simply because a needs-based distribution scheme may quickly eat up all the available resources and create the worst possible outcome: few, if any, salvageable survivors (case 2).

A clear conceptual distinction between conventional and mass-casualty triage makes room for disparate distributive principles to govern each and eases some of the moral dilemmas that arise as one is forced to choose between saving the worst off, saving the most lives, and saving those fit for duty. Conventional triage sorts patients to efficiently manage care and ensure that each patient receives timely and appropriate medical treatment. Conventional triage assumes that available resources are adequate if properly allocated. It is a logistical issue of the highest order but morally unproblematic. There is no clear consensus, on the other hand, about treating the wounded under conditions of mass-casualty triage. British and NATO guidelines instruct medical personnel to reverse the order of conventional triage and treat the least severely injured first in order to salvage the greatest number of soldiers. Others suggest a criterion of simple utility and using resources to save the greatest number of injured. American directives are ambivalent. The 1985 *Army Manual* emphasizes return-to-duty rates (that is, salvage), while the 1994 edition places return to duty behind saving lives (Beam 2003, 374–376). Although each criterion rests on different moral assumptions about the relative strength of collective and individual welfare and the rights of the wounded, it would certainly be difficult to condemn anyone working to save the greatest number of lives, particularly because the outcomes of using either principle are often similar.

Changing battlefield conditions further complicate the decision-making process, since military surgeons face enormous practical difficulties distributing medical resources on a case-by-case basis. Not only must they have some idea of the relative salvage value of each patient, military medical officers must constantly decide which sort of triage, conventional or mass casualty, applies—a decision requiring them to constantly monitor resources and the progress of the war—and how to switch over from one to the other without causing undue harm. Considering these difficulties, medical personnel do just as well expending their efforts on treating whoever they can, as best they can, with an eye toward saving as many as possible and in the hope that this will make a significant, if not efficient, contribution to their nation's war effort. This is certainly consistent with the training most health-care professionals receive.

None of this precludes, however, the imperative to use salvage as the distribution principle to govern *macro*allocation decisions. While surgeons in the field might not really think about salvaging soldiers but only about saving lives as the wounded pour in, policymakers and military commanders certainly consider allocating resources to improve the salvage capacity of military medicine.

Macrolevel Allocations: Simple Utility or Salvage Value?

Macrodistributors—politicians, policymakers, and military planners—often use utility as a criterion for distributing scarce resources. While these officials strive to allocate medical resources to maximize the health of the entire community, the definition of "maximum health" is the subject of continuous debate as values, priorities, and attitudes change and interests clash. During war, however, there is an unusually clear convergence of opinion to distribute all resources, medical resources included, to best further the "war effort." The underlying logic assumes that every other interest is subordinate to the integrity of the political community and the military effort to preserve it. And, indeed, this was the logic behind reserving the lion's share of available penicillin, 85 percent, for the armed forces in World War II.

Military interests also governed the allocation of the remaining stocks of penicillin among civilians as medical need ran second to military necessity: "COC [Committee on Chemotherapeutic and Other Agents, the committee responsible for rationing penicillin] chairman Chester S. Keefer stressed that clinicians should only treat civilians who suffered from penicillin-sensitive illnesses. Of these maladies, only those which would yield information useful to the war effort were to be considered" (Adams 1989, 198).

Since treating civilians could only aid the war effort indirectly (by yielding information that might possibly save the lives of salvageable combatants) while soldiers could aid the war effort directly (by participating in combat), officials reserved most penicillin for soldiers until mid-1944, when stocks were sufficiently plentiful to meet increasing demand. Until then, American and British officials made macroallocation decisions based on the salvage potential of an entire class of recipients likely to benefit from penicillin treatment. But by singling out an entire class for special treatment, they formulated policies that were inherently discriminatory.

Macroallocation and Medical Discrimination   Macroallocation decisions for mass-casualty triage are distinguished by selecting patients for treatment to save as many lives, particularly salvageable lives, as possible. These macroallocation criteria are inherently discriminatory and distribute resources based solely on some facet of social worth. In this way, the Geneva Protocols, like the World Medical Association, fail to fully consider the differences between peacetime and wartime bioethics. In times of peace, one does not ordinarily single out a specific group for preferred medical treatment. Any attempt to do so (during the early distribution of dialysis, for example) is roundly condemned as resting on morally dubious criteria of either intrinsic or extrinsic worth. Extrinsic worth or social utility measures the contribution an individual makes to society. Intrinsic worth refers to the value placed on people, by themselves or others, irrespective of their contribution to society.

There are serious problems with both of these measures and with any attempt to use them as distribution criteria. On the one hand, the utility of catering to a specific social class is largely indeterminate. Better-educated patients may not necessarily contribute more to society, assuming one can accurately measure contributions of this sort and assuming that society, rather than a smaller social unit like the family or ethnic group, is the proper unit of analysis. Intrinsic worth—largely a function of accidents of birth like intelligence, physical stamina, and socioeconomic status—is morally arbitrary, beyond the control and responsibility of the individual, and so should not influence medical entitlements, any more than it should influence the distribution of other important or primary goods. If anything, the intrinsic worth one accords to any human being demands that egalitarian principles govern the distribution of basic liberties, including access to medical care.

These are good arguments against using a principle of discrimination during peacetime. But what happens during war? Here the intrinsic argument does not hold either, and perhaps this was on the mind of those drafting the conventions. Morally innocent enemy soldiers are not intrinsically inferior to their adversaries, nor are one's own civilians intrinsically inferior to one's own soldiers. Extrinsically, however, the story is much different. Enemy soldiers have but negative social utility when they fight (that is, they are a danger to society) and zero utility once incarcerated. If one may invoke social utility during national emergencies and care first for medical personnel or important political figures so they may care for others, as Winslow (1982) and Beauchamp and Childress (1994, 385) suggest, one should also afford salvageable soldiers primary access to medical care before one's own civilians and before enemy soldiers. Similarly, contribution to the war effort rather than medical need should guide a civilian's access to scarce and militarily necessary resources. This rationale governed the distribution of penicillin. These distribution policies were never controversial, nor do they seem particularly offensive today, yet they fly directly in the face of the principle that medical personnel cannot discriminate in favor of their own troops.

Distinguishing between microallocation and macroallocation policies eases this tension. One suspects that physicians would like to treat all their patients as best they can without regard to a patient's status as friend or foe. This feeds the image of medical personnel as universal caregivers working beyond parochial nationalism and united in a common effort to rescue the sick and the wounded. But it also fulfills their obligation to save human life when they can. Should military medical personnel find themselves in a position where they can care for enemy soldiers or operate to save life rather than limb, then they are not morally remiss if they do so assuming that macroallocation principles direct resources where they will salvage the most combat personnel.

As a principle of macrodistribution, however, a nondiscriminatory policy could be a military disaster. When resources are scarce, any attempt to provide civilians or POWs with the same medical facilities one provides military personnel is, at the very least, counterproductive. No one ever suggested that authorities distribute penicillin based solely on medical need during wartime. Macroallocation policies distribute scarce resources to institutions, organizations, or sectors where they are most likely to serve the purpose that policymakers intend. These outcomes are largely unaffected by the idiosyncratic choices of individual doctors. Distributing penicillin or other similarly scarce drugs largely to outpatient military clinics, for example, will curtail access among critically ill soldiers, POWs, or civilians regardless of what medical personnel in the field may do in a given situation. Once policymakers allocate resources commensurate with salvage utility, they may then encourage medical personnel to treat their patients commensurate with simple utility and to save as many lives as possible by considering medical need and the efficacy of treatment.

While military necessity governed the decision to allocate 15 percent of available penicillin for civilian use, simple utility (the imperative to save as many lives as possible), governed allocation within this group. Two criteria, in effect, governed the distribution of penicillin—simple utility and military necessity—and while Keefer required clinicians requesting penicillin to pass both tests, it appears it was sufficient to pass one. The COC approved requests for penicillin from clinicians conducting clinical trials important for the war effort and from those treating desperately ill patients. Thus, it is not unusual to find macrolevel decisions based on salvage utility, while admitting microlevel decisions anchored in simple utility and medical need.

Some Problems of Macroallocation   Although generally uncontroversial, several aspects of salvage-based macroallocation polices may be troublesome. First, one encounters the same problem at the macrolevel that one faces at the microlevel, namely, the difficulty of determining the outcomes of one's actions. Second, there is a tendency to overplay the card of military necessity and distribute resources based on salvage utility when simple utility and saving more lives is a more appropriate criterion. At the same time, one cannot escape the impression that even at the macrolevel, military necessity sometimes gives way to the desire to save lives, as military medical personnel save more than are needed to simply salvage the maximum number of soldiers.

How do policymakers know whether their decisions will aid the war effort? The military grabbed most of the penicillin on the assumption that they could prosecute the war more successfully if they used penicillin to treat soldiers. Military planners distributed penicillin to units where military need was greatest and where doctors could use it best to ensure the integrity of the military's fighting force. Yet individual units make different contributions. Treating combat troops may contribute to the war effort more than caring for rearguard soldiers. Yet, in other instances, mechanics may be more important than the drivers of the tanks they maintain. While one might make general assessments about the relative contribution of various groups of soldiers, the wheels of policymaking do not always grind finely enough to draw this distinction. Moreover, when military surgeons used penicillin to prevent surgical infection, they were saving lives first and only then hoping their patients would return to duty. Both the inability to accurately calculate outcomes and the tendency of physicians to meet medical needs first can, unless monitored closely, work against the utility of salvage.

At the very least, salvage-based macroallocation policies require a clear distinction between soldiers and civilians, favoring the former to the detriment of the latter. But military planners themselves do not always observe this distinction when they continue to treat seriously injured soldiers who might not return to combat at the expense of similarly ill or incapacitated civilians. I argued in chapter 3 that severely wounded soldiers who are *hors de combat* revert to civilian status and merit the same treatment as any noncombatant. Thus, if there are good grounds for treating certain kinds of wounds to return soldiers to duty, there are no grounds for granting priority to seriously wounded but unsalvageable soldiers over seriously ill civilians. Once the social utility of each is equal—that is, neither has superior salvage value—simple utility to save more lives is the only acceptable criterion. Nor should merit skew our moral judgment. There is nothing in the obligation of citizens to die for their country to suggest that they are more meritorious than civilians who do not bear arms. To think otherwise is to misunderstand the reach of military necessity. It does not justify sweeping allocations of scarce medical resources to military personnel when this includes critically wounded soldiers who cannot return to duty. For the entire class of seriously ill soldiers and civilians alike, simple utility is the only equitable criterion for treatment.

Finally, one must consider that military necessity does not always guide macroallocation policies. I also described in chapter 3 how the United States devoted twice the manpower to medical care than the Germans were willing to muster. While this increased the number of combatant lives doctors could save, it did not return any more soldiers to duty. The resources necessary to provide forward surgical facilities could have easily been diverted to other civilian or military uses, yet policymakers chose, with little discord or uncertainty, to provide greater care than was necessary than if military necessity and salvage utility alone governed the distribution of scarce resources. One may speculate whether this concern stemmed from a cultural devotion to life at nearly any cost, certainly an attitude underpinning much of modern medical care in the United States, or a devotion to the lives of soldiers based again, and erroneously, on merit or gratitude due soldiers who fulfill their obligation to defend the state.

The macroallocation of medical resources during war is similar to the allocation of any other resource. Driven by military necessity, policy-makers publicly strive to distribute resources to maximize the war effort. Care, however, is not the only medical resource that authorities must distribute. They also control the flow of scientific knowledge. The atomic bomb and the mass production of penicillin were two of the most significant scientific developments during World War II and both were shrouded in secrecy. While no one ever thought to deliver the secrets of atomic energy to the Germans or Japanese, the decision to withhold medical information did merit brief discussion, if only because of the nagging thought that depriving others of knowledge that could save lives might be wrong.

Distributing Medical Knowledge to the Enemy

Neither the Germans nor the Japanese developed penicillin during the war. The Germans were largely content with sulfa drugs, and when the large German pharmaceutical companies resisted efforts to develop penicillin, the military did not pursue the project. The Japanese showed greater interest than the Germans and by the war's end successfully produced small amounts of penicillin (Sheehan 1982, 51–62). Neither government, however, realized the full medical potential of penicillin, and questions about the propriety of restricting scientific information surfaced once the Allies realized they would soon be able to mass-produce the drug:

Major General James G. McGee, Army Surgeon General, informed Harvey H. Bundy, Office of the Secretary of War (June 20, 1942), that neither international treaties nor the accepted rules of war allow for any distinction between friendly and enemy wounded personnel. "It would be shortsighted, however," McGee said, "to fail to recognize that knowledge in certain fields of medical science may bear more directly on the military situation than on the welfare of the individual." McGee was therefore against communicating penicillin information too widely. "The free dissemination of such information can be of very material aid to the enemy. It, therefore, becomes an instrument of warfare and its publication on the grounds of humanitarianism cannot be justified." (Sheehan 1982, 54–55)

The reasons for withholding medical knowledge cited by McGee are the same calculations of utility and military necessity that govern the macrodistribution of scarce resources. In each case, material aid is the pivotal concept. Distributing penicillin to one's own troops to salvage soldiers materially aids one's own effort; denying knowledge to the enemy cripples theirs. Just as military necessity governs the allocation of medical resources, it also regulates the distribution of scientific knowledge.

The argument is tidy but incomplete. Acts of providing medical treatment to enemy wounded and publicizing medical knowledge for the benefit of treating enemy wounded are not always analogous. Enemy soldiers have the right to receive medical care when they are *hors de combat* and no longer a material threat. They require treatment if, and only if, they remain incarcerated or do not recover sufficiently to return to duty. They cannot demand care when they maintain the wherewithal to threaten those who treat them. Yet this is precisely what will happen if the scientific community releases medical knowledge without restriction. Inevitably, it will make its way to enemy medical personnel who will use it for the same reasons Allied doctors did, namely, to return soldiers to active duty. The obligation to treat enemy wounded does not entail a blanket obligation to release life-saving scientific medical information if enemy soldiers continue to pose a material threat.

Yet this fact alone is insufficient to deny an enemy access to medical knowledge if one can distinguish between enemy combatants and noncombatants. The argument from material aid largely encompasses aid to enemy soldiers. But what of enemy civilians? What are one's humanitarian obligations to those who hold noncombatant immunity? John Sheehan calls penicillin "the secret weapon," but if it is a weapon, it is certainly a curious one. Penicillin cannot kill anyone; it can only save the sick and injured. It is, therefore, a weapon of omission: deny the enemy information to develop penicillin and they will die of preventable causes. Morally, it is not immediately obvious that allowing the enemy to die in this way entails any sort of culpability, particularly when they continue to pose a material threat. Yet if killing and letting die are equivalent in some cases, then allowing individuals to die of a preventable disease might be as morally reprehensible as killing them by biological or medical means. Withholding medical information therefore generates two problems that a straightforward appeal to military necessity does not capture. First, it glosses over harm to civilians whose interests sometimes override military necessity. Second, the utilitarian argument sets the stage for justifying biological warfare by allowing an enemy to die of preventable disease without paying a moral price.

Denying Scientific Knowledge and Harming Noncombatants

Penicillin successfully treats both life-threatening and non-life-threatening diseases. German and Japanese medical personnel might therefore have used it in the same way the Allies did and restrict civilian access while trying to return service personnel to duty. Inevitably, it would affect manpower significantly and materially aid an enemy. To take a different, hypothetical case, suppose that a devastating life-threatening plague broke out naturally among the belligerents and their civilian populations and only one side owned the antidote. Would there be an obligation to provide the antidote? Here the answer is less clear. Humanitarian duty might demand aid to civilians, while leaving soldiers to die. One might also ask about the course of the disease. Could affected soldiers return to duty? If not, then all affected persons should be treated on the basis of the humanitarian obligation to aid noncombatants and soldiers *hors de combat*. Here, one may go on to ask whether there are any reasonable ways to restrict the antidote to civilian populations. It seems unlikely. If so, does it matter?

This example helps flesh out the conditions of material medical aid. Material aid supports combatants as fighters and is a function of returning soldiers to duty, not saving lives. Moreover, the obligation to aid noncombatants is strongest when the benefits they gain are the greatest and the costs of providing aid are the smallest. Aid that saves innocent lives but does not augment the enemy's war effort, as an antidote might do if afflicted soldiers cannot return to duty, is morally obligatory. Aid that only eases suffering while ensuring that soldiers return to duty faster than not, as penicillin will do when used to treat venereal disease, is not obligatory. In this case, military necessity tempers humanitarian duty. Table 5.1 presents various scenarios. Difficult questions remain about what to do with the intermediate cases and whether the harder cases might be altered to mitigate the costs and allow aid.

Table 5.1
The moral obligation to provide medical aid or scientific information to prevent life-threatening disease during war

		Degree to which disease is life threatening	
		Low	High
Degree to which aid or scientific knowledge adversely affects a nation's war effort	Low	1. No moral obligation to provide aid or scientific information	2. Morally obligatory to provide aid or scientific information
	High	3. Morally obligatory not to provide aid or scientific information	4. Conflicting moral obligations to provide aid or scientific information

Cell 1   Cell 1 roughly corresponds to the status of foreign aid in peacetime. While one has an obligation to prevent catastrophic illness or disease when the cost is relatively low (either financially or in terms of security), nations do not have a prima facie obligation to provide aid to improve general health conditions in nations facing disease that is not life threatening on a catastrophic scale. To demand such an infusion of aid might obligate a nation to lower its own health-care standards to raise those of another nation to a more or less equal level. Whether nations incur this obligation sets "lifeboat" ethics against a unilateral obligation to provide significant aid to less developed nations (Singer 1972; Hardin 1974).

Cell 2   Cell 2 should be relatively unproblematic. It describes an enemy facing catastrophic life-threatening disease or injury. Knowledge of effective treatment will not adversely affect the war effort because many of those afflicted will not return to duty and/or noncombatants will be the chief beneficiary of treatment. Suppose penicillin was only effective for preventing surgical infection among the critically injured and could not cure gonorrhea, or that gonorrhea was nothing more than a minor problem for military authorities. In either case, penicillin would only help save soldiers undergoing major surgery, so that relatively few wounded soldiers would benefit and relatively few would return to duty. Alternatively, one might imagine an epidemic that was largely confined to civilian areas because of overcrowding, poor sanitation, and lack of sufficient clothing and shelter. In this case, divulging the knowledge to produce an antidote or vaccine would fulfill an army's humanitarian obligations while bringing significant benefits and incurring few military costs.

Cell 3   In cell 3 costs, particularly military costs, are high and the benefits are low. Should penicillin cure only gonorrhea and have no other uses, nations with access to pertinent medical knowledge have no duty to deliver it to their enemy. On the contrary, they have an obligation to guard it zealously. When nations are at peace, financial costs generally govern the allocation of medical care. Providers will fund expensive care when it offers clear benefits to a sufficient number of suffering individuals. Benefits, sometimes measured by quality of life and sometimes in terms of saving lives, however, are not always commensurable. This may sometimes bring health planners to fund expensive care for few people, premature neonates for example, or to forgo relatively inexpensive care that may improve the quality of life of many more, such as basic dental care. Although deciding among incommensurable goods benefiting conflicting interest groups occupies providers to no end, there is little doubt that economic efficiency drives decision making. If the costs are high and benefits, whether in terms of life or quality of life, are low, health-care providers do not generally incur an obligation to provide medical care. Conversely, when costs are low and benefits are high, a decision to deny care is difficult to justify. A drug that cures sexually transmitted disease at relatively little cost will generally obligate health-care providers to provide treatment. During war, however, military costs augment economic costs. These may easily overwhelm the benefits of treating a non-life-threatening disease that keeps soldiers from active duty. I will speculate in a moment whether this allows belligerents to *inflict* a similar non-life-threatening disease to keep enemy troops from active duty.

Cell 4   Cell 4 is the hardest case. Releasing knowledge of a vaccine that prevents a life-threatening disease carries costs and benefits that are both high. Rather than trying to decide how and what to distribute under these conditions, it is useful to defuse the dilemma by trying to move the case into a different category. To do so, one needs to distinguish carefully between combatants and noncombatants who will benefit from medical knowledge. One might therefore entrust the scientific knowledge to a neutral party who can develop and distribute cutting-edge medical care to acute-care centers serving civilians rather than to outpatient clinics serving military personnel. The International Red Cross, for example, often oversees and monitors medical care under adverse conditions of war and anarchy. Were they entrusted with the manufacture of penicillin for Germany and Japan, it is feasible that they could restrict it to Red Cross facilities caring for critically ill civilians and soldiers. In these circumstances, penicillin does not materially aid the enemy. This pushes the dilemma to cell 2 and elicits a moral obligation to disseminate scientific knowledge or provide aid.

In other circumstances, this might not be possible to do. Responding to an outbreak of plague, one would inevitably treat soldiers and civilians the same way, a cell 4 case that cannot be defused by allocating the knowledge to a neutral third party. Now one must ask whether one has an obligation to prevent soldiers from dying of preventable disease. The question turns on the importance of any distinction between killing and letting die. If one cannot kill enemy soldiers by infecting them with a life-threatening disease, how can one let them die of the same disease that may afflict them naturally? Or, alternatively, if one can allow enemy combatants to die of preventable illnesses, why not then use biological warfare to kill or disable them outright?

Killing by Bacteria and Letting Die of Disease

Arguments for not killing but letting die generally take the following form. First, the terms are defined to distinguish different roles an agent may play. "Killing" is accompanied by causality as an agent deliberately originates "a fatal sequence of events." "Letting die," on the other hand, allows the sequence "to run its course" (Foot [1975] 1994, p. 287–8). Second, agents that kill or let die each incur a different degree of moral responsibility. Most agents that kill deliberately and egregiously harm another human being commit morally reprehensible acts. Agents that permit others to die allow a fatal sequence to run it course, and while they may be able to prevent or mitigate the consequences, they are not responsible for initiating the wrong. As a result, their actions are less reprehensible than those of individuals initiating a chain of events that leads to another's death.

This line of reasoning does not get us very far, because the distinction between killing and letting die does not capture all the moral facets of the dilemma. It does not fully account for costs of action. Ordinarily, one has a prima facie obligation to prevent harm if the costs are reasonable. As I noted in the previous chapter, allowing someone to die is as morally blameworthy as killing if the costs of intervening are low. Nor does the simple distinction between killing and letting die account for the moral status of the victim. Allowing terminally ill patients to die is not equivalent to allowing healthy, treatable patients to die. Allowing soldiers to die might not carry the same moral implications as allowing civilians to die, and so on. For these reasons, the distinction between killing and letting die remains a false dichotomy that does not fully capture the scope of moral responsibility.

Instead of distinguishing between the agent's actions, it is, as I argued in the previous chapter, important to understand the agent's intent. Actions alone do not tell the whole story independent of the agent's motives, the rights and attitude of the victim, and the consequences that befall both the agent and the victim (Beauchamp and Childress 1994, 219–225). Certain forms of euthanasia that allow terminally ill patients to die by refusing treatment, for example, are often morally on a par with the forms of euthanasia that initiate a fatal sequence of events. But disconnecting a respirator need not carry the stigma of killing if a terminally or chronically ill patient consents and the patient's death does not benefit those who caused the death. Cases such as these require us to look closely at killing and letting die during war and force us to examine the motives of combatants, the rights and attitudes of civilians, and the consequences of different types of action. The complexity of killing and letting die during war is further compounded because there are two different victims: combatants and noncombatants.

Killing Civilians and Letting Them Die   With the exception of the double effect, there is a strict humanitarian duty to avoid harming civilians. That is, belligerents cannot harm civilians unless harm is the unintended consequence of a necessary military action. By the same token, belligerents must prevent or mitigate harm befalling noncombatants. Civilians may demand that military authorities maintain health, education, and welfare services for the benefit of an occupied population. Civilians may not be killed or allowed to die needlessly or excessively. These are two important qualifications central to the doctrine of double effect and proportionality. How do they affect the imperative to provide or censor medical information that will save lives?

The most difficult scenario, one not amenable to neutral, international supervision, requires us to sacrifice civilians—that is, let them die—in order to allow disease or infection to decimate an enemy force. May belligerents let civilians die in this way, assuming that this is tantamount to killing them if they might be saved at little cost? Civilians allowed to die of disease to destroy an enemy force are not killed with the express purpose of attaining a military goal. Instead, their deaths, although foreseen and unavoidable, are the byproduct or unintended effect of a necessary military operation. It is an operation of a very odd sort, an act of omission and not commission, but the logic of the double effect is the same. While belligerents cannot say that they did not *mean* to kill, they can mean, as Warren Quinn (1989) argues, that civilian deaths were irrelevant to the military's purpose. If the DDE holds for deaths caused by commission, it certainly holds for deaths caused by omission. The death of civilians that comes from denying the enemy medical information passes the test of failure, namely, the (o)mission depriving military personnel of life-saving medical care will succeed whether civilians die or not. Their deaths add nothing of military value. It remains, however, to determine whether civilian deaths are proportionate.

There are no firm guidelines to determine proportionality. Civilians have fallen victim to the DDE in increasingly greater numbers as the destructive power of war multiplies. Civilian deaths are disproportionate when they are excessive—that is, beyond what public opinion will bear at any particular time. This is a function of many factors: the ferocity of war, one's own casualties, attitudes toward one's enemies, and international public opinion. Nevertheless, one may, under some conditions, calculate the consequences of nontreatment. Penicillin undoubtedly saved

Allied lives and cost the enemy theirs during the short period the Allies maintained their monopoly. Yet its benefits are probably far less than those one might expect should one side maintain a monopoly on drugs necessary to treat a highly infectious and life-threatening disease.

During World War II, penicillin saved critically injured soldiers and returned to duty many soldiers suffering from sexually transmitted disease. Given its rationing throughout the war, it is difficult to determine how many civilians penicillin benefited or, conversely, how many lost their lives when it was not available. But because penicillin was not used to treat a deadly, contagious disease, enemy civilians did not suffer disproportionate harm if their suffering is compared with the lost mandays enemy forces experienced when an adequate means to treat venereal disease or surgical infection was unavailable. Contrast this outcome with the millions who could lose their lives to a disease similar to the virulent strain of influenza that shook the world following World War I. While a similar epidemic during wartime will doubtlessly cripple any army lacking a vaccine, one hopes that adversaries will understand that the massive civilian deaths that result should one side withhold life-saving scientific information are disproportionate regardless of how effectively disease decimates the ranks of enemy soldiers. But this hope, which directs one side to provide the other with life-saving medical knowledge, is probably vain. Few lost sleep over the estimated 800,000 German civilians who fell victim to Britain's blockade of Germany in World War I. Rampant disease would probably elicit no greater compassion. One might better console oneself, then, with the expectation that the conditions that fuel this dilemma—a deadly communicable disease, a therapeutic monopoly, and the inability of neutral agencies to treat civilians exclusively—rarely come together. Should they occur coincidentally there would be reasonable grounds to argue that proportionality demands that life-saving medical information belongs in the public domain.

Cases like penicillin, the plague, and influenza exemplify how the demand to release medical information when civilian lives are at stake often depends on local circumstances. To the extent that noncombatants may not be killed, they may also not be allowed to die. The prohibition is not absolute. The DDE and principle of proportionality teach us that much. Nevertheless, there is no moral tension between killing and letting die. One may not kill civilians nor may one let them die unless the benefits accompanying their deaths are very high and the costs measured by lost lives are relatively low. Otherwise, one is obliged not to kill civilians or let them die. The rule for soldiers, however, is quite the opposite. One may kill soldiers *and* let them die.

Killing Soldiers and Letting Them Die   Considering the status of soldiers, one immediately faces a moral puzzle. While one may kill soldiers, one generally may not allow them to die of their wounds. Thus, the moral ranking of killing and letting die is, as far as combatants are concerned, reversed: it is worse to let them die than to kill them. But this curious outcome is the result of mixing incommensurable classes, namely, combatants and noncombatants. Injured soldiers are no longer combatants but assume the status of noncombatants and are entitled to medical care as long as they stay that way, as either POWs or incapacitated invalids. The real test comes when we consider letting soldiers die who are neither seriously wounded nor POWs.

Soldiers at risk for contracting a deadly disease are no different than other combat soldiers; neither group enjoys any right to life from their enemy. Neither is *hors de combat*, neither regains the right to life following injury, and neither can invoke any obligation on the part of the enemy to save their lives. As long as soldiers remain soldiers, they may be killed and allowed to die. Whether killed or allowed to die, the status of the victim and motive of the killer remain the same. In each case, combatants are trying to end one another's life. There are very few limits on how combatants may take the lives of each other. Assuming that dying by infectious disease is no more excruciating than dying by high explosives, a question I will examine in detail in chapter 8, it seems to make no difference whether an enemy soldier is killed by initiating a fatal sequence of events or allowed to die from events that owe their first cause to acts of God. The outcome is the same in both cases. But if letting combatants die by infectious disease is equivalent to killing, and killing is permissible as an act of war, then may we push the argument one step further and suggest that adversaries may kill one another with biological as well as with conventional weapons?

Unless biological weapons cause unnecessary suffering or disproportionate noncombatant deaths, it certainly might seem that way. Of
course, the international community unequivocally bans biological
weapons for these very reasons. However, it is important to see that both
reasons are contingent; there are no inherent difficulties in using weapons
to kill enemy soldiers by biological means if one can avoid unnecessary
suffering or excessive death among civilians. I will leave this discussion
for chapter 8 and only note the challenge that *nonlethal* chemical and
biological weapons pose. If devastating consequences prevent adversaries
from killing one another with biological weapons, perhaps they can
simply disable one another by the same means, particularly if the foregoing discussion suggests that it is permissible to let combatants die or
suffer from disease, sexually transmitted or otherwise, that occurs naturally in the course of war.

Scientific Knowledge and Military Necessity

The distribution of the knowledge necessary to mass-produce penicillin
draws our attention to the ethics of publicizing medical information
during war. Without scrutinizing the outcomes of delivering medical
knowledge to one's enemies and drawing a distinction between the rights
of combatants and noncombatants, any sweeping generalizations similar
to those U.S. officials pronounced during World War II are unwarranted.
The dictates of military necessity together with respect for the immunity
of noncombatants compels one to carefully consider restricting access to
medical knowledge only when the military benefits are clear and noncombatants do not suffer grievous harm. Judging the issue solely on the
basis of material aid to the enemy skews the outcomes.

Similar thinking guides the flow of medical knowledge that may aid
bioterrorists. Echoing concerns of the scientific community (Selgelid
2003, National Research Council 2004), the *New York Times* reported
that advances in synthetic virus research might allow researchers to manufacture or genetically modify pathogens like smallpox that, in the wrong
hands, can infect vast numbers of civilians (Wade 2005). Should governments regulate or otherwise restrict this information? In this case, scientific knowledge does not prevent disease but may cause it. While a
therapeutic drug falling into enemy hands will not kill noncombatants,

virulent viruses can cause considerable harm to soldiers and civilians alike. Researchers will first ask whether it is feasible to restrict information in such a way that it promotes the welfare of ordinary civilians without harming military interests. Some researchers believe that "the machines and ingredients for synthesizing DNA should be controlled, with manufacturers selling supplies only to facilities whose DNA machines are registered" (Wade 2005). In other words, the manufacturing process *can* be controlled in much the same way a neutral party can oversee the distribution of a specialized drug and ensure that it will not aid an enemy (cell 2). The same is true if, as some believe, these advances in genetic science will be of little use to terrorists who "will find it easier to collect pathogens in the wild" If these assessments are wrong, however, one must confront medical and scientific innovations that hold the potential for considerable good and overwhelming harm.

As the development of nuclear power clearly demonstrates, the problem of dual-use technologies is not new. To meet this challenge, the world community has relied on control and deterrence rather than censorship. Rogue states and terrorists, however, might be difficult to deter and should genetic technology prove harder to control than nuclear technology, responsible states will have to weigh the relative costs and benefits of each new scientific advance. Innovations with the potential to bring great harm but little benefit face tight restrictions (cell 3). For those with the potential for great benefits and harm (cell 4), the same caveat governing the distribution of penicillin information applies: while military interests take precedence during war, restricting scientific information cannot disproportionately harm noncombatants. Unlike a single drug such as penicillin, genetic knowledge has numerous applications, most of which will benefit nonmilitary interests. This may then require authorities to be very selective about the information they censor, restricting scientific knowledge that harms military interests but has little effect on noncombatants and, at the same time, releasing information without which the civilian population suffers unduly.

If overstating the reach of military necessity harms civilians excessively, tunnel vision and the inability to draw on novel thinking also distort our ability to resolve moral dilemmas in wartime. One must seriously wonder whether the dilemma of penicillin triage, a paradigm case of distributive justice during wartime, is about medicine or simply about sex. Imagine that the disease incapacitating soldiers was not sexually transmitted but a debilitating, non-life-threatening, penicillin-sensitive respiratory disease. Would anyone be indignant about treating these soldiers with available supplies of penicillin before the critically wounded? I think not. Unencumbered by sexual mores, the preferences are clearly utilitarian. Officials regulating the distribution of penicillin, however, found themselves embroiled in two dilemmas at once, one social and one medical, leading us to ask which takes precedence when lives are at stake.

Alternatives to Triage

During wartime, triage presents a tragic choice to policymakers who must distribute resources in ways that will cause some patients to suffer. But bioethical dilemmas often lend themselves to creative solutions that may blunt the stark choice that face medical personnel and policymakers. Is there not a moral imperative to search for solutions that will mitigate the damage and reduce the number of individuals harmed?

Imagine again that a respiratory rather than sexually transmitted disease threatens Allied forces, and consider further that the routine use of an inexpensive surgical mask among troops could significantly reduce the incidence of this disease. Would authorities then be morally remiss if they did not enforce routine prevention? Certainly they would, insofar as the prophylactic means they propose did not significantly affect a soldier's ability to fight. Condoms, of course, are not surgical masks. While both can successfully prevent communicable disease, condoms are loaded with moral baggage. Regulating sexual behavior among troops entails regulating prostitution, a flight of moral imagination that neither British nor American authorities could exercise.

Both the British and the Americans put their war effort first. But this does not mean that they were not unencumbered by the force of other moral norms and attitudes that whittled away at their single-minded devotion to defeating the Germans and the Japanese. Sexual mores figure prominently here, for had a more "reputable" disease incapacitated troops, authorities would have expended considerable effort searching for alternative means to reduce the incidence of disease.

Regulations permitting physicians to treat civilians with penicillin offered an opportunity to conduct clinical trials with civilian patients suffering from venereal disease. While these trials yielded important clinical data, moral issues were always lurking in the background. In October 1943, a former congressional representative tried to obtain penicillin for a desperately ill physician and complained that penicillin was only available for "men who were careless in their lives." In response, A. N. Richards, chair of the Committee on Medical Research, one of the bodies overseeing penicillin testing, reiterated the guidelines for dispensing penicillin but nonetheless acknowledged that the "clinical information was obtained in treatment of civilian sinners and necessarily the penicillin used was taken from a supply inadequate for the treatment of more respectable diseases" (Adams 1989, 210).

Venereal disease was so morally loaded that it prevented any consideration of reasonable alternatives to tragic dilemmas. It set the stage for resisting an attempt to regulate prostitution among American and British troops while, at the same time, casts aspersion on infected men who required scarce medical resources. Should an issue like sexual behavior intrude on military and medical decision making?

The Alternative to Tragic Choice: Regulating Prostitution

During World War I, sexually transmitted disease caused 1.5 million casualties among Allied troops. The problem, of course, was not new and one solution was always to control the spread of venereal diseases by establishing supervised brothels for soldiers. During World War I, for example, both the French and German armies maintained medically supervised houses of prostitution, and strict control on the German side kept the incidence of disease to half that of the French and one-seventh that of the British. During World War II, the subject of regulating prostitution to control disease among troops was once again the subject of intense debate that played out in two forums: the U.S. Congress and military bases in Hawaii (Costello 1986, 212).

In the United States, the American Social Hygiene Association waged a relentless war against houses of prostitution. In July 1941, the May Act outlawed brothels near military bases and gave local military commanders the power to summon the FBI to close houses of prostitution.

While many commanders ignored prostitution, pressure increased as the public and press demanded that the administration take an active role in extinguishing prostitution. Abstinence was the solution of choice, a "shield" against venereal infection that decimated Allied forces in World War I. John Costello (1986, 86–87, 213) describes the campaign to enlist boxer Gene Tunney to admonish soldiers to wear the "Bright Shield of Continence" on their uniforms and display "moral bravery when confronted by the rouged challenge" of "motorized brothels" and "diseased harlots." The popular press asked ruefully, "Can our sailors and soldiers, as champions of democracy, afford to indulge in sexual promiscuities scorned by most prize fighters? Dare they forget that in the First World War 7,000,000 days of service were lost to the U.S. Army as a result of venereal infections?"

While the May Act significantly reduced the number of brothels and organized houses of prostitution, it did little to affect the rate of venereal disease as freelancers and amateurs took over much of the business. Similarly, prostitution among troops overseas flourished in unregulated brothels as commanders and chaplains turned a blind eye to illicit sexual activity lest they become unpopular with their troops. At U.S. bases in Hawaii, however, officials took a different tack, one that marked the only successful attempt to regulate prostitution and reduce the incidence of venereal disease among U.S. troops during the war. Largely immune from the May Act, military officials in Hawaii effectively decriminalized prostitution. While remaining illegal, houses of prostitution operated in specified districts under close supervision. The police registered and fingerprinted prostitutes, doctors oversaw periodic medical examinations, and military officials established prophylaxis stations to distribute condoms and advise service personnel about sexually transmitted disease. As a result, the rate of sexually transmitted disease in the Hawaiian military district was the lowest in the American armed forces (Bailey and Farber 1992, 65).

The effectiveness of regulated prostitution was, of course, only one aspect of the debate. Opposite the social utility of reducing the incidence of venereal disease stood the effects of prostitution on women. On the one hand, Costello (1986, 218) writes how "many of Honolulu's prostitutes made enough to move out of the red light district to smart houses

in uptown Honolulu." A more sobering account of this so-called vic-
timless crime comes from Beth Bailey and David Farber (1992), who
describe how prostitutes suffered from venereal disease, unwanted preg-
nancy, social ostracism, and drug abuse. Nevertheless, Bailey and Farber
also describe how many prostitutes believed they were making a vital
contribution to the war effort and how many could work for six months
or less and return to the mainland with considerably more money than
they could otherwise have earned. The debate over the relative merits of
regulating prostitution during wartime weighs conflicting rights, disparate social and military utility, and religious values. Most authorities,
endorsed an official ban on prostitution while unofficially turning a blind
eye and tolerating its practice. Hawaiian policy too, open-minded as it
may have been, fell in line with the rest of the country when military
rule ended in Hawaii in 1944.

Prostitution and Penicillin

This debate would have remained confined to the relative merits and
drawbacks of prostitution but for the coincidental fact that penicillin
could quickly cure most cases of venereal disease, and the drug was in
perilously short supply. This created, then, the unique situation of two
moral dilemmas impinging on one another: triage and prostitution.
Forcing a choice between aiding some patients while allowing others to
die, triage is the more tragic of the two. Regardless of how one ranked
men "wounded in brothels," soldiers "wounded in battle," and civilians
suffering from ordinary illness and injury, the shortage of penicillin led
to the death of some patients who could not obtain a supply of penicillin to save their life. Legalized prostitution, on the other hand, is the
less tragic of the two dilemmas. It forces a choice between regulating
sexual behavior and, in the opinion of some, condoning a moral evil.
Penicillin triage combines the two dilemmas, compelling policymakers
and legislators to choose between permitting prostitution and saving
lives, and between banning an unacceptable social practice at the cost of
curtailing life-saving treatment.

Regulated prostitution is a complicated issue. If the only outcome
worthy of attention is the spread of venereal disease and its effect on
fighting strength, at least during wartime, the preferred option is close

regulation. This was the policy of the U.S. military in Hawaii. If one is concerned with banning what one considers to be an immoral sexual practice regardless of its effect on actual behavior, or on the war effort, or on the spread of infectious disease, then one must absolutely prohibit prostitution and do one's best to stamp it out. This was the goal of American lawmakers in 1941. Finally, if one focuses on the harm women suffer as a result of prostitution, then the issue is less clear, compounded by problems associated with drug addiction, child prostitution, and crushing poverty that remain unaddressed by the simple question of regulating consensual prostitution.

I will not sort out these issues here. Nor do they require resolution to address the larger issue, namely, which of the two interconnected dilemmas—triage or prostitution—deserves prior attention? Answering this question does not require a solution for each dilemma but only that we see the essential differences between the two. Triage is a tragic dilemma. Any choice that forces one to choose one life over another when only a lack of resources prevents saving both, is a tragedy from any reasonable moral perspective. Regulating prostitution is neither tragic nor unambiguous. It neither forces a choice between lives nor presents choices that every reasonable person would consider morally momentous. The dilemma of regulating prostitution may reflect conflicting rights or present outcomes of contentious social utility, but only a minority would invoke an absolute religious injunction against "harlotry." However important the issue is, most observers would conduct their evaluation in terms of the relative costs and benefits alternative policies bring to different parties: the army, soldiers, women, and so on.

One need not, therefore, grapple with the intricacies of regulated prostitution before deciding that the entire issue is subordinate to the dilemma posed by triage. One must only note the interrelationship of the two dilemmas, which, to my knowledge, was never acknowledged during the penicillin crises. Given sufficient evidence that one could ease the dilemma of triage by reducing the incidence of venereal diseases through regulated prostitution, then the lesser dilemma falls before the graver. This does not detract from the merits of the regulating or prohibiting prostitution under different conditions, but when two dilemmas impinge on one another, the more tragic of the two deserves prior attention. One

wonders how the American and British public would have reacted if confronted with condoning regulated prostitution or accepting penicillin
triage as Beecher (1971) described it. They never faced this choice
because they continued to view each dilemma, triage and prostitution,
in isolation.

Tragedy and Triage: A Second Look

Recognizing two distinct and overlapping bioethical dilemmas may make
it easy to argue that prostitution is the lesser tragedy. But why is saving
lives a greater good than preserving important sexual or social norms?
Phrased in this way, the answer to most of us seems obvious. Tragedies
are always a function of death and privation. A scarcity of life-saving
medications always carries these tragic overtones; prostitution rarely
does. Given the general imperative to prevent more harm than less, there
should be little question that triage deserves our first priority. Triage can
save lives; regulating prostitution does not.

As neat and tidy as this sounds, one must keep in mind that war is
not about saving lives but about saving a way of life. Threatened by war,
nations sacrifice lives, particularly those of sturdy, young men. But lives,
in and of themselves, are of secondary value. Commenting above that
there is little practical difference between policies of triage that favor
salvage over the simple utility of saving lives when resources are scarce,
I glossed over the underlying, theoretical differences. Salvage utility is
instrumental: doctors save soldiers not because their lives are precious
but so they may return to duty and accomplish a specific task. In most
cases, this purpose reflects the overriding importance of a political community's norms, cultural values, and way of life. Simple utility, in contrast, aims to save lives because the value of life, independent of any
purpose this life will serve, is of supreme value. The difference is important. During war, human life is of but instrumental value. Biomedical
ethics usually assumes quite the opposite. Sometimes this difference is
insignificant, but sometimes it is critically important.

What at first may appear merely as a historical anecdote of only idiosyncratic value, the conflict between penicillin triage and regulated prostitution forces us to think twice about the different criteria of triage that

often defer to the bald instrumental value that salvage confers on human life. It is not enough to draw on bioethics for analytic clarity, to throw the two dilemmas into sharp relief and direct us to prefer tragic to less-than-tragic choice. We must ask whether bioethics is not constrained by principles that consider solely the instrumental value of human life, or in the very least, subordinate the intrinsic value of human life to super-aggregate interests, particularly those that dominate during war and tend to chew up human lives with abandon. That bioethics resists these principles is not surprising. Kant's maxim to treat others as ends guides bioethics. But it does not guide war. During armed conflict, there is very little compunction about using persons as means.

This should be kept in mind as we consider any problem of triage. Although neither American nor British lawmakers confronted triage and prostitution in tandem, it would not be unreasonable to expect them to safeguard significant sexual and religious values at the expense of saving more lives than less. "Harlotry," "sinfulness," and "disrepute" all characterize the men and women who visit or work in brothels. The spasm of indignation that gripped American legislators during the war reflects the fear that surrendering to "depraved" sexual behavior would indelibly stain their political community and undermine their way of life. Willing to sacrifice innumerable lives to protect these interests, many might agree that the prospect of saving lives by regulating prostitution and freeing up penicillin for other uses paled beside the certain damage sexual license would do their cause. One may take issue, of course, but doing so pushes the debate outside of medicine because the underlying principles of biomedical ethics that decry using persons only as means run up against attitudes that do exactly that. Penicillin triage puts this friction on the table. The laws of war do not respect the inherent value of soldiers' lives. These laws instead stress soldiers' instrumental value. Doctors providing medical care might ignore this as they treat their patients, but while they work to save lives, they cannot be oblivious to the fact that they are only saving their patients for an ulterior purpose. When it is impossible to do both, they are expected to save those whose lives can best safeguard a community's way of life, and allow those to die who cannot.

The incongruity of the underlying principles that characterize medicine and war will continue to plague us. It leads us to ask whether the disparate principles are ever compatible, whether medicine must, in the final analysis, simple renounce the norms of war and embrace pacifism. I will consider this question in chapter 9. In the meantime, the tension between medicine and war does not disappear as conventional wars become increasingly rare. On the contrary, unconventional war, insurgency, and limited war pose much more difficult problems. During conventional war, medicine will often content itself with conforming to the broad dictates of humanitarian law and the laws of armed conflict. Sometimes these laws also serve the principles of medical ethics. Other times, and triage is one example, they conflict and leave medical personnel to choose between the two. Unconventional war, particularly insurgencies, guerrilla war, and other forms of low-intensity conflict, however, raise the stakes and exacerbate the tension between medical and military ethics as the conventions of war themselves strain under their burden of protecting combatants, noncombatants, and political communities.

6
Medical Neutrality

Medical Neutrality and Armed Conflict

Medical neutrality suggests, in some rather odd way, that medical personnel are nonthreatening. Dedicated only to the care and welfare of the sick and wounded, doctors, nurses, and medics serve the injured. Medical personnel do not fight, do not bear arms but for self-protection, and, therefore, merit immunity from harm as they fulfill their duties impartially (Geneva Convention (I), 1949a, Article 22). The concept is odd because medical personnel clearly contribute to a nation's war effort by returning soldiers to active combat duty. They do not bear arms like ordinary soldiers, but individually and collectively, their contribution is significant. If the distribution of medical resources during armed conflict is subject to utility rather than medical need, and if it is permissible, indeed obligatory, to treat one's own soldiers and civilians before enemy soldiers and civilians, in what way, then, is medicine neutral during war?

Two Concepts of Medical Neutrality
Medical neutrality may mean either "impartiality" or "immunity." These are two distinct meanings, and in considering medical ethics in time of armed conflict, the WMA interprets neutrality in both senses. Emphasizing impartiality, WMA regulations first stipulate "The medical duty to treat people with humanity and respect applies to all patients. The physician must always give the required care *impartially* and without discrimination on the basis of age, disease or disability, creed, ethnic origin, gender, nationality, political affiliation, race, sexual orientation, or social standing or any other similar criterion" (World Medical Association,

2004, paragraph 4; emphasis added). Later, the WMA underscores the importance of neutrality as immunity or protection: "Physicians must be granted access to patients, medical facilities and equipment and the *protection* needed to carry out their professional activities freely. Necessary assistance, including unimpeded passage and complete professional independence, must be granted . . . Hospitals and health-care facilities situated in war regions must be respected by combatants and media personnel" (World Medical Association, 2004, paragraphs 12, 14; emphasis added).

It is no coincidence that the WMA precedes its appeal for immunity with an affirmation of impartiality. The same idea of impartiality animates many misconceptions of triage, and courses through military medical ethics as nurses and physicians hope to place medical need and the interests of individual patients above the demands of salvage and military necessity. I will return to this point throughout, for it contributes to the underlying tension that characterizes bioethics during armed conflict. The idea of medical neutrality is fraught with similar inconsistencies that can best be sorted out by preserving the distinction between immunity and impartiality.

Medical Neutrality: From Immunity to Impartiality

The immunity belligerents accord to medical personnel is considerably more sweeping than that extended to civilians. International law recognizes the absolute protection of medical personnel and medical facilities insofar as they are not used for hostile purposes. The international community shows little tolerance for attacks on medical facilities and personnel, however indignantly a belligerent appeals to the doctrine of double effect or proportionality—the same principles that diminish the force of noncombatant immunity. Why, then, do medical workers enjoy greater immunity than other players do during war? There are two answers, one that recalls the absolute, humanitarian obligation to care for the wounded and another that reminds us that medical neutrality is the product of slowly evolving conventions between warring parties, who have found it possible to help themselves by helping their adversary.

The humanitarian argument grounds medical immunity in the right of wounded soldiers to receive medical care. If combatants have an absolute right to medical care, then medical personnel deserve absolute protection to safeguard the means necessary to save the lives of the sick and wounded. Phrased this way, the argument for immunity overlooks a crucial question: Do combatants have an absolute right to medical care? If not, what then of the absolute nature of medical immunity?

Subject to various conditions, which I described in chapter 3, combatants and noncombatants enjoy the right to medical care during war. As importantly, medical neutrality is necessary to safeguard these rights. If the wounded are to have any rights at all, the parties to armed conflict must protect the medical personnel, ambulances, and hospital facilities responsible for providing care to the injured. Military medical personnel, therefore, gain their protection from rights of those they care for. Theirs is a derivative right, wholly dependent on the status of their patients and solely a function of the rights that others enjoy. This is an important point. Medical personnel are certainly not impartial in any meaningful sense of the word. They must violate confidentiality and denounce their patients as military conditions warrant, distribute medical resources for the benefit of their own forces, and toil to return soldiers to active duty. In and of themselves, they may be fair game. However, inasmuch as they may not suffer harm without irreparably jeopardizing the medical rights of both combatants and noncombatants, military medical personnel warrant considerable protection. But protection or immunity should not be confused with impartiality. There is a tendency to place medical personnel above the fray of war, a perception of medicine's role that is not accurate.

If medical neutrality is a function of the rights that others enjoy, then the normative force of immunity waxes and wanes with the relative strength of these same rights. If medical rights are not absolute, then medical immunity is likewise compromised. Recall that both soldiers and civilians command a fundamentally different right to medical care. Soldiers are entitled to medical care subject to their salvage value, enemy combatants receive care only insofar as they are nonthreatening, and civilians, including soldiers who cannot return to duty, warrant scarce medical resources subject to the dictates of military necessity and general welfare. None of these actors has an absolute right to medical care. This fact alone should compel us to take another look at medical immunity.

Military organizations provide medical care to return soldiers to duty, not because they have an obligation to save the lives of soldiers irrespective of their salvage value. At the very least, an uncomplicated calculation of utility demands that armies provide the medical resources necessary to enable their wounded soldiers to fight again. During conventional war, most belligerents concur and have good reason, therefore, to protect one another's medical assets. With this convention in place, violating medical immunity has severe consequences for each side. But this need not be the case; during insurgency warfare one side or another might find it advantageous to disrupt care or abuse immunity. Guerrillas violate medical neutrality when they know the costs are not high or when the benefits they gain outweigh the costs of being unable to care for their own wounded. Similarly, counterinsurgency forces violate medical neutrality when the benefits that come from thwarting a guerrilla or terrorist attack overwhelm the cost of violating the convention.

Considering the nonabsolute nature of medical rights during war, we see how the *norm* of medical *neutrality* more accurately signifies a *convention* of medical *immunity*. If the former is in some way abiding and absolute and encompasses both impartiality and protection, the latter is transitory, contingent, and limited to immunity. A historical analysis yields a similar result. In earlier periods of history, medical neutrality was more a matter of convenience than a principle of humanitarian law. Its primary function was reciprocity of protection. Only later did it move to embrace impartiality.

Medical Neutrality: Historical Perspectives
The principle of medical neutrality emerged in fits and starts as commanders found it prudent to allow medical personnel to offer first aid, and if necessary, evacuate the wounded from the battlefield. Given the sorry and sporadic state of military medical care prior to the twentieth century, there was little concerted action either to deploy medical personnel or to protect them. Early agreements were simply a matter of happenstance and benevolent leadership. As early as the siege of Metz (1551–1553), François de Guise summoned Ambrose Paré to care for the wounded and sick soldiers abandoned by Spain as their siege failed

and Spanish forces retreated from the city (Paré 1968, 37–50). De Guise's actions were unilateral and largely humanitarian, although he probably did not relish the prospect of sick soldiers flooding his city after the siege lifted. His actions marked a modest turning point in the treatment of the wounded. "During the next 200 years," writes L. C. Green (1998, 68), "it was becoming not uncommon for opposing commanders to sign binding agreements relating to the treatment of the wounded and sick." "Not uncommon," but not particularly common either. Garrison ([1922] 1970, 138), for example, notes only five such agreements between 1743 and 1864. By the American Civil War, Generals Jackson, Lee, and McClellan agreed to release captured medical personnel after allowing them to treat their wounded (Gabriel and Metz 1992, vol. 2, 194–195). In 1863, Francis Lieber incorporated these directives, together with regulations requiring treatment for sick and injured enemy soldiers, into the laws of armed conflict he prepared for the Union army. His code later served as a model for European conventions (Lieber Code, 1863, Articles 53, 79, pp. 115–116).

While the Lieber Code and similar agreements protected officers of the medical staff, nurses, and hospitals from attack, it remained for the Geneva Conventions together with the appearance of voluntary medical personnel to create the extensive concept of medical immunity *and* impartiality we understand medical neutrality to mean today. Throughout the nineteenth century, armies suffered terribly from the lack of medical personnel and the resources necessary to evacuate the wounded from the battlefield. In spite of the innovations that Larrey and Letterman introduced with their fledging medical forces, many soldiers received poor care or no care at all. Recognizing that European military commanders were reluctant to dedicate the personnel necessary to care for the sick and wounded properly, it was the genius of Henry Dunant to establish the Red Cross and call on the European states to permit *volunteers* to care for the wounded. Volunteer medical workers were often women. They were impartial, expected to collect and care for wounded and sick combatants "to whatever nation they may belong" (Geneva Convention, 1864, Article 6; also Geneva Convention, 1929, Article 1; Geneva Convention (I), 1949a, Article 12). Volunteer medical workers were not soldiers, not beholden to any army or nation, and neutral by definition. As such, they could not enter the battlefield without a guarantee of protection from the warring parties. This and little more was the basis for the first Geneva Conference (1863). Additional guidelines protecting *military* medical personnel were only recommendations:

Independently of the above Resolutions [protecting volunteer medical personnel], the Conference makes the following Recommendations: . . . that in time of war the belligerent nations should proclaim the neutrality of ambulances and military hospitals, and that neutrality should likewise be recognized, fully and absolutely, in respect of official medical personnel, voluntary medical personnel, inhabitants of the country who go to the relief of the wounded, and the wounded themselves. (Geneva Conference, 1863, Recommendation b)

These recommendations were adopted the following year with respect to land warfare and in 1868 to include naval warfare (Geneva Convention, 1864, 1868). These Geneva accords firmly established the conventions of medical neutrality. Nonmilitary medical personnel required immunity—that is, protection—because they were, in fact, neutral, unarmed, and incidental to the war.[1] They were also expected to administer medical care impartially with the understanding that "only urgent medical reasons will authorize priority in the order of treatment to be administered" (Geneva Convention (I), 1949a, Article 12). The immunity and impartiality we accord to medical personnel stem from their prior, objective neutrality as volunteers (and, most likely, as women as well), not from the medical task they performed. In other words, there was nothing inherent in providing medical care that conferred protection or demanded impartiality. Nuns tending religious needs would enjoy the same protection as nurses caring for the wounded, as might undertakers collecting the dead for burial. The fact that some serve a medical function does not, in and of itself, accord protection. However, because volunteer medical personnel worked closely with, and under the direction of, "official medical personnel"—that is, military surgeons—the two required and eventually came to enjoy identical protection. Neutrality passed seamlessly from nursing volunteers to military surgeons. As a result, the latter suddenly acquired a measure of objective neutrality as military medical workers came to be thought of as somehow incidental to war, impartially ministering to the sick and wounded and entitled to immunity and protection. By the twentieth century, volunteer medical personnel largely disappeared as modern armies expanded their medical corps significantly. The volunteers were gone, but the principle of medical neutrality they initiated remained behind and intact, a vestige of earlier circumstances.

Historically, then, the occasional agreement to allow military surgeons to treat the wounded unmolested gave way to blanket protection for corps of volunteers and later military medical personnel to provide medical care. Medical neutrality evolved from a descriptive term depicting the objective and impartial state of noncombatant volunteers into a norm governing the behavior of belligerents and medical personnel. As conventions turned to norms, absolute moral injunctions replaced rules of convenience and self-interest. While the philosophical basis for this transformation is thin, it did no harm to cover a desirable convention with the veneer of a moral absolute. If medical personnel and facilities can enjoy unconditional protection with little dissent from either side, so much the better for the warring parties. Medical neutrality, for all intents and purposes, is unassailable in conventional wars. Unconventional wars, however, particularly insurgencies, guerrilla wars, and other forms of low-intensity conflict, strip warfare of the veneer that protects medical professionals and lay bare the frailty of medical neutrality during armed conflict.

Medical Neutrality and Unconventional Conflict

Low-intensity conflict is an abiding feature of modern international relations, rapidly replacing conventional war between modern, sovereign nation-states. As the exigencies of contemporary geopolitics transform war, it is odd that many continue to think in terms of conventional war between two, more or less symmetrically armed, military forces fighting in a field that is largely clear of civilians. Warfare of this sort is increasingly rare. The last conventional war where both belligerents hoped to adhere to the laws of armed conflict sputtered for two and half months off the coast of Argentina more than twenty years ago. By the time Iran and Iraq fought one another from 1980 to 1988, warfare was already changing. Iran and Iraq were, to be sure, nation-states fielding conventional armies, but casualties were extraordinarily high as Iranian forces deployed "human waves" of children and the elderly to clear minefields and fortifications to pave the way for armored assaults. As Iranian forces violated Iraqi territory, Saddam Hussein responded with chemical weapons.

Low-intensity warfare dominates contemporary warfare. While these wars may be every bit as vicious as conventional wars and perhaps even more so as belligerents routinely violate the laws of conventional armed conflict and employ terror, they are low-intensity or limited conflicts because they do not overwhelm or generally threaten the international community of states. Two broad attributes characterize low-intensity conflict: asymmetry of international status and military capacity, and only a vague distinction between civilians and military forces.

The Asymmetry of Low-Intensity Conflict

The 1977 Protocols to the Geneva Conventions made note of CAR conflicts—that is, conflicts between state and substate actors and between internationally recognized nation-states variously characterized as colonial, alien, and racist (CAR) regimes. Among the defining features of CAR conflicts is military, economic, and juridical asymmetry. Most often these conflicts erupt in developing countries as a result of civil war, colonization, or occupation. Conflicts in Vietnam, Algeria, and Israel and the Palestinian Authority are three examples of low-intensity war regardless of the brutality that often prevailed. Of course, many other conflicts have racked nearly every corner of the world. In each of these three cases, however, a conventional nation-state fielding a modern army under democratic, civilian control faced off against relatively poorly armed militia and irregular forces representing the interests of a distinct ethnic or national group. Yet in these cases and many others, the weaker power defeated the stronger and gained a firm measure of international recognition.

There are many reasons for the success these emerging nations enjoy against stronger enemies and armies. In many ways, economic and military asymmetry works to the favor of the weaker power because military superiority can place the stronger states in a hopeless bind. Bound by the principles of European just war, the nations fielding strong, modern armies cannot bring the full weight of their military might to bear on their opponents for fear of causing excessive and disproportionate civilian casualties. Moreover, many of the weapons systems developed for conventional warfare prove useless in close-quarter fighting in built-up urban areas or against hit-and-run guerrilla tactics. This forces the stronger conventional armies to adopt local tactics, which often dispirit occupying troops so far from home. American soldiers in Vietnam despaired of fighting an enemy they often could not see, while Israelis fighting in the occupied West Bank face an unprecedented breakdown in morale when soldiers trained for conventional war man roadblocks and patrol densely populated areas as they search for terrorists or guerrillas. Time and time again, stronger Western powers have found themselves stymied by these quasi- and substate actors fighting for political recognition.

Part of the problem, no doubt, stems from the nature of the conflicts themselves, conflicts that are often futile and irresolvable by military means. Regimes that cherish democratic ideals find it difficult to fight a war that asserts military necessity and/or economic interests over another's right of self-determination. Many low-intensity wars assume the distinct moral dimension the term *CAR conflict* suggests and appeal to the same moral and political traditions venerated by the powers who find themselves on the wrong end of these wars. This stark incongruity saps military morale and undermines support at home because the justice of war, *jus ad bellum*, often lies squarely with the weaker party. While not all peoples command the right to territorial self-determination or political sovereignty and there are no clear guidelines about who deserves independence and who deserves lesser forms of autonomy, it is clear that the international community can ill afford to ignore the claims of those pressing for political recognition.

This is certainly true of the Palestinian-Israeli conflict. Few will deny that the Palestinians enjoy the right of self-determination and a state or national entity of their own. Nor will they decline to term their war one of national independence. But if the claims of just ends are apparent, many observers take issue with the means the Palestinians and other national groups employ to press their demands. The international community will never condone terror or other grave violations of *jus in bello*, the principles of justice in war.

The significance of *jus ad bellum*, therefore, does not belie the importance of *jus in bello*. Nations cannot wage just wars by unjust means. Nevertheless, many low-intensity conflicts bifurcate the two moral concepts common to just-war theory. *Jus in bello*, measured by the norms of humanitarian conduct incumbent on Western armies, often remains the purview of the conventional nation-state, while *jus ad bellum* remains on the side of the weaker party, who often violates humanitarian law, convinced in many cases that the justice of their cause allows them this prerogative. This divergence leads each side to seize different moral high ground and creates an irresolvable tension for traditional just-war theory, bringing many to speculate that low-intensity conflict requires an entirely different body of laws and conventions. Although this may well be, the tension plaguing just-war theory highlights an important characteristic of low-intensity conflict, namely, the reluctance or inability to observe humanitarian law or the canonical distinction between combatants and noncombatants.

Combatants and Noncombatants: A Fading Distinction?

Conventional war draws a clear distinction between combatants and noncombatants. Each enjoys an entirely different set of rights and obligations during armed conflict. Maintaining this distinction requires belligerents to recognize members of the two groups and afford each appropriate protection. Both of these requirements are difficult to meet in low-intensity war. As noted in chapter 2, the 1977 Protocols make several important changes to international and humanitarian law that bear directly on bioethical dilemmas during low-intensity war. First, the Protocols tighten the noncombatant protections that occupying forces must observe. These range from guaranteeing freedom of movement and access to medical care to an absolute ban on reprisals against civilians or their property. Second, the Protocols significantly relax earlier criteria that strictly defined combatants as uniformed members of a nation's armed forces. New criteria only require that combatants comprise part of a loosely organized hierarchical structure, carry their arms openly during armed combat, and generally respect humanitarian law. They no longer need to wear uniforms or identifying insignia (Protocol I, 1977a, Article 44).[2]

These changes place the stronger adversary in a bind. On the one hand, the they are obligated to protect, to an extent not previously required, civilian interests. On the other hand, the lack of identifying insignias coupled with the ease with which combatants can shed their status and attain civilian protection by simply leaving the battlefield has made it difficult to observe the distinction between combatants and noncombatants so necessary for the latter's protection. This difficulty is only exacerbated by the propensity of the weaker side to embrace terror and/or abuse civilian protections by masquerading as civilians, placing their armed forces in close proximity to civilian populations, or using medical facilities for hostile purposes. The difficulty of identifying combatants can seriously impinge on the implementation of humanitarian law in general and medical ethics in particular, as occupying forces battling insurgents jeopardize the protection that civilians enjoy.

The inability to identify and protect civilians is only part of the problem. Unrestrained use of terror is the other. While the stronger party to a low-intensity conflict often finds it difficult to distinguish between combatants and noncombatants, the weaker adversary does not, and may choose to intentionally harm innocent civilians. Terror is a particularly egregious and reprehensible form of fighting. Not all insurgents and guerrillas are terrorists. International law protects guerrillas as it does any other combatant who complies with humanitarian law. Terrorists, on the other hand, target innocent noncombatants with the express purpose of precipitating a disproportionate response that will increase solidarity for terrorist-backed causes among their own people and/or garner international support for their political aspirations (Kegley 1990).[3] The victims' innocence is a necessary condition for terror, without which its perpetrators fail to provoke moral outrage of sufficient intensity to elicit the response they desire.

The close proximity of combatants and noncombatants creates two sets of interrelated problems. In the best case, there is a clear distinction between the two groups, one of which is noninnocent and vulnerable to harm and another that is innocent and in need of protection. The only serious difficulty in this case is the close *physical* proximity of the two groups. Members of each group live, work, and fight among one another and are often outwardly indistinguishable. This makes it difficult for the armed forces of the stronger party to fight against combatants without harming noncombatants. In the worse case, it is not only difficult to distinguish the two by appearance or locale; it is equally difficult to draw a clear line between civilians who take no part in the conflict and those who actively assist insurgents. Active assistance may include providing food and shelter for guerrillas, smuggling arms, or providing reconnaissance, intelligence, and other forms of material, moral, and military support. But these civilians, as Louise Doswald-Beck (1999, 37) points out, lead mostly "normal lives" and only indulge in guerrilla activities "from time to time." In its current form, international law does not quite know how to treat civilians who support insurgents in this way. Do they have full immunity or only partial protection commensurate with the degree of military activity they maintain? Waging guerrilla warfare in crowded urban areas always entails civilian casualties. Are militarily active civilians more vulnerable than civilians who take no part in the hostilities, as humanitarian law consistently defines them? International law currently has no answers to these questions.

In this atmosphere, increasingly distanced from conventional warfare, military planners sometimes consider novel tactics that include targeted killing, infiltration, expulsion, siege, and detention without trial (Gross 2003). While international law prohibits many of these tactics, counterinsurgency warfare focuses on driving a wedge between guerrillas or insurgents and the civilian population that actively or tacitly supports their operations. Once they separate insurgents from their base of civilian support, military planners hope to isolate and eliminate guerrillas without harming civilians. Rarely do things work out this way, for it has proven remarkably difficult to separate the two populations without terrorizing the civilians one wishes to "pacify" or "rescue." Even then, civilian populations rarely succumb.

Counterinsurgency and Bioethics
Counterinsurgency warfare has profound ramifications for bioethics. In some cases, security officials turn to interrogational torture and aggressive means of questioning to elicit information to avert terror attacks on civilians. As they do, the authorities rely on physicians to provide

detainees with medical care. In quite different cases, military planners consider incapacitating nonlethal weapons to quell insurgencies. In contrast to conventional weapons, the development of many nonlethal weapons requires medical expertise. As a result, both nonlethal-weapons development and interrogational torture precipitate noncaregiving dilemmas that place medical personnel in a position of causing or facilitating harm. These are the subject of the following chapters.

Illustrated by Israel's conflict with the Palestinians and America's war in Vietnam, the commitment to medical neutrality, on the other hand, continues to raise caregiving dilemmas and draws our attention to two problematic aspects of providing medical aid during low-intensity war. The Israeli-Palestinian conflict highlights the difficulty of protecting medical facilities and personnel, and safeguarding their immunity. Trying to combat guerrillas or terrorists who take refuge among civilians and often use medical facilities for hostile purposes, Israelis routinely encircle Palestinian cities and hinder freedom of movement. Both sides disrupt access to medical care and seriously undermine the principle of medical neutrality as they attack medical facilities and personnel. If the Israeli-Palestinian case draws our attention to the fragility of *medical immunity*, inadequate access to care, and abuse of medical facilities, American policy in Vietnam underscores the dilemma of maintaining *medical impartiality* as officials implemented plans to provide medical care that could help American forces win the loyalty of South Vietnamese civilians. Medicine, in this case, becomes a critical component of counterinsurgency warfare. Though these cases are fundamentally different— medical care suffered in the Palestinian Authority as a byproduct of insurgency warfare, while U.S. forces deliberately used medical care as a carrot for military purposes—both significantly compromised the principle of medical neutrality.

Medical Immunity in the Palestinian-Israeli Conflict

We know relatively little about the provision of medical care and the protection of medical facilities among the weaker adversaries in low-intensity conflicts. One problem is certainly publicity. Many nations emerging from wars with colonial and occupying powers remain racked by instability, leaving little time for participants to publish their memoirs. The English publication of the first medical memoir from North Vietnam did not appear until 2004 (Dai 2004). Nevertheless, anecdotal evidence suggests that American bombers routinely attacked North Vietnamese medical facilities.[4] One reason was certainly that these facilities were difficult to identify; another was North Vietnamese unwillingness to make identification any easier for fear they would give U.S. pilots easier targets to attack (Zumwalt, n.d.). This vicious cycle made it very difficult to observe much less enforce the Geneva Conventions, conventions that each side felt the other violated with impunity. Nor did humanitarian law reign in places like Algeria to any significant degree. The French refused to recognize UN jurisdiction or participate as the UN debated the war (Horne 1977, 464).

For these reasons, the Israeli-Palestinian conflict is particularly interesting. The conflict is well documented and there is widespread consensus that the Geneva Conventions govern the behavior of the belligerents. Nevertheless, it is important to point out that Israel itself has not ratified the 1977 Protocols, nor does it always recognize the validity of the Geneva Conventions in the Occupied Territories (Shamgar 1977). Regardless, the United Nations has always taken an active interest in the conflict, frequently judging the actions of the belligerents by the standards of humanitarian law.

The current phase of the conflict dates to 2000. Following the collapse of President Clinton's peace initiative, widespread unrest erupted in Israel and the Palestinian Authority (PA) in October 2000. While the Palestinians certainly sought deeper concessions from Israel, many observers argue that Arafat exploited the strife to extricate himself from a "strategic predicament" (Sayigh 2001, 49). Unable to either turn down the U.S. initiative or take the offer back to the Palestinians, the uprising afforded Arafat an opportunity to sidestep the peace talks and intensify the conflict to his advantage. Hoping to internationalize the conflict and bring additional pressure to bear on Israel, Palestinians sought to escalate the fighting by provoking a massive Israeli military strike against Palestinians. Mass demonstrations, sometimes violent, and armed attacks against military targets and settlements formed an integral part of this strategy. At the same time radical groups launched terror attacks against Israeli civilians (Schulze 2001).

In response, Israel tried to quell the violence using limited means that many hoped would avoid the civilian casualties that marked early confrontations between Israelis and Palestinians. While these means fell well short of conventional warfare, they included sieges of civilian populations, the destruction of homes and infrastructures, targeted killing, deportation, and expulsion. These measures were particularly provocative and all flew in the face of international law. As the situation deteriorated and terror attacks in Israeli territory took increasing numbers of lives, Israel invaded the previously autonomous and self-governing areas of the Palestinian Authority in March 2002. Limited in scope, this action too failed to stem the tide of terror attacks and Israel reoccupied the entire West Bank in late 2002.

As the conflict drags on, Israeli military planners have taken what can best be described as a holding strategy as they work to minimize terror so that political leaders can conduct peace negotiations when they consider conditions most favorable to do so. It is easy to see that as an operational goal, this aim is extremely vague and open-ended, both indeterminate and interminable. It lacks the precision of an identifiable military goal and the criterion by which to judge successful implementation of a mission. "Minimizing terror" in hopes of some vague timetable from the political echelon is a novel assignment for conventional military forces. There is no ready military goal forces can seize to end the conflict, no firm end is ever in sight, and while there are always more steps to take, they are often controversial. Though Israel might easily defeat the Palestinians in a conventional war, there are few guidelines to prevent terror from emerging in a large, hostile population where distinctions between civilians and terrorists are difficult to make. In this climate, intelligence and interdiction are alternatives to conventional war.

Interdiction and the Obstruction of Medical Care

Intelligence is often the product of collaboration and interrogation. Intelligence gathering presents special problems for medicine, as noted in the following chapter, but it does not generally affect the provision of medical care to the civilian population.[5] Interdiction, on the other hand, is commonplace and necessitated blockades of Palestinian cities to disrupt communication between terrorist cells. Troops stationed in and around major population centers slow traffic as they check ID cards and search residents, turning back many civilians at roadblocks that cut off entire villages from one another. Physical obstructions, concrete blocks, trenches, and pits make internal movement difficult, as do frequent curfews and closures.

Blockading Palestinian cities to prevent terrorism also disrupts access to medical care. B'tselem, the Israeli Information Center for Human Rights in the Occupied Territories, cites an appeal by the Palestinian Red Cross to Israel's High Court of Justice in February 2001 on behalf of 121 sick or injured patients whose transportation to medical facilities was delayed by military forces. Their report describes how closures adversely affect the functioning of Palestinian hospitals and reiterates the Red Cross's concern that the failure to provide timely treatment aggravates individual medical conditions (B'tselem 2001a; B'tselem 2002–2004).

Sustained military actions exacerbate these hardships. Following a vicious wave of terror attacks against Israelis in 2002, the Israeli Defense Forces (IDF) systematically entered Palestinian cities to destroy terrorist infrastructures. The fighting in some areas was fierce and troops sometimes fired on ambulances and killed medical personnel. In the most serious incidents the director of the Red Crescent in Jenin, a medic, an ambulance driver, and an UNRWA employee were killed by gunfire as troops attacked their ambulances. The director of a Bethlehem hospital was shot dead by troops unaware that he had received permission to collect medical supplies. Intense fighting also impeded the timely evacuation of the wounded and made access to medical care precarious. B'tselem, the Public Committee against Torture in Israel (PCATI), and Physicians for Human Rights (PHR) document cases of hospitals blockaded and closed, of wounded who died unable to reach medical facilities, and of dialysis patients and pregnant women unable to receive treatment after being turned back at roadblocks and checkpoints (B'tselem, 2002; Physicians for Human Rights, 2002; B'tselem and Physicians for Human Rights, 2003).

As the fighting and the occupation continue to impede access to medical care, human rights organizations such as B'tselem, PHR, and the ICRC call on Israel to fulfill its obligations under international law. As an occupying power, these obligations require Israel to safeguard access to medical facilities. As a party to an armed conflict, Israel—like the Palestinians—must also respect the protected status of medical personnel and medical facilities, and provide care for the wounded, the sick, the infirm, and expectant mothers.

In response to the charges leveled by Palestinians and by human rights organizations, Israel draws attention to Palestinian violations of medical neutrality as guerrillas have booby-trapped the wounded, used ambulances to transport terrorists, and taken refuge in hospitals. Under these circumstances Israel responds by invoking exceptions provided by international law together with the more generalized defense of military necessity. Israel presents two different arguments in response to charges of violating medical neutrality and obstructing medical care. One argument reaches to the conventional and reciprocal nature of medical immunity and suggests that once one side violates neutrality, the other side is no longer bound to respect it. The other argument accepts the overwhelming importance of medical immunity but argues that the obligation to respect medical neutrality is not absolute and may be overridden by military necessity in exceptional cases.

Each of these arguments is already part of international law. Hospitals and medical facilities lose their protected status if used for hostile purposes (Geneva Convention (IV), 1949d, Articles 19, 20). Indeed, Israel has documented cases of Palestinians using ambulances to transport men and matériel while, in other cases, healthy guerrillas and terrorists have taken sanctuary in hospitals. In each case, there are grounds to argue that reciprocity breaks down as one side violates the immunity of medical facilities. In other cases, military necessity may override access to medical care when, during combat, international law allows exceptions to the timely evacuation of the wounded if military considerations do not enable medical teams to enter an area and evacuate the wounded (Protocol I, 1977a, Article 15; Protocol I, 1977b, Article 15, paragraph 634). The key of course is "during combat" and "military considerations." Unlike conventional warfare, low-intensity conflict is a simmering and continuous engagement rather than a series of discrete battles. It is this same interminable indeterminateness that not only wreaks havoc on conventional military tactics but complicates international and humanitarian law as well.

Consider, for example, attacks on ambulances. Ambulances are marked clearly and designated solely for the transportation of the sick and wounded. While it might be tempting to abuse this protection for military purposes, significant costs usually preclude using military facilities in this way. These costs reflect the immediate harm to those whose ambulance is stopped and searched, as well as long-term harms that destroy the very institution of medical immunity. Obviously, any side abusing protected facilities would like to limit its costs. To this end, one side violating medical immunity may argue that the other's response must be proportionate. Critics of Israeli guidelines restricting ambulance traffic point out, for example, that while the few Palestinian violations of medical neutrality necessitate careful searches of suspected ambulances, they cannot justify a sweeping policy of indiscriminate attacks on medical facilities. In other words, the convention has collapsed in part, not in whole.

Unfortunately, it is sometimes difficult to see how this is possible. Violations of medical neutrality are not confined to a specific theater of operations or specific engagement but are part and parcel of the way the conflict is managed. The abuse is particularly egregious when terrorists use ambulances to transport material for attacks on civilians. Under these circumstances, Israeli military planners try to weigh the costs and benefits of stopping, searching, or even attacking ambulances. Hampered by uncertainty, however, this assessment is difficult to make. Once one ambulance is used to transport arms or terrorists, what are the chances another will be used in the same way? Human rights activists call on Israel to show restraint because the probability is not high. In fact, most ambulances *are* utilized for their intended purpose. Israeli responses echo rational choice: under uncertainty, the odds of abuse are even. And if the odds are even and the potential harm posed by terrorism pales beside the potential harm to a single patient in an ambulance, then simple utility demands stopping each and every one. Palestinians complain that harm accumulates to their detriment; Israelis fear that the next ambulance may be a car bomb. In this environment, civilians and the wounded suffer as medical care is disrupted in precisely the way the Red Cross hoped to prevent. Here we see how clear, traditionally honored guidelines are upended by insurgency warfare, creating acute dilemmas for commanders in the field—dilemmas for which international law and custom offer no ready solution.

Dilemmas of Medical Neutrality

Low-intensity conflict endangers the convention of immunity as belligerents place civilians at risk. Guerrillas wage war against enemy forces in heavily populated areas and often violate medical immunity in a way that can jeopardize the medical care available to local civilians. Terrorists wage war against enemy civilians, often prompting military authorities to take actions that may curtail access to medical care. In these circumstances, reciprocity dissolves as each side violates neutrality. Nevertheless, parties to armed conflict must consider their obligation to respect noncombatant immunity and avoid intentionally harming noncombatants. Should a medical facility lose its immunity, the doctrine of double effect continues to restrain belligerents from causing more harm than necessary.

Consider the following case:

On Friday 22 August [2003], at approximately 17:00, three Palestinian militants, defined by the Israeli army as "wanted men," escaped from Israeli forces into Rafidya Hospital in Nablus. Once inside, they went up to the hospital's roof. According to testimony given to the AP, the militants "ignored pleas from the staff to leave." On the roof a firefight broke out between the militants and Israeli soldiers, who were stationed on another rooftop, some 300 meters from Rafidya Hospital. One militant was killed and the other two wounded. These were then hospitalized in Rafidya.

According to Rafidya hospital staff, today, 26 August, at approximately 2 AM, large forces of the Israeli army surrounded the hospital and shortly after, entered it by force and arrested the two wounded men, who were both apparently still in the intensive care unit following extensive surgery. According to the hospital staff the patients were still in grave condition. The men were taken by the Israeli army into Israel and hospitalized. (Physicians for Human Rights 2003)

Now consider the response of Physicians for Human Rights (2003)

According to Article 19 of the Fourth Geneva Convention: "The fact that sick or wounded members of the armed forces are nursed in [a] hospital" shall not terminate the protection granted to the hospital. PHR-Israel condemns in the strongest language both violations of medical neutrality: both the disregard of the armed militants for the safety of the patients and medical staff in Rafidya hospital, in deciding to position their shooting point on the hospital roof; and the blatant disregard for medical neutrality and human rights on the part of the Israeli army when entering a medical facility and arresting patients in grave condition. The participation of Israeli medical personnel in this process—if indeed this was the case, is a grave breach of medical ethics.

Physicians for Human Rights highlights two independent problems. First, it claims that Israeli forces violated medical immunity by forcibly removing combatants from a medical facility, and second, it condemns physicians who breached medical ethics for lending a hand to a gross violation of international law and unnecessarily endangering a patient's welfare. The charge against the physicians is partially dependent on the first claim, namely, that counterinsurgency forces violated medical immunity by forcibly removing patients from a protected facility.

Violating Medical Immunity: The Reach of Combatants' Rights   The claim that Israeli forces violated the principle of medical immunity when they removed combatants from a hospital by force requires closer scrutiny. In the case just described, Israeli forces violated medical immunity twice: first when they attacked guerrillas firing on them from the roof of a hospital and second when they entered the hospital to capture wounded insurgents. Few would find the first violation contentious. It would be a reasonable response should any combatant exploit a medical installation for hostile purposes. An installation is vulnerable to attack as long as military action is proportionate and necessary. The latter conditions are important. The hospital was filled with civilian patients and any action that unduly jeopardized their well-being would violate the principle of noncombatant immunity and proportionality. By all accounts, the Israeli action did not cause civilian casualties or place noncombatants at unnecessary risk.

The second violation of medical immunity is more difficult to assess. A medical facility caring for wounded combatants does not lose its immunity. To think otherwise guts medical immunity of any force whatsoever. This does not change during guerrilla war unless patients are illegal combatants or suspected war criminals. Combatants, innocent of wrongdoing, are not subject to arrest or trial for their wartime activities. Subject to the conditions described in previous chapters, combatants enjoy rights to medical care and respect for dignity and self-esteem. Subject to capture, their incarceration lasts only as long as hostilities continue. War criminals, those suspected of war crimes or grave breaches of international humanitarian law, and illegal combatants, akin to common criminals, enjoy no such rights. To arrest either, authorities may enter a medical facility just as police may enter a hospital to arrest a common criminal. Insurgents suspected of terrorism either join the ranks of suspected war criminals or relinquish any recognition whatsoever as combatants. War criminals are wayward combatants, while suspected terrorists have no legal status to bear arms. Unattached to any military hierarchy that enforces compliance with international law, guerrillas belonging to terrorist organizations are illegal combatants, little different from common criminals and subject to arrest as conditions merit.[6]

Apart from the difficulty of distinguishing between combatants and noncombatants during low-intensity conflict, it is equally difficult to draw a line between legitimate combatants, guerrillas, insurgents, and irregulars, or between terrorists and other criminal elements. Arresting terrorists as they recuperate from their wounds does not violate medical immunity. It does, however, obligate troops to follow guidelines of law enforcement, a paradigm entirely different from armed combat. Law-enforcement officials do not recognize the immunity of medical installations, may arrest suspects with sufficient cause, and may resort to lethal force only as necessary to protect their lives and the lives of innocent bystanders (Rodley 1999, 182–188).

The inability to clearly define the conventions of low-intensity conflict coupled with the willingness of the belligerents to put medical immunity aside when it suits their interests, only makes it more difficult to sustain the convention of medical neutrality and safeguard the protection of medical personnel and the facilities they work in. The PHR makes an important point, namely, that during a conventional war a hospital and its patients, whether combatants *hors de combat* or civilians, are inviolable. However, they do not, and, perhaps, cannot, consider whether the rules of law enforcement apply in this case. While medical personnel assisting troops violate international law if, indeed, arrestees are combatants, the issue is less clear-cut if they are criminal suspects or terrorists. As international law confronts the challenges of low-intensity conflict, insurgency, and terror, a number of issues defy agreement and continue to stymie legal scholars. The once clear distinction between combatant and noncombatant rights and between the laws of armed conflict and the rules of law enforcement are but one example. An armed force considering nonlethal weaponry (chapter 8) is another as military planners and politicians try to decide whether they are fighting a conventional war, waging a "military operation other than war," or enforcing domestic or international law. Each case governs the use of lethal force differently. Given the complexity of these issues, the question for physicians remains whether they must, or even can, sort through these questions when instructed to provide medical care during a military operation. In the absence of an obvious and egregious breach of humanitarian law, should physicians simply follow their orders on the assumption that the legal and military authorities assessed the situation properly, or should they turn to independent bodies for an alternative viewpoint? Like any citizen and soldier, they should probably do both. While time constraints may prevent them from properly evaluating all but the most obviously unlawful or immoral orders, there is certainly room for public discourse to draw lessons that may change future behavior.

Violating Medical Immunity: The Reach of Medical Ethics   If there is room for medical personal to equivocate on questions of military law, there is less room to maneuver when principles of medical ethics are at stake. This is at the heart of PHR's second claim, namely, that physicians removing a patient from intensive care violate the canons of medical ethics regardless of how one interprets international law governing the status of the suspects. The principle of nonmaleficence demands that medical personnel put the interests of their patients first. In this case, it might mean refusing to move them until their condition stabilizes. Unlike questions of legal status, this remains a medical judgment and the sole purview of medical personnel.

It would be easy enough to argue that medical personnel should not lend their hand to any action that harms their patients. In peacetime medicine this is usually the case. For this reason, the PHR condemns the physicians present during the military operation on the assumption that they endangered the suspects that troops removed by force. During war, however, the question often arises whether military medical personnel may subordinate their patient's welfare to the interests of others. Physicians will violate confidentiality when it serves military purposes, just as they will distribute scarce resources with an eye to the war effort rather than patient welfare. This is a recurring and troublesome question, particularly as we consider whether physicians may ever facilitate interrogation or participate in weapons development. I will defer a full discussion until the following chapter and now only suggest that in the case PHR describes, physicians may consider whether the harm their patients could suffer is offset by the benefits to others (such as civilians who might be saved by information obtained from an arrestee about an impending terrorist attack). In many ways, this question is no easier to answer than those concerning a suspect's status in international law. Here, too, the same caveat applies: physicians may find it prudent to assist in what they have good reason to believe are legitimate military operations and then, in their aftermath, reassess their actions in the hope of drawing lessons for the future. In doing so, they must consider the harm their patients suffer, the necessity of evacuation under difficult conditions, and the potential benefits their actions may bring. In time of peace, we do not ordinarily ask these questions; in war, they become crucial.

Low-intensity conflict presents the stronger adversary with a constant challenge to wage war while limiting civilian casualties. This is all the more difficult because war in close quarters is often stymied by the inability to distinguish between combatants and noncombatants. Terror further undermines humanitarian law. Terrorism is not, however, a feature of every struggle against a colonial or occupying power. In Vietnam, for example, neither side employed terror in the way insurgents do in the Middle East. Nevertheless, the Americans found themselves in a war complicated by asymmetry of arms and obscure distinctions between combatants and noncombatants. Like other nations fighting counterinsurgency wars, the United States encountered a pressing need to isolate the guerrillas from the civilian population they depended on and lived within. Achieving this end required that the American armed forces nurture goodwill and foster reliable sources of information. Providing medical services seemed an ideal way to do this. This raises the altogether novel question whether using medical care as a tool to wage war constitutes an egregious violation of medical neutrality or of the ethics of medicine more generally. Both demand that medical personnel remain impartial and avoid using medicine for any other purpose than caring for the sick and injured during armed conflict.

Medical Impartiality in the Vietnam War

During the Vietnam War the Medical Civic Action Program (MEDCAP) treated more than 40 million Vietnamese civilians at a cost of $500–750 million (1960s dollars). There were two MEDCAP programs. Under the aegis of MEDCAP I, the U.S. government provided material assistance and advisors to establish medical facilities administered and staffed largely by South Vietnamese personnel. MEDCAP II, on the other hand, organized American medical personnel to care for South Vietnamese civilians directly. MEDCAP II organized personnel into small teams to make the rounds in the countryside and set up makeshift clinics. MEDCAP I and II were part of a larger medical aid program that also included hospital-based programs: Military Provincial Hospital (later "Health") Program (MILPHAP) and Civilian War Casualty Program (CWCP). Each of these programs stationed American medical personnel in local Vietnamese hospitals to train personnel, organize supplies, and institute public health programs (Wilensky 2001, 815–819).

The goals of all the medical-aid programs were both medical and political. The medical goals elicit no controversy. Medical care in South Vietnam was abysmal; only 300 physicians served a population of more than 17 million. Hospitals were few and far between and chronically short of supplies and equipment. Ninety percent had no running water. With most physicians practicing in these provincial hospitals, care in the countryside was left to midwives, nurses, and native healers. The overriding medical goal of MEDCAP and other aid programs was to build a relatively efficient and modern public health system to provide basic medical care, contain rather than eradicate communicable disease, bolster manpower, increase the number of medical facilities, and instill a measure of fiscal planning and responsibility. It was a gargantuan undertaking in a country plagued by poverty, superstition, inadequate health education, and a crumbling, century-old infrastructure. It would require extensive training programs, including schools for nurses and paramedics, public health and education, sanitation, vaccination, and ambulatory and acute-care facilities. The medical goals of MEDCAP and its related programs are not provocative. On the contrary, they are laudable, running only the risk of overambition and of raising expectations they could not meet. The political-military goals of medical-assistance programs, however, remain contentious and highlight conflicting medical and military interests (Humphreys 1968; White 1968).

Military Medical Operations

War wracked Vietnam long before the Americans arrived, as North Vietnamese guerrillas, the Viet Cong, sought to destabilize the South and unify the country under Communist control. The 1954 Geneva accords partitioned the country into northern and southern districts, each under separate leadership and subject to an agreement to hold unifying elections within two years. Although relative calm prevailed for several years, elections never materialized and by the early 1960s, Viet Cong were attacking government troops in the South and gradually pushing them from the countryside. By 1964, the South Vietnamese government was in disarray, already destabilized by an American-backed coup the previous year. At the same time, North Vietnam deployed large numbers of regular troops to assist guerrillas fighting in the South. The United States, already mired in South Vietnamese politics, decided to commit large numbers of troops in 1965 (Tuchman 1984, 289–474).

Apart from the military and political aims of the Vietnam War, which I will not discuss here, medical personnel in the American army began to ask themselves an interesting question: What special role should medicine play in counterinsurgency warfare? It was a question few had ever asked before. Throughout the modern era, military medical care was driven by one overriding concern: to maintain a fighting force by providing care to wounded combatants and expeditiously returning them to duty. As they performed these duties, military medical personnel treated civilians and often earned immeasurable goodwill. But Vietnam was different. At first, there was no large fighting force to maintain. Instead, there were advisors—that is, military personnel stationed in Vietnam to advise the Vietnamese. Might there not also be a role for medical advisors? This, in fact, was the idea behind MEDCAP I. But apart from the medical goals, there were also political goals: military planners wanted to use medical care to win the "hearts and minds" of the Vietnamese and thereby break the influence and control of the Viet Cong.

Writing in 1967, Spurgeon Neel, Surgeon of the U.S. Military Assistance Command in Vietnam, commented on the importance of "stability operations" designed to prevent insurgency "by assailing latent or incipient turbulence in emerging nations at the earliest possible stage" (p. 605). This led Neel to think in terms of "*medical* stability operations," which

concentrate on the pre-insurgency phase of operations in order to produce maximum results with minimum resource investment [and] employ medical treatment programs for immediate impact, and preventive medicine projects to produce short-term improvement in the emerging nation's health. The keystone of the program is the development within the host nation's army of a medical training program which eventually will yield a permanent increase in the degree of medical self-sufficiency. . . . In South Vietnam today, the [U.S.] Army Medical Service is actively engaged in stability operations of both counter-insurgency and limited war types. (p. 605)

Citing the work of MEDCAP, Neel pushed way beyond its medical function to succinctly describe it strategic importance: "MEDCAP I . . . is the epitome of medical stability operations in counterinsurgency. . . . Emphasis is placed upon improvement of the image of the GVN (Government of Vietnam). The effort concentrates on peripheral areas where security problems preclude function of civilian medical activities, and where pacification is most important to stabilization" (p. 607).

Using medical care specifically to pacify and stabilize a war-torn nation is quite novel (Zajtchuk 2003). With facilities so sorely lacking among the Vietnamese peasants, military medical planners reasoned that modern medical care provided in the name of the central government would generate immeasurable goodwill and "create ties of loyalty essential to the strengthening of the government and consolidation of the nation" (Webb 1968, 391). Failure to pursue medical care and other stabilizing measures would only leave the field open for guerrillas to "usurp" popular support.

Using medicine to nurture allegiance and devotion to a corrupt and unstable regime that commanded precious little of either quality imposed a formidable task on medicine. No less demanding was the role medicine might play to win the war: "The real objective [of MEDCAP and related programs] is to do those things which have a sharp impact upon the people *now*, in order to convince them that their government is trying to help them and thus contribute to an early end of the war. Great national or regional programs which bear fruit only with the passage of time can wait a little" (Humphreys 1968, 205).

The "tactics" of medical stability operations, therefore, eschewed long-range medical programs and focused instead on providing basic care and treating a small number of "high-impact" cases. MEDCAP provided basic care as they set up improvised clinics, or "sick-call patrols," in remote villages. But basic care was extremely limited. Doctors and nurses examined patients until nightfall or until medications simply ran out. They had no provisions for simple surgery. There were no medical records. Personnel could neither schedule follow-up treatment nor monitor compliance (Wilensky 2001).

Military planners knew that sick-call patrols only offer rudimentary medical care. But this was not their intent. Instead the patrols were an important tactic in an ongoing medical stability operation. Noting that "people under treatment are frequently very cooperative in revealing information about the guerrilla force" (Webb 1968, 393), planners understood that a system of local medical care could yield useful intelligence. But the primary impact remained psychological, not physiological. Admitting that sick-call patrols were less medicine than "medical show business," MEDCAP personnel would often refer high-impact cases—cleft palate, burn contractures, and orthopedic deformities, particularly among children—for corrective surgery. Predictably, villagers were awestruck and presumably grateful when "after treatment, the individual returns to his village as living proof of the good intentions of his central government" (p. 394).

In retrospect, it is difficult to assess the success of these programs. Understanding that MEDCAP and related programs could only produce, at best, short-term effects, planners also sought to institute long-term programs devoted to training, education, and preventive medicine. But "long term" was not in the offing. Neel (1967) concluded his thoughts about the medical role in stability operations by noting the close connection between medicine and wars of insurgency. "Prevention of war," he wrote, "makes equally good sense as prevention of disease. Actually the former can be facilitated by the latter" (p. 608).

No one, of course, prevented war in Vietnam, so it still remains to test the validity of Neel's prediction. Conceptually, however, it raises a number of questions associated directly with MEDCAP operations in Vietnam. Do MEDCAP-type programs represent a cynical use of medicine? Do they violate principles of medical neutrality or other principles of medical ethics?

The Ethics of Medical Stability Operations

Images of medicine as a psychological weapon of modern warfare, of "warriors in white," and of medical stability operations place medicine in a new and different role from the one it normally assumes in conventional warfare. Nor does one expect this imagery to be confined to Vietnam. Israelis were quick to set up medical shop in South Lebanon during their long occupation there, and the United States and coalition forces can be expected to do likewise as the war on terror in developing countries continues. Currently, there are MEDCAP programs in Southeast Asia, Africa, and South America to promote medical care and political stability (Baker and Ryals 1999, 619–625; Ritchie and Mott 2003; Zajtchuk 2003).

Although the Vietnam War was the focus of harsh condemnation, few criticized American medical policy in Vietnam. Among those who did, the juxtaposition of "medicine as a weapon" was the most unsettling and led critics to charge American military medical policy with a fundamental violation of international law and medical ethics. E. A. Vastyan (1974, 337) emphasizes "an explicit separation of the healing from the wounding roles" that he believes is inherent in the rights and obligations that the 1949 Geneva Convention grants to medical personnel. Rights include immunity from attack and prompt repatriation after capture, and these rights, Vastyan suggests, generate obligations that forbid medical personnel to engage in acts of war, require them to treat the sick and wounded solely on the basis of medical need, and prohibit physicians from coercing patients to obtain information. Immunity and impartiality go hand in hand and the latter, for many, is paramount.

This criticism raises several interrelated questions. First and foremost: Was MEDCAP an act of war? Second, if it was, what is its relationship to the other norms that obligate or constrain medical personnel? In each of the other obligations Vastyan cites—needs-based triage, noncoercion, and confidentiality—the relationship between obligations, rights, and military necessity is fundamentally different. Needs-based triage signifies a common misunderstanding that I examined in the previous chapter. There is no duty to distribute scarce military resources during wartime based on need. Rather, the overriding goal of triage is salvage utility and the obligation to return soldiers to duty. Confidentiality, as I argued in chapter 4, is nonabsolute and often falls before military necessity. Coercion, the subject of the following chapter, sometimes prompts authorities to enlist medical assistance when a significant number of innocent lives are at stake. In general, Vastyan suggests that MEDCAP-type programs entirely undermine the norm of neutrality that animates many medical duties during war, such as those of the WMA described at the beginning of this chapter. A more accurate assessment, however, takes into account that medical rights and obligations may conflict with military necessity, and often with one another. Sometimes impartiality defers to military necessity and other prima facie rights and duties, and sometimes not. This is true of medical stability operations.

Medical Care as an Act of War   If the defining criterion of "weapon" is its ability, generally in the hands of a trained person, to cause harm, then we must ask whether MEDCAP-type programs cause any harm. Harm may by physical or psychological and may affect one's life, quality of life, and human or civil rights. Alternatively, or in conjunction, it may affect the life of the community, state, or any other significant collective.

Certain aspects of MEDCAP are particularly problematic. If officials use medical care to coerce patients to divulge information, it is wrong. Violating confidentiality alone to reveal important information is less offensive and is justifiable subject to an assessment of relative harms and benefits. While chapter 4 considered patients who were, without doubt, enemy soldiers, MEDCAP care focuses on patients who *may* be enemy soldiers or sympathizers. Given the exigencies of guerrilla warfare, I would suggest that similar guidelines apply in both cases. Doctors may, and often must, divulge confidential information, but may not withhold medical care to obtain militarily useful information. But beyond these isolated cases of using medicine to gather intelligence, what are we to make of the charge that using medicine as a tactic of counterinsurgency warfare is to turn medicine into a weapon and irretrievably blur the line between its wounding and healing roles? What is it about a MEDCAP-type program that makes medicine a weapon or a party to an act of war? What harms can the program cause?

By all accounts, it is difficult to see how, beyond creating expectations that sometimes cannot be fulfilled, sick-call patrols and high-impact interventions cause material harm to patients or to their communities. Nevertheless, one can also speak of other kinds of harms, particularly if MEDCAP is a tactic of psychological warfare. Designed to nurture support for the government, the program might be humiliating and manipulative, if indeed its goal was to use medical care solely for political purposes. But this is not entirely clear. Two divergent views characterize the aims of MEDCAP: "One view assumed the major goals as winning the confidence and loyalty of the people to the GVN by using MEDCAP as psychological tool, and secondarily improving the health of the people. The other viewpoint was that the major effort should be to improve the health and relieve suffering with the winning of the people to the GVN as a possible bonus effect" (Bishop 1969).

While Vastyan dismisses these as little more than two sides of the same coin, intentions and effects play a central role in medical ethics. Emphasizing the importance of delivering medical care to an impoverished population while acknowledging the beneficial side effects can dispel a complex moral dilemma plaguing health-care professionals. This is particularly true when one considers that from either perspective, medical care remained an important component of the program and there is nothing to indicate that personnel did not deliver compassionate and professional care. Care was not substandard or faked or phony.

Yet something still rankles our moral sensibilities. Of course care was compassionate and professional; otherwise it could not accomplish its political goals. Moreover, the political side effects appear to be more than good fortune and happenstance. They were, by many accounts, one of the intended benefits of medical care among civilians. Could it be that medicine was used in a way that was manipulative, paternalistic, and humiliating? Military authorities did not deliver medical care for the sole benefit of ill patients but to consciously influence their political decision making. At best, this sounds like a serious infringement of personal autonomy. Is a program that provides medical benefits while, at the same time, affecting patients' political attitudes tainted or exemplary? Is it one we should curb or encourage?

To answer, it may help to distance MEDCAP from Vietnam. Reports of MEDCAP programs in Cambodia are free of moral controversy. In 1997, a small team of ten doctors, dentists, and medics visited Cambodia and provided medical and dental care to more than 3,000 patients. This program followed on the heels of a similarly successful program in Thailand the year before. Apart from providing acute medical care, participants hoped to care for an ailing society as well. Recalling that one controversial goal of MEDCAP Vietnam was to "consolidate the nation," proponents of other MEDCAP programs laud their larger purpose, namely, "nation building":

Nation building can be broadly defined as those activities that assist nations to develop their own unique institutions and infrastructure to address the needs of their citizens. In health care, this may include strengthening and refinement of the existing public health care network, improving communication between nations regarding health care and evaluating the populations. . . . It should also focus on patient teaching and improving simple public health factors such as clean water, sanitation, and healthy livestock. (Baker and Ryals 1999, 624)

Military Medical Care and Nation Building Divorced from the Vietnam conflict, this description of nation building sounds eminently sensible. MEDCAP activities in Cambodia or Thailand are entirely consistent with the duty to provide humanitarian aid to developing nations desperately in need of modern medical care. But medical care not only serves patient welfare; it benefits their community as well. Shouldn't medicine be charged with protecting individual and collective interests alike? If so, this dilemma, unlike many others, dissolves when placed in neutral and less emotionally charged setting. Ensuring medical health to strengthen the political health of the community points to a different good that medicine does not ordinarily provide in developed nations. But there is nothing ethically amiss about using medical care in this way, particularly because the health of an individual and the health of his or her community are intimately related.

The aim of ensuring collective health and well-being were, in fact, the early goals of MEDCAP in Vietnam, when policymakers thought they could prevent war by stabilizing the country. They, like the French before them, failed to grasp, however, that the war had never ended in Vietnam. And, unfortunately, long-simmering warfare is a constant feature of the new wars Western nations now confront. Few of the third-world nations where humanitarian aid is being provided are stable if, by political stability, one means universal recognition of political authority, a state monopoly on the use of armed force, and freedom from political violence. There is no clear line separating a state of war from one of peace, nor the medical care one might provide during peace and or offer during war. Medical care to a developing nation will always transpire in the context of nation building and "stability" operations. Its goal is to shore up local medical infrastructures and improve the welfare of the local population, often in the face of armed insurrection and insurgency. But in doing so it must inevitably lend strength and credibility to local political institutions. MEDCAP-type programs do not blur the line between humanitarian-like operations that focus on healing and military-like operations that focus on wounding, for no such line exists. Often it is very difficult to separate humanitarian medical aid from medical stability operations. This was particularly true when the United States sought to implement medical-aid programs in nations such as Honduras and El Salvador, when each nation was threatened with insurgency from within and armed aggression from without. American medical aid provided care to local civilians and military personnel and improved infrastructures for care and training, but, at the same time, aid also improved relations between the military and civilian population it governed and helped to "stabilize and further relationships between the United States and its allies" (Zajtchuk 2003, 778).

Apart from those instances of medical workers withholding care to obtain military intelligence, MEDCAP does not present a moral dilemma that sets norms of medical neutrality or obligations to avoid harming patients against military necessity. In practice, neither patients nor their communities are harmed by medical care or by the manner in which it is provided. Nor does MEDCAP blur the line that purportedly separates medicine and war. MEDCAP programs provide humanitarian aid in developing nations suffering from political instability. Unless the result of natural disaster, the need for humanitarian aid stems directly from war and conflict. One may, for example, take issue with medical show-manship and high-impact interventions because they are an inefficient use of medical resources. But this, too, may be off the mark, particularly if showmanship creates a well of goodwill that facilitates the implemen-tation of long-range programs designed to bring medical self-sufficiency and, with it, political stability.

Nevertheless, providing aid in a hostile, unstable, and foreign envi-ronment brings many problems of its own: often military medical workers are unable to establish an effective and trusting relationship with their patients owing to language and cultural differences, short tours of duty, and lack of modern equipment; military goals often dictate short-term assistance at the expense of long-term follow-up; direct aid to women may inadvertently place them at risk as men seek control over food and supplies; and host nations find it difficult to meet medical expectations when American or European troops depart (Palmer and Zwi 1998; Ritchie and Mott 2003). For some of these reasons, it may prove advantageous for civilians rather than military medical personnel to assume the duty of providing medical care. Insofar as many wars are fought by either the nation directly threatened or by those offering aid, medical personnel are generally part of military forces. As the interna-tional community, however, considers multinational efforts to undertake wars of humanitarian intervention, a development I examine in chapter 9, some of the problems attending MEDCAP may disappear.

The Challenge of Medical Neutrality

MEDCAP, or any other aid program that inextricably links medical aid for one country with another nation's military interests, raises two important questions about the moral relationship between medicine and war. The first, alluded to just above, speaks to the juxtaposition of medicine and war, between healing and wounding roles. Critics accuse physicians party to MEDCAP of crossing the line, of using medicine to wage war. But this line is blurred; MEDCAP programs exist in areas of the world where this distinction is difficult to maintain and where humanitarian aid also aids a regime fighting for political stability. And yet, practical difficulties aside, one still asks whether and to what degree medicine can or should be used to prosecute a war, and whether the functions of healing and wounding are *conceptually* distinguishable during armed conflict.

MEDCAP, particularly in the context of the Vietnam conflict, also raises the question whether medical personnel have a duty, perhaps even a greater duty than others, to consider *jus ad bellum*, the ends of war. MEDCAP is a program that is part of an overall policy to bring aid and stability to developing countries racked by war, devastation, and poverty. Humanitarian aid, in general, is never without conditions. Often, donors demand political change: representative, if not democratic, practices, guarantees of human rights, law and order, and an equitable system of justice. These demands overcome disrespect for autonomy that may cloud a MEDCAP-type program, as recipients of aid build institutions guaranteeing self-determination. Medical care that fosters respect for a regime that exemplifies self-critical values can enhance rather than undermine personal autonomy. However, when donor nations do not make demands for reform and support corrupt regimes, they are—or should be—justly criticized. Criticism, rebuke, and condemnation come in the form of democratic dissent. Ideally, Western nations face the court of local public opinion when their governments or those they support deviate from norms of democracy and decency. We are rankled with MEDCAP Vietnam, more than Cambodia or Thailand, because we now know, and believe many knew then, that stability operations in Vietnam did nothing but prop up a corrupt regime. U.S. policy ultimately failed when American democratic institutions rebelled.

For these reasons, the place of medicine's role in counterinsurgency warfare does not turn entirely on whether MEDCAP serves politics by other means. In spite of its political overtones, medicine can justifiably form part of a program to enhance the political health of a distressed nation. Rather, the question should focus on whether the aim of securing the political health of a distressed nation is pursued consistently. When it is, and when a developed nation uses its resources to instill political well-being, self-determination, and a sense of national esteem, then medical care will form an important part of this effort, regardless of a developing nation's need to fend off insurgents with armed force. When these aims are neglected, the entire idea of "stability" operations falls into disrepute and, with it, the role that medical care plays.

The two questions raised at the beginning of this section—whether healing and wounding roles are separate, and whether medical personnel must question the ends of war—are interrelated. The first highlights a strict separation between medicine and war, between healing and wounding. The second draws them together, making the justice of providing medical care in some sense dependent on the justice of the war itself. The first suggests that medical personnel remain aloof from the practice of war; the second demands they carefully consider the justice of war as they practice medicine. The first implies that MEDCAP programs are misguided and, perhaps, dangerous, the second that medicine is an important component of just war that cannot and should not be ignored. Not only do these two questions affect neutrality, they color every issue of bioethics in armed conflict. Medical neutrality, patient rights, and triage during war push our intuitions in two directions. Are physicians, nurses, and medics unique actors on the battlefield and beholden to the norms of their profession, or do they differ little from other soldiers who command a particular form of expertise and must answer to military necessity? Must doctors consider the welfare of their patients exclusively, or should they weigh the interests of other members of their political community threatened by war and armed conflict? While military commanders may view medical neutrality as a matter of convention or agreement that collapses when one side or the other no longer finds it advantageous to comply, medical personnel face a difficult challenge when unconventional war threatens neutrality. Whether immunity or impartiality is at stake, the dilemma of medical neutrality suggests that physicians have an obligation to serve their patients' interests and, at the same time, make every effort to answer to utility, military necessity, and the common good. While it is sometimes possible to do both, the two often clash during war and may force one to reevaluate the norms of medical conduct and civic responsibility. This tension becomes particularly acute when physicians consider the noncaregiving roles they must play as they are called upon to participate in military interrogation and weapons development.

7

Torture, Ill-Treatment, and Interrogation

There are many indictments of torture and the physicians who practice or facilitate ill-treatment. Anthony Zwi's (1987, 649) statement is characteristically unequivocal:

The involvement of health personnel in torture is perhaps the most explicit violation of the basis of medical practice. Here such personnel are directly contradicting every dictum which forms the basis of their practice—their task has been transformed from caring and relieving suffering, to inflicting pain and suffering. Direct involvement in torture must be seen in a political context; the doctors and other health workers who participate in such activities are performing repressive acts.

Zwi raises two arguments. First, it is always wrong for physicians to support torture. Second, torture is repressive—that is, always wrong in and of itself. Although related, these are two independent claims and I will examine each beginning with the second: Is torture always wrong, or are there rare circumstances, often associated with terror, "ticking bombs," and low-intensity conflict, that might warrant "aggressive" interrogation? The second half of this chapter addresses this possibility and questions the role of medical personnel: Should physicians participate in or facilitate ill-treatment during interrogation in any way? Ordinarily, this question is not posed separately from the first. Most observers hope to bar physicians from participating in torture and ill-treatment because torture itself is inexcusable (British Medical Association, 1992). Nevertheless, authorities in some democratic nations continue to hold out for harsh interrogation techniques and, at the same time, require a physician's presence before, during, and after questioning. This presents medical workers with a difficult noncaregiving dilemma when they are asked to facilitate harm to others.

The Dilemma of Torture

Torture comprises any act that intentionally inflicts grievous physical or psychological pain and suffering to either elicit information from an individual (*interrogational* torture), or to silence dissent and force citizens into strict compliance with government policy by brutalizing political opponents (*terroristic* torture) (Shue 1978).[1] The 1984 Convention against Torture and Other Cruel, Inhuman or Degrading Treatment or Punishment (CAT) condemns torture in terms of undefined "severe" pain and suffering (CAT, 1984, Articles 1, 16). This leaves torture open to conflicting operational definitions. In 2002, American officials, for example, identified "severe" with "excruciating and agonizing" pain "equivalent in intensity to the pain accompanying serious physical injury, such as organ failure, impairment of bodily function or even death" (Gonzales 2002, 1). By December 2004, the U.S. Justice Department broadened its definition of torture to include physical and mental suffering in addition to extreme pain or unusually cruel practices (U.S. Department of Justice, 2004). At the same time, U.S. officials, like CAT, distinguish between "acts of torture" and less severe forms of "inhuman and degrading treatment." Similarly, Israeli officials draw a distinction between torture and "moderate physical pressure," and they, like the Americans, forbid the former but permit the latter in some circumstances. This distinction is difficult to maintain in practice: moderate physical pressure or aggressive interrogation techniques can easily culminate in torture and cause the pain and suffering that policymakers hoped the distinction between torture and ill-treatment would prevent. Moreover, it is of little significance for medical personnel who are called on to provide medical supervision as investigators interrogate prisoners using a variety of techniques that can cause significant pain and suffering.

Historically, opposition to torture rose in the wake of the Enlightenment. While torture complemented the rampant nationalism of the late nineteenth and early twentieth centuries, it was again the focus of international concern as the savagery of the Second World War led to a succession of postwar treaties prohibiting torture under any circumstances (Peters 1996; Rodley 1999, 18–176). By 1984, the international community resolved the issue unambiguously. Today, torture is nothing less than a grave breach of international humanitarian law: "No State may permit or tolerate torture or other cruel, inhuman or degrading treatment or punishment. Exceptional circumstances such as a state of war or threat of war, internal political instability or other public emergencies may not be invoked as a justification" (CAT, 1984, Article 2).

International codes of medical ethics prohibit physicians and other medical personnel from participating in torture or facilitating ill-treatment. Following a recommendation by British officials that doctors be present at all times in interrogation centers in Northern Ireland, the British Medical Association appealed to the World Medical Association for guidelines to regulate physician behavior. Issued in 1975, the Tokyo Declaration decreed that "the doctor shall not countenance, condone, participate, [or] . . . facilitate torture or other forms of cruel, inhuman or degrading procedures" or "be present" where these behaviors are used or threatened (World Medical Association, 1975).

Were one to condemn torture and ill-treatment unconditionally, the entire question of medical participation would be moot. An alternative view, however, finds that the prohibition of torture, while compelling, is not morally absolute in all cases. In his critical analysis of torture, Henry Shue (1978) explains how torture is permissible only when it is the least harmful means available to secure a supremely important moral goal. Adding that this is almost *never* the case, he nonetheless concludes: "An act of torture ought to remain illegal so that anyone who sincerely believes such an act to be the least available evil is placed in the position of needing to justify his or her act morally in order to defend himself or herself legally. The torturer should be in roughly the same position as someone who commits civil disobedience" (p. 143).

This is an odd analogy, to say the least, but what could this "supremely" important moral goal be? Perhaps it is the life of the political community, so that the threat of genocide is a legitimate exception to the prohibition of torture. Yet this exception is problematic. Nations prohibit torture precisely in those situations when it might prove a useful expedient during war. Torture is repugnant because the vast majority of enemy soldiers are innocent by convention, leaving no cause to brutalize or punish them for participating in armed conflict. Torture is wrong whether the information one seeks saves numerous lives or forestalls an existential threat. In other words, the prohibition against torture appeals to a deontological imperative unimpressed by utilitarian outcomes. Utilitarian outcomes, moreover, are decidedly mixed. While short-term effects may save lives, torturing soldiers may undermine the war convention entirely. Calculations of utility run afoul of the slippery slope. Once we permit torture when a nation's life is as stake, why not condone it when the lives of many innocent individuals are threatened?

It is noteworthy that contemporary discussions of permissible interrogation do not invoke genocide or defeat in war, but turn on the threat to innocent lives that terror presents. Neither Israel nor the United States, two nations facing an onslaught of terrorism, faces any immediate threat to their political community. Instead, the dilemma of torture arises when the lives of some individuals confront the dignity of the torture victim, circumstances tied directly to terror and "ticking bombs"—massive explosive devices designed to kill and maim innocent civilians.

While ticking bombs pose an immediate and grievous threat to innocent life, there must be something peculiar about them that they bring otherwise conscientious individuals to think twice about torture and ill-treatment. It cannot be simply that many lives are at stake. Many lives are at stake during war when vital information may prevent the death of soldiers. Yet we do not tolerate the torture of captured enemy soldiers. Could it be the identity of those whose lives are threatened? Unlike soldiers, the victims of ticking bombs are innocent and nonthreatening. Nor have they lost their right to life. Yet we do not torture mass murderers or those with knowledge of heinous crimes in order to save their victims. Might the identity of the torture victims themselves drive our intuitions? Only terrorists plant ticking bombs. Have they somehow forfeited their claim to human dignity in a way that distinguishes ticking bombs from all other threats to innocent human life?

To better grasp the ethical quandaries that torture and ill-treatment pose for both ordinary citizens and the health-care professionals of a democratic nation, it is important to see how various nations cope with terror. Britain, Israel, and more recently the United States face difficult choices as they confront the threat of terror and consider the need for aggressive interrogation. Once officials consider aggressive questioning techniques accompanied by torture and ill-treatment, health-care professionals find themselves on the spot as they are called on to lend their medical expertise to facilitate effective interrogation.

Torture, Ill-Treatment, and Terror

Many nations struggle with the question of permissible torture. Following complaints raised by the press, the courts, and human rights organizations in Israel, a state commission of inquiry, the Landau Commission, reviewed the use of torture in 1987. Weighing military necessity against the harm inflicted on an individual by interrogational torture, the committee hoped to regulate torture and, in defiance of all international norms, suggested that Israel set standards for using "moderate physical pressure." The commission's position rests on several salient points: terrorism threatens the security of the state, it cannot be subdued without some measure of physical force, and moderate physical pressure is distinct from torture (Landau Commission, 1989a, paragraphs 2.9–2.10, 2.20, 3.17, 4.6).

Although the international community absolutely forbids torture and inhuman and degrading treatment, firm definitions remain unspecified. Convinced that moderate physical pressure "must never reach the level of physical torture . . . which deprives [the suspect] of his human dignity," the commission tried to discriminate between torture and other physical means of interrogation by drawing on British attempts to publicly defend torture to interrogate suspected IRA terrorists in 1976 (Landau Commission, 1989b, paragraph 3.16). At a hearing of the European Court of Human Rights, judges heard sufficient evidence to conclude that the combined use of five particular techniques—hooding (covering a suspect's head with a filthy, opaque sack for long periods of time), wall standing (a stress position that forces a suspect to stand spread-eagle against a wall for an extended time), powerfully loud noise, sleep deprivation, and starvation—constituted inhuman treatment and torture (*Ireland v. the United Kingdom*, 1976, paragraph 96; Rodley 1999, 90–95).

These were the same techniques the Israeli commission approved in 1987 when it accepted the European Court's distinction between the *combined* use of the five techniques, which constitutes torture, and the *techniques themselves*, which, while inhuman and degrading, are free of the "stigma" attached to "deliberate inhuman treatment causing very serious and cruel suffering" (*Ireland v. the United Kingdom*, 1976, paragraph 167). With this in mind, the Landau Commission concluded that British techniques did not "occasion suffering of the particular intensity and cruelty implied by the term 'torture'" and decided to sanction the use of "moderate physical pressure."

But the effort to carve out relatively benign interrogation techniques was an odd argument then and remains so today, ignoring the fact that the international community unequivocally prohibits both inhuman treatment and torture. Both significantly undermine dignity and self-esteem, and inflict physical and mental harm (Rodley 1999, 92). Nor did interrogation methods remain static. B'tselem (the Israeli Information Center for Human Rights in the Occupied Territories), describes additional techniques that later came into play, including forcefully shaking a victim's upper torso, causing the neck and head to "dangle and vacillate rapidly," seating suspects in painful, contorted positions on low chairs during interrogation, and excessively tightening handcuffs to impede blood flow (*Public Committee against Torture in Israel v. The State of Israel*, 1999, paragraphs 8–13).

Similarly, America's experience in Iraq and Afghanistan has brought officials to consider the merits of "exceptional" interrogation techniques. Faced with an organized counterinsurgency of Islamic militants, deposed Baathist politicians and military officers, and common criminals, the United States faces coordinated attacks against the local civilian populations at the same time that it confronts the ongoing threat of international terror aimed at its own citizens. In the wake of the September 11 attacks, U.S. security forces adopted techniques identical to those Israel and Britain used. In November 2002, the U.S. Secretary of Defense, Donald Rumsfeld, approved several categories of interrogation techniques, including yelling, deception, "good cop–bad cop" routines, stress positions (wall standing, crouching, and so on), isolation, hooding, light and auditory deprivation, and "using detainees' individual phobias (such as fear of dogs) to induce stress." Techniques such as "exposure to cold weather or water" and "use of a wet and dripping towel to induce the misperception of suffocation" would remain "legally available" but without blanket approval (Haynes 2002). Rescinding permission to use many of the more aggressive methods in January 2003, the secretary of defense nonetheless left room to approve additional interrogation techniques on a case-by-case basis.[2] In spite of these memoranda, which apply solely to the interrogation of unlawful combatants held by the United States in Guantanamo Bay, Cuba, Amnesty International and the Red Cross report that U.S. forces in Iraq regularly utilize harsh interrogation methods that include hooding, physical abuse, prolonged standing and other stress positions, sleep deprivation, loud music, and bright lights (Amnesty International, 2004; International Committee of the Red Cross 2004; Lewis 2004).

Whether these techniques used alone or in combination constitute torture remains the subject of intense debate in nations facing terrorist threats. The European Court of Human Rights, as noted earlier, regards these techniques as torture when used in combination. But this court binds neither Israel nor the United States. In 1997, the Committee against Torture stated to the UN General Assembly that methods including stress positions, hooding, loud music, sleep deprivation, shaking, and exposure to intensely cold air are, in the committee's view, breaches of CAT Article 16 (prohibiting ill-treatment) and also constitute torture as defined in Article 1 of the Convention. "This conclusion," they write, "is particularly evident where such methods of interrogation are used in combination, which appears to be the standard case" (United Nations, 1997). The United States, however, does not recognize the categorical authority of CAT, because U.S. lawmakers reserve the right to apply Article 16 only insofar as it is consistent with Article 8 of the U.S. Constitution, prohibiting "cruel and unusual punishment." With little case law in the United States to define "cruel and unusual punishment," officials currently interpret torture to prohibit egregious physical and psychological pain and suffering inflicted in the most extreme, sadistic, and malicious circumstances. Inflicting any other harm or deprivation on detainees is permissible if used in good faith to protect the legitimate interests of the government (U.S. Department of Defense, 2003b, 39). This reflects precisely the use of force CAT wishes to prevent, but one that draws our attention to the arguments nations raise to justify torture and ill-treatment when fighting terror.

Justifying Torture and Ill-Treatment

The distinction that nations like Britain, Israel, and the United States draw between torture and other forms of ill-treatment does not always take them very far. While CAT, the reigning paradigm, acknowledges the distinction, it has made every effort to condemn extraordinary interrogation techniques as torture. Practically, neither Israel nor the United States avoids using these techniques in combination; in fact, both countries augment them with increasingly severe practices. Over the years, B'tselem, Amnesty International, and the Public Committee against Torture in Israel published numerous reports on Palestinian detainees who were killed, beaten, crippled, and psychologically abused by interrogational methods similar to the five British techniques, precisely the kind of interrogation the Landau Commission wanted, but ultimately failed, to prevent (Gordon 1995; Pacheco 1999; B'tselem 2000). It therefore makes little difference whether a nation defines abusive or aggressive interrogation techniques as torture, ill-treatment, or moderate physical pressure. Once a nation chooses to employ them, it finds it must justify its actions to the international community and to its own people.

It is noteworthy, then, that when Israel's Supreme Court considered permissible interrogation techniques in 1999 it glossed over the distinction between torture and ill-treatment, writing that a "reasonable investigation is necessarily one free of torture, free of cruel, inhuman treatment of the subject and free of any degrading handling whatsoever" (*Public Committee against Torture in Israel v. The State of Israel*, 1999, paragraph 23). But if reasonable interrogations are the rule, a starting point the Landau Commission did much to erode as it lent authority to the notion of moderate physical pressure, exceptions nonetheless remain. Emphasizing Israel's commitment to international conventions prohibiting torture and ill-treatment, Israel's Supreme Court reiterated its stand that torture is illegal. Nevertheless, torture may be *defensible* if necessary. Aptly, this is called "the necessity defense." Necessity may *exempt* a person from criminal responsibility when violating the law in the face of imminent harm, if an individual acts "in order to avoid consequences which could not otherwise be avoided and which would have inflicted grievous harm or injury [and] provided that he or she did no more harm than was reasonably necessary [nor] disproportionate to the harm avoided" (Israel Penal Code, section 22). Necessity demands that five conditions be met: the threat of (1) grievous and (2) unavoidable harm and a (3) proportionate, (4) effective, and (5) last-resort response. The term *exempt* is subject to conflicting interpretations. Most legal scholars agree that the necessity defense "excuses" rather than "justifies" an action, so that the law one overrides retains its force and demands some degree of punishment, regret, or restitution (Cohen 1987/8).

While Israel's Supreme Court decision sharply reduced complaints of ill-treatment, it did not unequivocally ban torture. In February 2001, Israeli officials approached the justice ministry and complained that the inability to use moderate physical pressure hindered their investigations. This led the State Prosecutor to declare, "as long as interrogators act in a *reasonable* manner they will not be tried on criminal or disciplinary charges for their actions even if jurists define these actions as unjustified" (Benn 2001, Harel 2002). "Reasonable," which just two years earlier meant an investigation free of torture and ill-treatment, shifted subtly to embrace moderate physical pressure as a last resort to elicit information from suspects planning to kill large numbers of civilians. Given the preference that militants have for suicide bombs together with the government's lax attitude in spite of the best efforts of the judiciary, it is not surprising that torture and ill-treatment are again on the rise in Israel particularly as the conflict with the Palestinians intensifies (*Public Committee against Torture in Israel*, 2001a). Things appear little different among American forces struggling to maintain security in Iraq.

Necessity, Torture, and Ticking Bombs

The necessity defense is not simply an exercise of post hoc justification but a serious attempt to allow an investigator to weigh the evil of torture against the evil of terror. Ticking bombs are the often-cited example. Consider the following news item:

A suicide bombing was narrowly averted in Haifa [Israel] yesterday morning when the would-be perpetrator was arrested shortly before carrying it out. The drama ... began when police, acting on *specific intelligence information* about a planned attack in Haifa, arrested a number of Palestinians who had been staying in the city illegally. One 18-year-old from Samaria was arrested ... and *when questioned*, he admitted that he had hidden explosives for use in a suicide attack [and] directed [police] to an abandoned building where they found a belt containing several bombs that the Palestinian had planned to strap to his body and set off. (Harel 2001, emphasis added)

Typical of the many cases that become public knowledge, many details of this one are obviously missing. Nevertheless, I will use it to paint several scenarios to illuminate the dilemma of torture and ill-treatment democratic nations face as they confront terror. If moderate physical pressure or exceptional interrogation techniques can avert ticking bombs and prevent grievous harm to innocent individuals why, ask some, should anyone including medical workers think twice about protecting a suspected terrorist's dignity and self-esteem? For others, the answer is obvious: torture is an inexcusable affront to human dignity.

Torture: An Affront to Human Dignity?

Dignity, as noted in chapter 1, reflects an overarching moral principle that designates an individual's intrinsic worth as a human being. The right to life and respect for self-esteem are crucial components of dignity, and both are among the first casualties of armed conflicts. In the aftermath of World War II, the universal prohibition against torture and ill-treatment grew from the obligation of world bodies to shield weak, unprotected citizens from rampant human rights abuses that included every affront to human dignity imaginable: torture, experimentation, rape, murder, and enslavement. While international conventions make a strenuous effort to safeguard life *and* self-esteem as fundamental, primary goods, the contemporary dilemma of torture and ill-treatment sets the lives of some against the self-esteem of others. Considering that "war, the threat of war or other public emergencies"—that is, events that threaten the lives of innumerable individuals—can never justify torture, the international community comes down firmly on the side of self-esteem. Torture and ill-treatment are repugnant because they are an affront to human dignity. Torture inflicts enormous pain and suffering, destroys self-esteem, and robs people of their capacity for free will. Utterly dehumanizing, torture, like wanton rape and murder, destroys the conditions necessary for any form of social or political interaction.

These are powerful arguments that bring many to conclude that the "ticking-bomb" case described above is no different from any other that endangers the lives of innocent human beings. Terrorist suspects are no different from cold and deliberate mass murderers who stalk and kill their victims. Yet few proponents of aggressively interrogating suspected terrorists would agree to question ordinary murder suspects in the same manner.[3] To overcome the obvious charge of inconsistency, they must argue either that terrorists constitute an especially heinous and morally unique class of suspects that somehow forfeits their right to respect for self-esteem, or that death and indignity force a tragic choice between two evils that only utilitarian outcomes can decide.

Do Terrorists Forfeit Their Right to Self-Esteem?

Turning to the logic of ordinary self-defense, some observers argue that terrorists lose their right to respect for self-esteem in the same way that some aggressors lose their right to life. When they present a serious, material threat, aggressors are vulnerable to harm once they create a situation "in which someone must be killed, either [the aggressor] or his intended victim"—a harm that the intended victim "can now only redirect but not eliminate." This may then "forfeit, override, or specify out of existence the aggressor's right to life" (Moore 1989, 321–322). Michael Moore uses this argument, prominent in the self-defense literature, to justify torture and ill-treatment on the assumption that aggressors forfeit their dignity—that is, respect for their self-esteem—in the same way that they may lose their right to life (Montague 1981; McMahan 1994a; Thomson 1996).

Attractive to proponents of interrogational torture, Moore's argument is overly elastic because it permits one to kill or torture any mass murderer or common criminal whose actions put others at risk. This, of course, few wish to do, nor is there any indication that they want to extend the argument in this way. However, one might tighten the argument by distinguishing between forfeiting the right to life (which Moore explicitly accepts) and forfeiting self-esteem (which is only presumed if the lessons of self-defense apply to torture). While criminals may indeed lose their right to life by threatening others, it is not as clear that they lose our respect for their self-esteem. If the argument from self-defense leads to loss of respect for self-esteem, then we could torture criminals (which we do not); if it does not affect respect for self-esteem, then we cannot torture anyone. So an additional claim, beyond defending oneself against a criminal whose action puts others at risk, is needed to justify loss of respect for self-esteem. This might come from the nature of terrorist acts themselves.

Criminal acts are fundamentally different from acts of terror. However heinous, crimes against persons fall within the framework of recognizable human interaction, so that the net of human dignity protects both perpetrators and victims. Proponents of interrogational torture will not torture a mafia hit man to find his potential victims, victims of avarice, greed, rage, desire, and envy. However innocent his victims, they are not dehumanized but murdered and robbed as men are wont to do to one another. There remains a link between the criminal and his victim. The link may be immoral, corrupt, and perverse but one we recognize within the constellation of quotidian human passion. As such, all the parties retain some semblance of human dignity even as they are hated, feared, envied, and despised.

Terrorist crimes are entirely different and beyond the minimal norms of human interaction. Terrorism, by definition, targets innocent civilians for political gain, whether to weaken civilian morale, derail prospects for peace, place a national cause firmly on the international agenda, or garner support for militant groups at home. To attain these goals, innocence is an indispensable condition of victimhood, without which it is impossible to further the political aims terrorists espouse. Terrorists reduce civilians to the basest of means. The abomination of terrorism rests precisely on the conviction that its victims are innocent of any wrongdoing. The terrorist who recognizes no intrinsic value to the life of his victim, who takes advantage and intentionally abuses his victim's innocence for his own purposes, forfeits his own moral status as a human being.

In response, one might object that this argument ignores "intrinsic" human traits that bestow respect for an individual's dignity and self-esteem regardless of his or her behavior. Avishai Margalit (1996, 70), for example, finds promise in the "capacity of reevaluating one's life at any given moment [and] the ability to change one's life from that moment on." As a result, "even the worst criminals are worthy of basic human respect" (p. 71), and this, of course, protects them from torture. Two difficulties, however, come to mind. First, the argument requires an empirical foundation. "Thus respecting humans," writes Margalit, "means never giving up on anyone since all people *are capable* of living dramatically differently from the way they have lived so far" (p. 263; emphasis added). This is certainly contingent, particularly because living "differently" means, in this context, living a better moral life, a change dependent on conditions that Margalit does not specify but that must include an alternative and normatively superior worldview and probably better socioeconomic conditions as well. While criminals live in a society that can offer them morally preferred norms together, in many cases, with a higher standard of living, this is not true of terrorists. Terrorists are often "home-grown" and find normative, social, and financial support among those in whose midst they operate. Second, it is not clear why the ability to change overrides actual behavior. Actual behavior, at least, is entirely tangible and under some circumstances, particularly those characteristic of terrorism, might entail *dis*respect.[4]

Accepting arguments like Moore's means that while human dignity offers powerful protection for ordinary criminals, it carries little force among terrorism suspects. Terrorists may suffer torture but the common criminal cannot. The strength of this argument lies in its distinction between two classes of criminals and the ascription of different rights to each. But this is also its weakness. It is not always clear, for example, whether heinous criminals are categorically different from terrorists. The former may kill those entirely innocent, while the latter may ascribe some measure of guilt to their victims. More importantly, it is difficult to conclude that a person may forfeit one's dignity or respect for self-esteem without undermining the very idea of *human* rights that we generally assign solely on one's status as a human being. For these reasons, advocates of interrogational torture may turn to utilitarian arguments for support.

Death and Indignity: The Utilitarian Argument

Utilitarians present the dilemma of torture as a tragic choice that only a careful evaluation of competing utilities can resolve. Terrorists retain their right to respect for self-esteem; innocent civilians retain their right to life. In some cases, most notably ticking bombs, the good that comes from saving many innocent lives outweighs the harm that comes from torturing or ill-treating a small number of suspected terrorists. In this case, torture saves many lives while costing few, if any at all. Consider the ticking-bomb case in Haifa described earlier. Commenting on this case, a utilitarian might argue that authorities prevented a suicide bombing by eliciting crucial information at two stages. Before the arrest of the bomber, undisclosed sources provided authorities with the bomber's identity and plan to attack civilians. While this allowed authorities to locate and arrest a suspect, it did not necessarily defuse the threat. Perhaps the suspect had already planted his ticking bomb. Authorities then "questioned" the suspect until he revealed that he had hidden an explosive belt that he only intended to use later. Given these circumstances, a utilitarian might argue that interrogational torture and, with it, the medical care necessary to facilitate a successful interrogation, were justified at each stage because they successfully saved many innocent lives at relatively little cost. Anyone questioning the actions of the authorities would then demand that interrogators defend their actions, and they might do this with arguments that utilitarians find persuasive.

To invoke the necessity defense, however, interrogators as well as physicians who facilitate aggressive interrogation must demonstrate that their actions were, in fact, a proportionate, effective, and last-resort response to a threat of grievous and otherwise unavoidable harm. Even as Israel's Supreme Court weighed the merits of the necessity defense, the justices adopted the stringent conditions of efficacy suggested by some commentators that the threat of terror attacks cannot justify interrogational torture unless there is a firm assurance that the suspect is morally and causally responsible for imminent acts of terror. This unpacks to mean that the suspect is telling the truth, that his information is complete, that he will talk in time to locate and defuse an explosive device, and that there is no chance a confederate will reprogram the device or simply move the attack to some other time or place (G. E. Jones 1980; Kadish 1989; Human Rights Watch 1994; Tindale 1996; Statman 1997).

These conditions push beyond the immediate question whether torture, harsh interrogation, or moderate physical pressure elicits the truth from detainees and demand, in addition, that information, however true, is also sufficient to save lives. If it is impossible to fulfill these conditions, then the argument stops here and interrogational torture is never justified. If the chances are only very low but, as Israel's justices believe, realistic nonetheless, then it remains to examine the long-term consequences of interrogational torture. Satisfied that interrogational torture will elicit the information necessary to save many innocent lives does not absolve one from considering its other effects on society or on the rights of innocent civilians.

Ticking bombs focus our attention on short-term costs and benefits. Putting aside harm to self-esteem, an attribute of humanness that is difficult to compare with any other, it is likely that any attempt to weigh the lives of many against the suffering of relatively few will always favor the former. Death will always trump discomfort as long as the probability that torture will save lives is relatively high. This is not always obvious. The courts can set the bar very high, but the day-to-day decision making falls to operatives in the field, who tend to lower the bar whenever the lives they swear to protect are in danger. Costs extend to everyone affected by torture and ill-treatment and include those who suffer tortured but cannot supply necessary information as well as those responsible for terror who nonetheless endure something more than moderate physical pressure. Moreover, ad hoc decision making by investigators in the field rarely takes into account the long-term consequences of torture. This is the slippery-slope argument, and many consider it decisive: once the door opens to ill-treating suspected terrorists, then innocent individuals or common criminals will eventually suffer, and torture will become the interrogational tool of choice when lesser means are available, will erode other civil liberties, and will grow to embrace terroristic torture.

Victims of Torture   Proponents of interrogational torture demand that the suspects authorities question by exceptional means must be responsible for the acts of terror officials are trying to prevent. Others insist that only the need to question a suspect who can provide the information necessary to avert a catastrophic attack warrants torture. A cogent argument must combine these two criteria; otherwise, an innocent person harboring critical information may suffer. Yet it is not clear how utilitarians can avoid extending interrogational torture to those who happen to be in possession of useful information. Consider, once again, the ticking bomb in downtown Haifa: "Police, acting on *specific intelligence information* about a planned attack in Haifa, arrested a number of Palestinians who had been staying in the city illegally. One 18-year-old from Samaria was arrested."

How did authorities obtain *specific intelligence information*? After having tried more benign methods, utilitarians may not object to using sleep deprivation, stress positions, or powerfully loud music to elicit the information necessary to avert an attack. But we do not know how many individuals suffered ill-treatment before investigators realized that they knew nothing of value, let alone necessary to prevent a suicide bombing. The ticking bomb is only persuasive if the harm that befalls some individuals from interrogational torture pales beside the number of lives saved. This assumes that authorities can zero in on appropriate suspects. Inevitably, however, this requires precise information that can only come, at least at one point early on, from sweeping interrogation of the usual suspects. Circularity is inevitable: while only those responsible for terror may be tortured, only torture can tell investigators who is responsible. For this reason, authorities had to arrest "a number of Palestinians." Were they all reasonable suspects, although only one "18-year-old from Samaria" was responsible? Here, too, utilitarians face a difficult calculation of utility. How many of those *not* responsible for terror acts may suffer harm in the interest of protecting the lives of innocent civilians?

Apart from those who bear no responsibility and know little, what of those who bear no responsibility but know something? May one torture the cook or passerby who chances on information of an impending attack solely because she holds vital information? Those who believe that terror suspects forfeit their right to self-esteem can resist this question because innocents remain protected from torture by their inviolable claim to dignity. Utilitarians, however, have a harder time, for utility seems to demand that anyone may suffer harm if the information he or she can provide will prevent a ticking bomb. To prevent torturing innocents to save the lives of others, some have suggested that innocents are blameless but become a party to a threat when they can reveal information *at no cost to themselves* (Moore 1989). While this saves us from torturing a terrorist's child to force a suspect to talk, it endangers others who may fear costs that investigators consider irrelevant. Who is to say, for example, that a cook who knows something of an impending attack but fears reprisals against his family can reveal information at no cost to himself? Innocent of any wrongdoing, he may yet suffer torture if his interrogators consider his fears trivial. Given that terrorists and insurgents are well embedded within the local community, harm to "knowledgeable" innocents is a possibility that utilitarians cannot always prevent.

The Means of Torture   Apart from those not responsible but who may hold valuable information, what of those who are responsible for planning an impending attack? After detaining and questioning "a number of Palestinians," authorities believed that they had sufficient information to identify the suicide bomber, whom they then arrested and who *"when questioned, . . .* admitted that he had hidden explosives." What kind of interrogation techniques are permissible once security officials have tolerable grounds to suspect a person of terror activity and have decided to forgo "reasonable" questioning? Most advocates of torture try to distinguish between moderate physical pressure or exceptional techniques, and between sadistic, mutilating, and brutal torture. While each is a form of physical abuse, the distinction emphasizes the difference between uncomfortable and painful conditions of interrogation, and the outright abuse of a person's body. Hooding, cold, hunger, sleep deprivation, squatting, and wall standing all make victims suffer but in a way that is different from shaking, beating, burning, electrocuting, and sexually abusing them. But if the purpose of torture is to save innocent lives as quickly as possible, then why avoid any technique that will elicit information? Utilitarianism has no answer other than utility: for most purposes, the former techniques are sufficient while the latter are gratuitous. Perhaps, but what if the former are not sufficient? May investigators then inflict severe and overwhelming pain on a suspect?

While utilitarians have no ready answer to this objection, deontologists who place terrorists in a moral class of their own may invoke the conditions necessary for a terror suspect to forfeit the right to respect for self-esteem. Here, they might consider the window of opportunity that justifies harsh interrogation. One violates a suspect's self-esteem because, for a certain time, he or she can provide information to avert a catastrophe and prevent the death of many innocent civilians. The grounds for interrogational torture hold only during this window and prevent harm that extends beyond the period where it no longer serves any purpose. This would preclude any interrogation accompanied by mutilation, physical or sexual abuse, or severe psychological trauma. Insofar as one can evaluate this accurately, the trauma of torture should not exceed, for example, the trauma one suffers from ordinary incarceration.

Long-Term Social Consequences   How does interrogational torture affect democratic society? During France's war in Algeria, Pierre Vidal-Naquet warned of the dangers torture posed to French society: sadism and indifference among soldiers, disrespect for laws prohibiting torture, and a steady erosion of judicial protections as "emergency measures" gained ground and as authorities set secretive rather than transparent public policy (Vidal-Naquet 1963). While many in Israel and the United States fear similar consequences, some seem content with the fact that many democratic regimes practicing interrogational torture successfully limit ill-treatment to those belonging to a clearly defined and hostile out-group that often resides beyond their territorial boundaries and constitutional protections. French abuses in Algeria did not penetrate metropolitan France. The British limited their five techniques of interrogation to IRA militants. In spite of increasing reports of interrogational torture among Palestinian Arabs, there are no instances of ill-treatment among Israeli Jews. Nor are all observers convinced that the abuses at U.S. facilities in Guantanamo Bay or in Iraqi prisons will affect law-enforcement procedures in the United States. The institutions of democratic society, by these accounts, appear to hold human rights abuses at bay, preventing the slide down the slippery slope that many fear.

The resilience of democracy to stand firm against the slippery slope is by no means certain. In spite of what may be their best intentions, many democracies still lack a transparent and accountable regulatory mechanism to supervise interrogational torture. The Israelis have worked at it the longest, as each branch of the government has broached questions about the limits of permissible torture and ill-treatment on the assumption that rare cases of ticking bombs justify hooding, sleep deprivation, loud music, and stress positions. While the utilitarian arguments they have raised are not entirely without foundation, Israel's civilian authorities have failed to institute the necessary oversight mechanism to prevent a slide down the slippery slope. Torture grew increasingly severe and savage in the years following the Landau Commission report. Following an outbreak of violence, the police and army may have recklessly endangered lives of Israeli Arabs during street riots in October 2000 and abused the rights of minors suspected of incitement, a process of deterioration that cannot be unrelated to the ill-treatment of Palestinian detainees (Public Committee against Torture in Israel, 2001b).

Whether these brutal social consequences are more than sufficient to repudiate torture or highlight, instead, the need to proceed with extreme caution as legislators, public officials, and ordinary citizens consider the necessity of interrogational torture in conflicts plagued by terrorism remains, of course, at the center of the debate. Utilitarian arguments, by their very nature, remain contingent and, to some extent, indeterminate. In July 2002, for example, newspapers in Israel reported that security services used extraordinary means of interrogation, including moderate physical pressure and sleep deprivation, in ninety "ticking-bomb" cases (Harel, 2002). Undoubtedly, some jurists and legislators believe that some of these cases are defensible despite the many difficulties utilitarianism presents. As a result, some advocates focus their attention on regulating rather than preventing interrogational torture and envision judicial or public oversight committees of the kind only a democratic regime can provide to stem the worse excesses of ill-treatment (Zamir 1989). While proponents of the necessity defense claim that only rare and extenuating circumstances warrant any deviation from "reasonable" investigation, they also remind us that interrogators must defend themselves before their fellow citizens, up front and in public.

If there are legitimate and compelling grounds to permit interrogational torture in isolated cases, what are a physician's obligations? Do medical personnel who accept the inevitability of interrogational torture have a civic duty to comply and assist their government, or must they fulfill a professional duty to desist and oppose torture and ill-treatment regardless of any convincing arguments to the contrary? Physicians called on to facilitate interrogational torture may face an excruciating dilemma. Some may evaluate the deontological and utilitarian arguments and conclude that interrogational torture is never permissible. For others, the unique moral status of terrorists or the exceptional circumstances of ticking bombs and grave threats to human life they pose may lead them to conclude that the injunction against ill-treatment and moderate physical pressure is not absolute. While they may believe, like Shue, that there are few justifiable violations, conditions remain contingent. These doctors then face a dilemma more acute than the judges who must weigh the lives of some and the dignity of others, for unlike jurists, health-care professionals who accept the inevitability of interrogational torture must use their medical expertise in a way that facilitates harm to certain individuals.

Torture and the Role of Physicians

Whatever role medical personnel *may* play, we know the role they *do* play. Physicians are present in interrogation centers to supervise a prisoner's health before and after interrogation and may sometimes certify a suspect's fitness for various forms of questioning.

The Role of Physicians in Interrogations
Doctors may fulfill one or more central, facilitating roles in interrogational torture.

Certification Physicians may evaluate a prisoner's fitness to endure certain forms of interrogation including slapping, chaining, hooding, and prolonged standing. Based on prison medical forms found circulating in

1993, human rights groups charged that Israeli doctors certified prisoners for torture. Condemned by the Israel Medical Association, these medical forms were reportedly removed from circulation (Human Rights Watch, 1994). American doctors in Guantanamo Bay also certified the fitness of detainees for questioning as they helped tailor interrogation plans for specific prisoners (Miles 2004; Bloche and Marks 2005).

Medical Supervision Physicians provide regular and routine medical care in detention facilities as they treat detainees suffering from illness or injury. Detainees are examined on admission and monitored throughout the course of interrogation. In some cases, physicians provide less-than-comprehensive treatment. Describing the interrogation procedures in an Israeli police station, B'tselem (2001b, 2) notes the place of physicians providing medical care:

Most of the detainees were taken for a medical check-up immediately upon their arrival at the police station. According to the testimonies, the physician performed a superficial examination, based in some cases on a quick glance, after which the physician signed a form confirming that they were healthy. At times, the detainees were handcuffed and blindfolded during the medical check-up. Some detainees were taken to the physician after being tortured during interrogation, were treated, and were returned for further interrogation.

In the United States, directives from senior officials impose similar duties on American medical personnel serving in detention facilities. Attached to each of the secretary of defense's memoranda authorizing aggressive interrogation techniques are provisions for medical certification and supervision:

Application of these interrogation techniques is subject to the following general safeguards: . . . the detainee is *medically evaluated as suitable* (considering all techniques in combination); . . . a specific interrogation plan (including reasonable safeguards, limits on duration, intervals between applications, termination criteria and the *presence or availability of qualified medical personnel*) has been developed." (U.S. Southern Command, 2003; emphasis added)

Participation While there are few reports of doctors taking an active or direct part in interrogations, medical personnel sometimes move beyond certifying detainees or supervising medical care to what I will refer to as *passive* torture:

American officials acknowledged that such techniques (sleep and light depriva-tion and the temporary withholding of food, water, access to sunlight and medical attention) were recently applied as part of the interrogation of Abu Zubaydah [a high-ranking Al Qaeda leader known to be involved with the 9/11 bombings]. Painkillers were withheld from Zubaydah, [or "were used *selec-tively*," in some reports], who was shot several times [in the groin] during his capture ["until he agreed to cooperate more fully," in some reports]. (Bonner, Natta, and Waldman 2003, 1; also Priest 2004)

Medical personnel who administered emergency care to stabilize Zubaydah but then withheld painkillers until security officials completed their interrogation were parties to torture and ill-treatment. While "passive" torture suggests a difference between acts of omission and commission, there is no significant difference between withholding stan-dard medical care and inflicting pain and suffering by other means. While the omission-commission distinction is central to many fundamental debates in ethics, it is irrelevant in this case. There is a prima facie duty to care for an injured person unless a patient refuses care, or care is futile or accompanied by overwhelming pain and suffering. None of these conditions applies when someone requires immediate medical care for gunshot wounds to the groin. Withholding medical care, particularly selectively withholding care to maintain the detainee in a state of extreme but not life-threatening distress, is nothing but another form of torture and ill-treatment. Nevertheless, it places physicians in a far more visible and central role than certifying prisoners for interrogation or providing medical supervision does.

Medical conventions prohibit physicians from participating in any of these activities. They should not certify prisoners for interrogations that employ torture, they should not be present in facilities where investiga-tors use moderate physical pressure, and they should not be parties to passive torture. In each case, physicians have an overriding commitment to the health and welfare of their patients and, in most circumstances, could refuse to offer medical treatment unless it met the standards of acceptable care in a detention facility free of inhuman or degrading treat-ment. Interrogational torture cannot succeed without medical assistance, and doctors play a crucial, facilitating role that many claim would allow them, at the very least, to hamper an investigation, seriously obstruct the system, or compile documentation of abuse. I pursue these claims in the sections below, first by considering the position of the international medical community and then by asking whether physicians who acknowledge defensible instances of interrogational torture should facilitate the efforts of military authorities and security officials to obtain information.

Medical Ethics and the International Community

After torture came to the attention of the British public in 1969, a parliamentary delegation reported to the British Parliament that "if torture has become inevitable, it is necessary to humanize it and have an attending physician to moderate it, and even stop it if, in his medical opinion, it became physically dangerous" (Wilson 1983, 237). In response, the British Medical Association turned to the World Medical Association for direction and, in 1975, the WMA issued the Tokyo Declaration, unequivocally prohibiting physicians from participating in torture. The international community soon followed suit. Modeled after the Tokyo Declaration, which bars physicians from condoning, facilitating, or participating in torture and bans their presence in any facility that uses torture, the United Nations Principles of Medical Ethics (1982) prohibit physicians from engaging "actively or passively in acts which constitute . . . torture or cruel, inhuman or degrading treatment or punishment, or certifying the fitness of prisoners for any form of treatment or punishment . . . *not in accordance with the relevant international instruments*" (United Nations, 1982, Principles 2, 4; emphasis added).

Commentators continue to wonder whether the final reference to "relevant international instruments" undoes the blanket injunction that prohibits physicians from certifying a prisoner's health prior to ill-treatment and softens the Tokyo Declaration's unequivocal denunciation (Rodley 1999, 373–377). Because medical certification and supervision are the primary roles physicians play during interrogation, the contingent international injunction is less than entirely helpful. How should physicians behave? Nations often interpret relevant international instruments at their own discretion. The American government, for example, defines its international obligations to refrain from torture consistent with its interpretation of the U.S. Constitution, which, in the opinion of some administration officials, allows the United States considerable latitude as it interrogates certain suspects. The Landau Commission leaned heavily on two contentious assumptions as it approved moderate physical pressure: treaty law protecting occupied peoples does not apply in the territories administered by Israel since 1967 because these are not technically occupied (Shamgar 1977), and "moderate physical pressure" is legally and morally distinct from torture as proscribed by international law. Regardless of the merits of these claims, one can hardly expect local physicians to adjudicate them when legal scholars in their own countries continue to disagree. This leaves medical personnel between a rock and a hard place. International legal instruments, including international guidelines on medical ethics, are of little help when physicians must consider their role in state-sanctioned interrogational torture. Instead, it might be more helpful to appeal to the underlying norms of biomedical ethics.

Medical Ethics and Interrogational Torture

International prohibitions against ill-treatment reiterate the principle that "it is the privilege of the physician to practice medicine in the service of humanity and restore bodily and mental health . . . to comfort and to ease the suffering of his or her patients. The utmost respect for human life is to be maintained . . . and no use made of any medical knowledge contrary to the laws of humanity" (WMA 1975, Preamble).

This phrase, which recurs in other WMA declarations including those prohibiting physician participation in the development of chemical and biological weapons (see the following chapter), masks two general principles of biomedical ethics. The first commits physicians to beneficence and nonmaleficence and the second subordinates medical practice to the laws of humanity. By laws of humanity, the WMA clearly has in mind the many international instruments that prohibit or limit torture, ill-treatment, and degrading or cruel punishment: the Fourth Geneva Convention, the Convention against Torture, and the UN Declaration of Human Rights, and UN Principles of Medical Ethics. These do not, however, offer firm or unambiguous guidelines. The instruments themselves conflict. Some stipulate unilateral guidelines, while others are contingent on local interpretations. But beyond the instruments themselves, the WMA has in mind the *idea* of humanitarian law, an ideal that protects the lives and dignity of innocent human beings caught up in the violence of war and conflict. Historically, humanitarian law has protected noncombatant victims of war and, to a lesser extent, combatants themselves.

While these protections are proper, terrorist activity poses a unique challenge for humanitarian law that now force it to rank the relative harms of death and indignity in a way never before contemplated. When Winston Churchill, for example, condemned the excesses of World War I, he famously observed, "when all was over, torture and cannibalism were the only two expedients that the civilized, scientific, Christian States had been able to deny themselves." In the past, nations rarely thought to torture enemy soldiers or civilians to save the lives of their own. Torture was not expedient because torturing enemy soldiers would expose their own soldiers to equal danger. Nor would torture do much to save innocents who were, at least through the First World War, kept from the line of fire. As World War II shattered the illusion of noncombatant immunity, the international community reiterated its stand against torture and, at the same time, directed considerable efforts toward protecting civilians from the ravages of war. This is the corpus of norms we define as humanitarian law. Confronting terror—that is, grave breaches of humanitarian law–the international community faces a dilemma. Humanitarian law forbids torture *and* terror. But *if* torture is necessary to prevent terror, something has to give; one cannot unequivocally condemn both. Physicians who accept the inevitability of interrogational torture, then, must find alternative arguments to justify their reluctance to certify suspects for questioning or provide medical supervision in detention facilities. As they do, physicians confront a conflict between civic and professional duties.

Civic Duty and Professional Obligation   In a rare discussion of a physician's role in torture independent of the morality of torture itself, R. S. Downie (1993) sidesteps the question of legitimate torture and moves directly to the quandary of physician involvement. Because a doctor's professional role demands that she relieve suffering and promote healing, a physician may never participate in or facilitate torture, however justified or necessary one believes it to be. This is the argument from beneficence and nonmaleficence and one that Downie, as well as most physicians I imagine, accept. R. M. Hare (1993), responding to Downie, considers the argument long enough to make the important point that Downie fails to account for a conflict of duties as a doctor's obligation to heal collides with any person's moral duty to do the greatest good. Pushing on, however, Hare (1993, 139) confronts the dilemma the old-fashioned way, by denying any justification for torture with an argument that might now seem naive. "It is hard to believe," writes Hare, "that the litter bin [ticking-bomb] case would ever occur, that is, a case in which there was no way of locating a bomb except by torture. It is even more unbelievable that the skills of the doctor would be of much use in torturing the terrorist; torture is not all that difficult in such a case; a crude, quick and effective means would be what was needed."

Neither argument is necessarily compelling. Even Hare stops short of claiming that it is *impossible* to believe that there is no way of locating a bomb except by torture. Moreover, while physicians rarely apply their skills to torture, Hare entirely fails to consider their facilitating role, without which torture and aggressive interrogation cannot succeed. Although Hare highlights the conflict between civic and professional roles, neither he nor Downie offers a successful resolution of the difficulties this conflict causes. Coming down on the side of professional obligations, Downie presumes to leave interrogation and torture to someone other than a physician. Surely this creates some difficulty for any self-reflective person and does little to remedy the dilemma of interrogational torture that physicians may face.

Hare's argument turns on actions that bring the greatest good and is one that many raise to defend interrogational torture. After evaluating the cogency of utilitarian as well as deontological arguments, one will hopefully reach a decision: torture is either defensible or it is not. But a judgment one way or the other may not quiet a physician's conscience. Torture may remain indefensible, but leave one to still ask whether some good may come from providing medical care in a detention facility. Alternatively, one may envision defensible instances of torture and question the level of care (or lack thereof) necessary to facilitate a successful interrogation.

Passive Torture and Beneficent Care in Detention Facilities   Passive torture, of which there are few reported instances, is the least defensible of any medically related involvement in interrogation.[5] I have already suggested that passive torture is no less problematic simply because it is an act of omission. On the contrary, because standard medical care is readily available and presents little or no risk to the provider, passive torture is tantamount to inflicting any other harm to elicit information from a suspected terrorist. Is it, then, permissible? In the case described earlier, it does not seem that withholding medical care causes greater suffering than other techniques. Nor does it necessarily cause permanent harm. As we consider whether passive torture may be permissible, it is important to keep Shue's admonishment in mind: torture must be the *least harmful* means available. Passive torture, if by this we mean leaving someone to suffer without readily available medical care, cannot be the least harmful means available. Rather, it is an opportunistic means; one does not consider passive torture after first attempting to use less harmful means of interrogation. Instead, one exploits an arbitrary turn of events that makes torture, however passive, the first rather than the last resort and, therefore, unjustifiable by any standard.

The case, however, is instructive for a different reason. Passive torture fails for reasons unrelated to physicians' obligations to their patients. That is, it does not fail because it requires physicians to cause harm but because it is not the least harm necessary to save innocent lives. But other forms of harsh interrogation may represent the least harmful means available, and should an effective interrogation technique require direct medical participation, physicians will find it difficult to opt out. Administering psychotropic drugs to detainees might be one example of physician-assisted torture and leaves one to reasonably ask whether physicians should participate if their active assistance is necessary to secure crucial information. I will not pursue this question here if only because instances of direct physician involvement, particularly in the nations surveyed in this chapter, are rare.[6] However, the question whether and to what extent a physician may cause harm to others figures prominently in the following chapter, as we consider their role in the development of modern weaponry.

In most cases related to interrogational torture, physicians will consider the care they can deliver rather than the harm they can cause. Nevertheless, it is important to keep in mind that doctors in a detention facility are not serving their patients' interests by providing medical care and/or certifying prisoners for questioning. Torture is a noncaregiving dilemma. Although they may not necessarily cause harm, doctors who facilitate torture facilitate harm. While physicians may rescue patients from some degree of avoidable harm by offering medical treatment or evaluation, they are setting their patients up for greater pain and suffering. If asked, I would further imagine that doctors in detention facilities know this. Those who reject the inevitability of interrogational torture may be divided because they realize that any attempt to prohibit doctors from working in detention facilities will deny care to detainees. While some may believe that this protest will eventually force authorities to forgo exceptional means of interrogation, others must be aware that security officials are likely to continue their interrogations in the absence of medical care. Many physicians may then consider their obligation to provide care to those in need. Under these circumstances, can physicians limit themselves to beneficent care and avoid care that facilitates interrogational torture?

Beneficent care is the first concern of physicians. It precludes "superficial" medical examinations and requires physicians to treat detainees in need of medical care unrelated to the interrogation process. This may include treatment for disease or injuries incurred in prison. Facilitating care allows security officials to conduct their investigations. It may mean certifying a detainee for a particular kind of interrogation or reviving an unconscious suspect for further questioning. Often the two overlap. When they do, physicians will find it difficult to fall back solely on the duty of beneficence to provide care. Some may quit the facility or do their best to thwart interrogations, as some human rights organizations advise. Others, perhaps the majority, will believe that the harm their patients suffer is necessary to achieve a greater good. They will ask whether a physician or other medical worker may facilitate harm to a patient in the interests of the common good of the political community to which they belong.

Liberal Bioethics and the Common Good

Any physician who accepts the need for interrogational torture must consider the duty to provide facilitating as well as beneficent care. Israeli physicians, for example, invoke Hare's utilitarian imperative and take refuge in the firm conviction that their aid is essential to preserve the public good. While human rights groups charge compliant physicians with acquiescence to torture (Public Committee against Torture in Israel, 1993, 60–61), the Israel Medical Association (IMA) stands firm in the face of criticism that its members violate the basic duties of medicine. Before the 1999 Israeli Supreme Court ruling, the IMA denounced torture but tacitly supported interrogations restricted to using moderate physical pressure. By 1999, the IMA welcomed the Israeli Supreme Court's ban on torture, hoping that the "dark days" of widespread moderate physical pressure would not return but again acknowledging support for physical measures—as distinct from torture—in "ticking-bomb" cases (Blachar 1997, 1999). The IMA's underlying message is clear: collective well-being and civic duty complement, if not supercede, a physician's responsibility to a patient's well-being when interrogational torture is necessary to prevent ticking bombs. In these cases, which the IMA believes inevitable, physicians must provide beneficent *and* facilitating care in detention centers. One must assume that American guidelines that direct medical personnel to certify detainees for interrogation and provide medical supervision in interrogation facilities, in direct contravention of most international agreements as the medical community understands them, draw on similar arguments.

But do physicians act morally when they allow their duty to society to override their duty to their patients? There is no doubt that humanitarian law gives overriding weight to the rights, welfare, and dignity of individuals at the expense of the interests of the state or political community. Codes of medical ethics, too, remain dominated by an abiding injunction to "do no harm" and to protect patients' welfare; whether and how physicians' actions affect individuals other than their patients are often secondary questions. Increasingly, however, this outlook is beginning to change.

At the same time that the Tokyo Declaration proscribes torture and ill-treatment, it also prohibits physicians from force-feeding hunger-striking prisoners (World Medical Association, 1975).[7] This is an odd juxtaposition for such seemingly incommensurable harms, but each prohibition subordinates human life, whether of others or of the patients themselves, to the iron axioms of liberal bioethics: self-esteem, informed consent, respect for autonomy, and self-determination. As the duty of the state to safeguard life falls before the pillars of liberal morality, patients gain the right to forgo life-saving medical treatment and to obtain a physician's help to commit suicide. These are the logical outcomes of a medical ethic anchored in self-determination and respect for individual autonomy. They are the same principles that forbid force-feeding hunger strikers and prohibit torture, ill-treatment, and cruel, inhuman, or degrading punishment. The prohibition is absolute: there are no exceptions whatsoever for any emergency threatening collective well-being.

It is noteworthy that in recent years and in contexts other than war, reemergent communitarian concerns and soft paternalism have blunted an overriding concern for individual welfare. In some ways, the effect is local as the idea of the "patient" expands to include family and community. The decision to care for a critically ill neonate, for example, might depend on the financial, social, and emotional impact this has on other family members, a factor considered irrelevant if not immoral not long ago. Similarly, parents may deny hearing-impaired children cochlear implants in the interest of preserving the integrity of the Deaf community. In other cases, the effect is global, pushing beyond the family to society at large. Resource allocation, for instance, may demand that we restrict services to the elderly or certain classes of critically ill patients to preserve resources for the entire community (Callahan 1990; Emanuel 1991).

These trends devalue norms that trumpet individual interests and solidify claims to collective welfare. Physicians who force-feed hunger strikers knowingly violate their patients' dignity, and right to self-esteem and autonomy to save their lives (Glick 1997), just as those who provide medical care in detention facilities sacrifice the same liberal norms in the hope of saving the lives of others. This less liberal but increasingly communitarian perspective does not merely place an individual's life ahead of self-esteem and autonomy, but anchors a person's life in the integrity of the community. Failure to do whatever is possible to save the lives of these individuals rends the fabric of the entire community.

As an individual's responsibilities to collective well-being gain strength, a physician's duty to "do no harm" expands to embrace the interests of actors and entities beyond the individual patient. This allows, and may in fact demand, physicians to weigh the effects of their actions on others. A physician who is part of an interrogation team faced with a ticking bomb may consider the welfare of others beyond a single patient in trying to decide what to do. Collective interests focus on concern for the immediate safety of a large number of individuals and are oriented toward the long-term welfare of society. The moral duty of physicians rests on the prima facie obligation of any human being to bring about more good than harm when this does not entail unreasonable personal risk. In this case, all citizens, including physicians, must consider the harm done to every agent affected by their actions. If doctors remain convinced that interrogational torture could save more lives than other forms of interrogation, avoids unnecessary harm, and only targets those who have forfeited their right to respect for self-esteem, they may consider providing facilitating medical care during an interrogation. Then the physicians, like the interrogators, will have to defend themselves. They will have to convince their peers that physical force met the test of necessity and was the least harmful means available to secure a higher moral good, namely, the welfare of innocent people. If interrogators must defend themselves, so must physicians. Torture requires medical assistance, and the decision to use physical force always requires a physician's consent. Doctors, like investigators, are not simply acting under orders. They are part of the decision-making process and must later defend themselves in public.

There is no doubt that the position of the medical community depends, to a large degree, on the general assessment of the world community that torture is not justified. That is, a physician's first line of defense refutes the premise. If torture is not justified, then the question of a physician's participation is moot. Moreover, physicians have a duty, as does anyone else, to oppose torture when used for repressive purposes. If, on the other hand, ticking bombs make interrogational torture defensible in some instances, it is inconsistent to permit physicians to shun a facilitating role. No argument, however, denies the shame of torture.

The Shame of Torture

In his exhaustive study of torture, Edward Peters (1996, 178) ridicules the "classic" attempt to justify torture, one that hangs on "the possibility of the heroic, unemotional torturer in the service of the state on behalf of innocent victims," While it is true that the need to protect the lives of innocent victims sets the stage for interrogational torture, torture remains subject to strict conditions: grave threats, properly identified subjects, quality intelligence, the efficacy of physical pressure, and the lack of alternative means of avoiding catastrophe. These conditions will limit interrogational torture to exceptional circumstances and ensure that it is almost never the case that torture is the least harmful means to secure a supremely important moral goal.

None of this, however, makes the torturer heroic or unemotional. Because of the horrific nature of terror, many reasonable individuals grasp both the need and the shame of torture: needed for safety and security, shameful because torture compels us to divest others of their moral status as human beings. The extenuating circumstances that make interrogational torture defensible, however, carry no weight with the world community, and the UN expressly rejects them. From an atomistic, individualistic perspective, this makes sense. The modern state, constituted primarily to protect the civil liberties of its inhabitants, loses its raison d'être when it grossly offends a person's dignity and self-esteem. But protecting self-esteem, however significant a primary good it is, is not always the overriding function of every state, and some liberal states may subordinate some individual interests to the common good. Defensible interrogational torture, like force-feeding or coerced medical treatment, mirrors this concern. In these cases, the onus cannot rest entirely on interrogators or on facilitating physicians, or on some hardened core of security agents. The duty to confront the horror of torture is the burden of all citizens. No one can say he or she did not know. This plays out as interrogators, no less than physicians, must defend themselves publicly so the community may hear them out and pass judgment.

In extreme circumstances, interrogational torture and ill-treatment tests a physician's intuitions, her duty to her patient, and her obligations to the state. In the wake of indiscriminate terror, liberal democratic states are sitting on the horns of a dilemma that places life and well-being against respect for self-esteem. Unlike questions of assisted suicide or force-feeding, it is not the life and self-esteem of the same person that is at stake, but the lives of some and the self-esteem of others. These circumstances upset the traditional doctor-patient relationship, which rarely considers interests beyond those of the individuals physicians must treat. The threat of terror, however, throws this traditional perspective into disarray, as fidelity to the principles of beneficence and nonmaleficence may harm others. A similar predicament arises when physicians are called on to develop biological and chemical weaponry.

8

Chemical and Biological Warfare

It is the privilege of the medical doctor to practice medicine in the service of humanity, to preserve and restore bodily and mental health without distinction as to persons, to comfort and ease the suffering of his or her patients. The utmost respect for human life is to be maintained even under threat, and no use made of any medical knowledge contrary to the laws of humanity.

Therefore, the World Medical Association considers that it would be unethical for the physician, whose mission is to provide health care, to participate in the research and development of chemical and biological weapons, and to use his or her personal and scientific knowledge in the conception and manufacture of such weapons.

—World Medical Association 1990

The World Medical Association's (WMA) 1990 Declaration offers an appropriate starting point for investigating bioethics and the development of chemical and biological (CB) weapons. Underlying this declaration are a number of claims that speak to the physician's role and duties as a healer, the laws of humanity, and the permissible limits of participating in the development of CB weapons in a hostile international environment.

Historically, chemical and biological warfare (CBW) was the subject of reciprocal agreements rather than humanitarian norms, because early conventions banning chemical and biological warfare permitted retaliation in kind. Fears of first strikes coupled with the right to retaliate raised claims then, and continue to raise them now, that some nations require a deterrent capability in parts of the world where warring nations have not agreed to dismantle their CB arsenals. Yet any attempt to permit nations to develop a deterrent capability must confront the compelling claim that CB weapons cause "unnecessary suffering and superfluous injury" and/or constitute weapons of mass destruction. As such, CB weapons contravene the laws of humanity regardless of any strategic value they afford. While this claim underlies the WMA Declaration, it remains the subject of more than a century of debate, especially as one contemplates the unique ethical challenges that new generations of nonlethal weapons pose.

CBW creates overwhelming tension between military necessity and humanitarian obligations, particularly from the standpoint of the ever-increasing need to rely on medical expertise to develop chemical and biological weapons. Beginning with the First World War, nations first developed CB weapons for their offensive potential, later for their defensive and deterrent capabilities, and most recently for their nonlethal capabilities. Supporters of CB weaponry invoke both the military necessity of deploying chemical and biological weaponry and the prospect that these weapons may advance rather than retard the humanity of modern warfare. Regardless of how one assesses these arguments, some of which carry weight in certain geopolitical circumstances, the WMA unequivocally prohibits physicians from participating in the development of CB weapons in any way. In doing so, the WMA leans heavily on what it characterizes as humanitarian obligations and, indeed, these are often overwhelming. The very idea of physicians contributing to the development of weapons of any kind is problematic, for every sort of chemical or biological weapon utilizes medicine to harm rather than heal. For this reason alone, it seems reasonable to conclude that a physician's duty to shun chemical and biological weapons remains absolute.

This discussion opens with an overview of chemical and biological warfare and the attempts of the international community to control each type of weapon. The discussion then turns to the ethical arguments that underlie support of and opposition to CBW since its first appearance in World War I. Opponents of CBW emphasize the very long-standing aversion to poisoned weapons, the century and a half–long drive to banish weapons that cause unnecessary suffering or superfluous injury, and recent attempts to control indiscriminate weapons of mass destruction. Proponents underscore the deterrent value of chemical and biological weapons—an argument reinforced by the behavior of the belligerents in World War II—and the emerging value of nonlethal weapons to fight low-intensity wars in the post–Cold War era. If mutual deterrence held the superpowers at bay, nonlethal weapons offer the possibility that warfare in built-up civilian areas might bring far less devastation than using high explosives, however "smart" they are. Not all of these arguments are as relevant today as they were during the Cold War. Deterrence survives only in those parts of the world, particularly the Middle East, where adversaries have not ratified the conventions against CBW. For the rest of the world, however, nonlethal weapons—including chemical and biological incapacitating agents, acoustical munitions, and optical weapons—pose a more significant challenge. Deterrence and nonlethal CB weapons present hard dilemmas for physicians who stake their professional duty on beneficence and nonmaleficence.

Historical Overview

It did not take long to realize that if medicine can cure, it can also kill. If, prior to the twentieth century, disease posed the greatest danger to the health of a nation's armed forces, it stood to reason that once effectively harnessed, infectious diseases might also prove war's most effective weapon. History, therefore, is dotted with stories of armies poisoning one another's wells, catapulting the plague-ridden carcasses of farm animals into besieged towns, and leaving disease-infested garments or blankets to decimate enemy ranks (Wheelis 1999). In periods when the mechanics of disease transmission were not understood, these tactics were not always successful, nor, when they were, were they easy to control. By World War I, however, the idea of using bacteria, germs, plague, and noxious chemicals to kill or injure one's enemy had taken hold.

Prior to World War I, the specter of chemical weaponry together with the havoc many military planners feared it would wreak on the battlefield led the European nations to prohibit the "use of projectiles the sole object of which is the diffusion of asphyxiating or deleterious gases" (Hague Convention, 1899, Declaration IV, 2). In April 1915, the Germans promptly violated the ban and gas warfare remained a major feature of the First World War. While there was little moral compunction about using gas in the trenches, poison gas did not allow either side to mount a decisive offensive or quickly end the stalemate on the

Western front. Rather, gas was an attritional weapon, far more incapacitating than lethal, but readily sowing fear among troops while
forcing soldiers to don burdensome suits and masks simply to hold their
positions.[1]

Following the war and in response to concerns that chemical weapons
are difficult to control, impede military efficiency, threaten civilians, and
inflict fearsome suffering, the Western powers (with the important exception of the United States) again banned chemical weapons, together with
fledging "bacteriological" weapons, in 1925 (Stockholm International
Peace Research Institute, 1971–1975, vol. 1, 250; Jones 1980; Slotten
1990). The ban was not absolute, because most nations reserved the right
to retaliate against belligerents who initiated chemical warfare (Sims
1987). The Protocol, therefore, only banned the *first use* of chemical
weapons among its signatories. It did not prohibit the research, development, or stockpiling of weapons or the right to retaliate in kind, and
by World War II, France, Britain, Germany, Russia, Japan, and the
United States made significant strides in chemical-weapons development.
As France and Britain refined and stockpiled armaments filled with chlo-
rine, phosgene (choking gases), mustard gas, and Lewisite (blistering
agents), the Germans were developing potent forms of nerve gas. Considerably more lethal than either choking gases or blistering agents, small
amounts of nerve gas inhibit the action of enzymes that regulate muscle
behavior. Without medical treatment, victims die of respiratory failure.
During the interwar period, Britain, Japan, and France would allegedly
employ poison gas to suppress unrest in their colonial territories,
while Italy used mustard gas to rout Ethiopian troops hiding in
caves (Stockholm International Peace Research Institute, 1971–1975,
vol. 1, 141–146; Croddy 2002; Harris and Paxman 2002, 45–52).

Although both sides entered World War II with large stockpiles of
chemical weapons and worked aggressively to develop increasingly lethal
weapons during the war, neither side deployed them. The nonuse of CB
weapons in World War II is one of the most impressive displays of mutual
deterrence during war and owes its success to a variety of military and
nonmilitary circumstances (van Courtland Moon 1984; Harris and
Paxton 2002). Despite the role gas played in the First World War, military commanders never warmed to the use of chemical weapons. Weather

dependent, chemical weapons were unpredictable, logistically complex, and offered only questionable superiority if enemy defenses were difficult to overcome. Nevertheless, and on rare occasions, both Allied and Axis commanders considered chemical warfare (CW) to reduce their casualties during fierce fighting in France and in the Pacific. In each instance, however, military leaders balked, fearing the military disadvantage of fighting a chemical war for which they were ill-prepared, as well as the prospect of gas attacks on vulnerable civilian populations (Stockholm International Peace Research Institute, 1971–1975, vol. 1, 294–335; van Courtland Moon 1984, 1989). Interestingly, each side grossly miscalculated the other's CB capabilities. Contrary to what the Germans believed certain, the Allies never developed nerve gas during the war. The Allies, on the other hand, were astonished to discover that the Germans had no biological warfare (BW) capability whatsoever.

Unlike the Germans, however, the Japanese diligently pursued biological warfare. In contrast to chemical weapons, biological weapons utilize living microorganisms or toxins to infect or poison their target. Biological agents may be lethal or incapacitating, contagious or noncontagious, and directed against plants, animals, or humans. Toxins include ricin and botulinum toxoid (BT). As much as 100,000 times more powerful than sarin nerve gas, BT blocks neurotransmitters, inducing paralysis and respiratory failure. Living organisms include infectious bacteria such as anthrax, plague, glanders, cholera, and tularemia as well as such virulent viruses as smallpox (Wright 1985; Croddy 2002, 204–216). To develop and test their weapons, the Japanese erected a notorious facility in China. The horrors of this facility, the infamous Unit 731 in Ping Fan, rivaled Nazi medical experiments. Researchers injected toxins and biological agents into live subjects, vivisected patients to study the effect of infection on the human body, and tested biological weapons in populated areas. Nevertheless, the Japanese never produced an effective biological weapon. At the war's end, Ishii Shiro, a medical doctor by training and director of Japan's BW program, escaped trial for war crimes by agreeing to make his data, which proved relatively useless, available to the United States (Harris 1999; van Courtland Moon 1999; Moreno 2001, 104–114).

In Britain, researchers turned to weaponizing anthrax and BT and soon raised a number of incipient questions that thrust medical personnel to the forefront of weapons development:

Paul Fildes [director of BW research at Porton Down in Britain during World War II] consulted with the Porton staff on the means whereby chemical warfare agents could be disseminated from weapons and then considered how such means could be applied to BW. Obviously, the respiratory tract was the best portal for the entry of micro-organisms into the body in the BW context. While the gastrointestinal tract was eminently susceptible to infection by a considerable number of pathogens, the military use of food and water contamination in biological warfare was considered to be logistically complex. . . . The eyes and skin were not particularly vulnerable, unlike the situation in chemical warfare. Clearly, the possibility that a biological warfare agent could be aerosolized from a munition or spray, and be shown to initiate an infection through the respiratory tract, was the best basis for assessing the reality of biological warfare. (Carter and Pearson 1999, 176)

Relying on medical expertise, research proceeded apace, and by the end of the war Britain had developed and tested prototypes of anthrax cluster bombs, 100–1,000 times more potent that any comparable chemical weapon. Lacking resources for large-scale production, the British ordered a half million antipersonnel anthrax bombs from the United States to use should Germany initiate biological warfare. This order was never filled, but in 1943 the British stockpiled five million anthrax-laced cakes they manufactured to infect livestock and destroy Germany's food supply.

Following World War II, chemical and biological weapons lost some of their luster as the major powers focused their efforts on nuclear weapons. Nevertheless, they continued to develop and stockpile chemical and biological weapons but in the absence of any well-developed strategy of mutually assured destruction, the superpowers could only stake their deterrence policy on massive stores of CB weapons, small numbers of specially trained troops, and crude means of delivery (Christopher et al. 1999; Balmer 2002). At the same time, unlike nuclear weapons, CB weapons, proved vulnerable to effective defensive measures, forcing researchers to develop antidotes, gas masks, warning devices, and protective suits. Aware of these limitations, the United States unilaterally decided to destroy its stock of biological weapons in 1969 and limit its chemical-weapons programs in an effort to jump-start arms-limitation talks with the Russians. These measures induced the Soviets to accept biological-weapons disarmament and, by 1972, most nations ratified the Biological Weapons Convention, (BWC) agreeing "never in any circumstances to develop, produce, stockpile or otherwise acquire or retain" biological weapons (Biological Weapons Convention, 1972, Article 1). With the ratification of the Chemical Weapons Convention (CWC) in 1993, the United States halted offensive-weapons research and committed itself to destroying its chemical arsenal by 2007. Lack of funds hampers similar commitments by Russia.

Throughout the twentieth century, physicians participated in the development of chemical and biological weapons as part of the scientific staff at facilities in Britain, the United States, Japan, Germany, and the Soviet Union (Rosebury 1949, 1963; Handelman and Alibek 2000, 252; Moreno 2001, 126, 192–198, 203ff.; Hammond and Carter 2002, 221). Following the conventions prohibiting CB weapons, medical scientists today play a central role in the development of "defensive" and "nonlethal" chemical weapons. Moreover, there are a number of nations, particularly in the Mideast, that have not ratified either convention banning CBW, continue to stockpile weapons, and call on medical personnel to lend a hand in the development of CB weapons in much the same way as their Cold War–era colleagues (Croddy 2002, 23–35, 43–50).

In spite of, or perhaps because of, these developments, the international community and the World Medical Association in particular condemn chemical and biological weapons as "contrary to the laws of humanity." In doing so, the WMA prohibits physicians from participating in the development of chemical and biological weapons or using their scientific knowledge to build such weapons. The laws of humanity, therefore, are the first line of defense for medical workers contemplating the development of unconventional or nonlethal weaponry. If chemical or biological weapons indisputably violate humanitarian law, then the argument stops here. There are no grounds for thinking that physicians or anyone else may build CB weapons for any purpose whatsoever. Yet a careful look at the laws of humanity that govern chemical and biological weapons, together with the need for deterrence in some parts of the world and the promise of nonlethal weapons in others, brings us to reconsider whether unconventional weaponry remains beyond the domain of medical participation.

The Inhumanity of Chemical and Biological Weapons

The laws of humanity prohibiting chemical and biological warfare reflect three distinct concerns: ancient prohibitions against using poison during war, nineteenth-century hopes to avoid weapons that inflict unnecessary suffering and superfluous injury, and twentieth-century fears of annihilation at the hands of weapons of mass destruction (Stockholm International Peace Research Institute, 1971–1975, vol. 3, 90–99).

CB Weapons and Poison

The long-standing prohibition against using poison in warfare reflects the repugnance toward a weapon that is treacherous. Like treachery, poison is a "concealed" weapon, transported in stealth and secrecy, and a popular means of assassination: the archetype of "perfidious" warfare.[2] Morally repugnant in their own right, perfidious weapons also undermine the fragile trust necessary to ensure the conventions of war. Agents carrying and using weapons covertly, whether emissaries ostensibly on peace missions or soldiers who lay down their arms only to attack their unsuspecting captors, jeopardize conventions of safe passage, peace negotiations, and surrender so necessary to end war short of total annihilation.

Chemical weapons are tarred with the same stigma of any poison and, as such, remain beyond the pale of civilized warfare. It is important to note, however, that the aversion to poison rests not on the way it kills, but on how it is used. Chemical and biological weapons, therefore, are not perfidious in the same way as poison. Far from using them covertly, adversaries deploy CB weapons openly and in ways that allow detection and enable soldiers to take protective measures. In spite of the occasional attempt to assassinate political dissidents with bacteriological agents, CBW remains a doctrine of open warfare. Recognizing that the ban on perfidy would do little to dissuade belligerents from employing CB weapons, lawmakers did well to invoke the principle of unnecessary suffering. Chemical weapons are unlawful and repugnant not because of the way they are deployed in battle but, primarily, in light of the way they kill.

CB Weapons, Unnecessary Suffering, and Superfluous Injury

The Geneva Conventions make their point clearly:

In any armed conflict, the right of the Parties to the conflict to choose methods or means of warfare is not unlimited.

It is prohibited to employ weapons, projectiles and material and methods of warfare of a nature to cause superfluous injury or unnecessary suffering. (Protocol I, 1977a, Article 35)

Of particular concern to any scientist is the prospect that weapons that require their expertise will cause unnecessary suffering. "Unnecessary suffering" is a function of both military and medical criteria. Militarily, the emphasis falls on *unnecessary* suffering and connotes any means beyond those required to disable or disarm enemy combatants, rendering them unable to fight and no longer a threat. The means necessary to disable adversaries are, however, situationally dependent. In some cases, one may inflict great harm and suffering to dislodge a well-entrenched or particularly tenacious enemy, while at other times anything beyond minimal force may be unnecessary. Unnecessary suffering, in this sense, has no bearing on the level of pain combatants may suffer. On the other hand, unnecessary suffering also connotes "unbearable" or "frightful" suffering. Asphyxiating gas, often deployed with the intent to incapacitate and disable rather than kill, is "unnecessary" if it causes appalling suffering regardless of its military benefit. In this sense, the emphasis falls on unnecessary *suffering* and precludes intense suffering whether necessary to disarm an enemy or not.

Finding it difficult to define "unnecessary suffering" with any precision, most international conventions make do with prohibitions on certain kinds of weapons: dumdum bullets, poisoned weapons, asphyxiating gas, bayonets with serrated edges, and lances with barbed tips. But without clear criteria for defining the limits of unnecessary suffering, it is increasingly difficult to formulate workable guidelines to govern permissible forms of warfare and weapons development. To remedy this difficulty, the International Committee of the Red Cross (ICRC) has sought objective measures by proposing that any harm or suffering

beyond that which ordinarily occurs in conventional warfare is unnecessary and superfluous. Based on data similar to those presented in
chapter 3, the ICRC recommends that weapons cause "superfluous
injury and unnecessary suffering" when they bring about:

1. Specific disease, specific abnormal physiological state, specific abnormal
psychological state, specific and permanent disability or specific disfigurement,
or
2. Field mortality of more than 25 percent or hospital mortality of more than 5
percent, or
3. Grade 3 wounds as measured by the Red Cross wound classification.
4. Effects for which there is no "well recognized and proved treatment." (Coupland 1991, 1996, 1997a, 1999; International Committee of the Red Cross,
1997, 23)[3]

The last requirement is reminiscent of the "fighting-chance" argument
that guides conventional warfare: soldiers should have a reasonable
chance to repel an attack and recover from the injuries they suffer.
Weapons of mass destruction, together with those inflicting novel diseases, belie this condition.

These guidelines are not without conceptual difficulties. The
proposal contains two criteria to judge unnecessary suffering and superfluous injury. One criterion is quantitative and based on the combined
casualty rates of conventional war. The other is qualitative, based on
the ICRC's understanding that weapons should not kill or maim in
certain ways. But these criteria beg the question: Why is the suffering
of conventional war an adequate baseline? Robin Coupland, principal
architect of the ICRC guidelines, argues that the ICRC criteria are
ultimately based on what "most people" are prepared to accept in
the context of conventional war. Most people will not accept, on this
view, a combined casualty rate in excess of 30 percent or weapons
that cause lingering death, disease, disfigurement, or severe disability.
But why is this so? Are these kinds of death somehow worse than those
that other weapons cause, or is it simply that most people accept this
as inevitable, inured, as it were, to a certain level of pain and suffering
that is caused, perhaps necessarily, by the way most nations choose to
wage war?

Unless one assumes that the casualties caused by conventional
weaponry represent, by definition, the minimal harm necessary to pursue

the just aims of war, the ICRC criteria are unrelated to military necessity. Regardless of the potential benefit some weapons bring in certain situations, those that cause the kind of harm outlined in the proposal remain prohibited. Ultimately, the ICRC proposal turns on a vague understanding of suffering and injury that is inhuman and beyond that which people should have to bear as they wage a just war. Yet criteria are clearly elusive. To identify unnecessary suffering and superfluous injury with what "most people" accept assumes that most people, on careful reflection, will tolerate the harm that conventional war causes. Some may not, while those that do probably tell themselves that this harm is militarily necessary. But once unnecessary suffering is linked again to military necessity, none of the criteria suggested by the ICRC are absolute in the way it wishes. Instead, the criteria will change relative to military needs. As such, there will be times when a 30 percent casualty rate is too high, and other times when it is too low.

Avoiding relativism returns us to a vague criterion of inhuman, excessive, or unbearable suffering. This is apparent from the first criterion the ICRC proposes, which from a bioethical perspective might be the most important: any weapon causing *disease* inflicts, by definition, unnecessary suffering and superfluous injury. Unlike the other criteria, which designate varying degrees of harm, disease draws our attention to the physiological processes or, more generally, the *means* that injure a healthy person, irrespective of the harm it ultimately causes. This viewpoint is probably widespread, and it underlies the prohibition of poison as well as chemical and particularly biological weapons. But it is not an outcome-oriented, quantitative argument. CBW, by many accounts, will kill far less than one in three of those affected.[4] Nor does it necessarily cause a lingering death, permanent disability, or disfigurement. Detection and protection also offer combatants a fighting chance to survive. Nevertheless, Coupland (1996), writes, "*Most people* consider warfare waged with weapons developed in laboratories by biomedical scientists unacceptable. ... The primary effect [of weapons] should not be to target a specific part of the human anatomy, physiology or biochemistry." The repugnance associated with biological weapons echoes Martin van Creveld's (1991, 85–87) observation that "the distinction between chemical and other weapons exists solely in man's mind"; and reflects a "cultural" aversion to killing people by choking them to death. The aversion to killing by disease runs deeper still. Anchored, perhaps, in a primordial fear of disease or a genuine concern about tampering with the physiological systems of the human body, armed adversaries remain wary about using poison, pathogens, and toxins to disable enemy combatants.

These fears forge a sharp contrast between killing by illness and killing by injury that warrants closer scrutiny. Both illness and injury harm individuals in the same way, either by killing or by impairing physiological functions. Both bullets and bacteria are sometimes, but not always, amenable to treatment and/or protection. What difference there is, if any, may stem from the role that physicians play in illness but not injury. While physicians are called on to cure both, they can only inflict disease. This casts a pall over the role we commonly cede to physicians as heathcare providers. Weapons that bring death by disease may require physicians to act maleficently, a dissonance modern society may be unable to bear. "It is a crime against humanity," wrote Professor Pfeiffer of the University of Breslau to the League of Nations in 1923, "to think even of attempting to use the achievements of modern medical science for the destruction of life and health" (Stockholm International Peace Research Institute, 1971–1975, vol. 4, 54). While using medical expertise for weapons development certainly presents formidable problems for the medical profession, a claim I will take up as I consider the role medicine plays in the development of nonlethal weaponry, it certainly does not follow that it is a crime against humanity. Using disease or chemical compounds developed with medical expertise to inflict illness is not qualitatively different from using high explosives to inflict injury and unless they breach the quantitative measures that define unnecessary suffering, neither violates the laws of humanity. Therefore, scientists and physicians should be free to develop both, unless the CB weapons pose the threat of mass destruction.

CB Weapons and Mass Destruction

Neither the Biological nor Chemical Weapons Convention refers to poison or unnecessary suffering when they prohibit the development of each type of weapon. Instead, each strives to eliminate "all types of weapons of mass destruction." "Mass destruction" calls to mind a dimension of devastation that is somehow distinct from that caused by high explosives. Most obviously, mass destruction is associated with nuclear war and denotes "total" destruction, in this case, of the entire human race. Any weapon capable of such devastation contravenes, by definition, the laws of humanity. The specter of CBW, particularly biological warfare and the deadly pathogens it weaponizes, often presents this image because it holds the potential to cause vast numbers of military and nonmilitary deaths that far exceed anything necessary to disable an enemy. The issue is not unnecessary suffering, but unnecessary death.

Nevertheless, various means of defense that are unavailable in nuclear war—vaccines, antidotes, gas masks, and sealed rooms—can mitigate the devastation of chemical and biological warfare. "Mass destruction," then, does not necessarily mean "total annihilation" but signifies the "indiscriminate harm" noncombatants will suffer should belligerents lose control of their CB weapons or decide to target civilians intentionally. In nations with well-developed civil defense systems, the devastation unleashed by CBW may be no more than the overwhelming destruction that high explosives, incendiary devices, and other means of modern warfare can inflict on combatants and noncombatants alike (Steinberg 1993). The threat of chemical or biological war has then led some nations to consider the merits of deterrence.

Deterring Chemical and Biological War In spite of, or again because of, the deep-seated repugnance and destructiveness associated with CB weapons, many nations have found cause to develop, and later abandon, the means to deter others from starting a chemical or biological war. The success of mutual chemical and biological deterrence during World War II offered compelling grounds for maintaining an unconventional arsenal in the postwar years. But as development continued, there were growing misgivings about the tactical value of chemical and biological weapons, their use during battle, and fear of accidents during manufacture and delivery (Harris and Paxman 2002, 222). Moreover, the superpowers realized that deterrence would remain unaffected by chemical and biological disarmament if nuclear weapons could fulfill the promise of retaliation should another nation start an unconventional war. Once the

United States decided to disarm unilaterally, the major parties of the then-ending Cold War agreed to ratify the Biological and Chemical Weapons Conventions and destroy their stockpiles of CB weapons.

The picture remains less rosy in the Middle East. None of the parties to the Mideast conflict has ratified either the Chemical or Biological Weapons Convention and each continues to develop and stockpile chemical and biological weapons. Relying on the experience of World War II, Israel, Egypt, and Syria each expects to deter the other from the first use of chemical and/or biological weapons by posing a credible threat and developing passive (gas masks, vaccines, and sealed rooms) and active (anti–ballistic missile systems) defenses. Israel's nuclear program complicates matters further. In a twist of Cold War logic that led many to hope that nuclear weapons might deter others from using chemical and biological weapons, some Mideast nations have adopted the opposite strategy. Unable to match Israel's resources to develop and deploy nuclear weapons, Egypt and Syria pursue the "poor-man's" option and turn to chemical and biological weapons to deter Israel from ever using nuclear weapons (Barak 2003). More significantly, both the Chemical and Biological Weapons Conventions allow any nation to withdraw from its provisions when "extraordinary events have jeopardized the supreme interests of its country" (Biological Weapons Convention, 1972, Article 13; Chemical Weapons Convention, 1993, Article 16). As a result, parties to the Middle East conflict, as well as any other nation threatened by extraordinary events, will continue to develop CB weapons to protect vital national interests. And, as they do, they will call on the medical community to provide expertise. Given the exigencies of the Mideast, do chemical and biological weapons developed for *deterrent* purposes violate the laws of humanity?

The Ethics of Unconventional Deterrence   An effective deterrent policy demands a credible threat to retaliate in kind and raises difficult ethical issues for any citizen regardless of profession. To adequately protect one's own assets, a deterrent force must be capable of targeting both civilian and military targets. While retaliatory strikes against military targets are no cause for special moral concern, there are considerable misgivings about threatening civilians. If civilians are not proper targets—that is, if one may not intentionally harm them—how then may one *threaten* to harm them? The horns of this dilemma weigh military necessity and humanitarian imperatives. From the perspective of humanitarian norms one must ask whether anyone can ever threaten a civilian population with mass destruction—that is, intend to violate the principle of noncombatant immunity by deliberately killing large numbers of noncombatants should one's adversary launch a nuclear, chemical, or biological attack. The debate over the morality of deterrence has persisted since mutually assured destruction first guided American and Soviet policy during the Cold War. These arguments also bear on the ethics of biological and chemical deterrence and, at the same time, on the participation of physicians and other medical personnel.

Opponents of nuclear deterrence focus on the utter immorality of a policy that not only contemplates, but also formulates plans to destroy civilian population centers in retaliation for an unconventional first strike. Stated in this way, the argument ignores the effectiveness of deterrence and focuses solely on the intentions of armed adversaries to harm noncombatants. Nuclear, chemical, or biological deterrence, argue its opponents, requires its advocates to threaten noncombatants with egregious harm and, thereby, act in a way that is grossly immoral. In its most unyielding form, the argument is rigidly deontological, refusing to weigh potentially beneficial consequences and highlighting instead the immorality of the actors' intentions. Targeting noncombatants, like intentionally harming them, is always evil and indefensible regardless of any benefits it may bring.

To work around this problem and support unconventional deterrence nonetheless, some deontologists claim that policymakers do not, in fact, target civilians. This argument falls back on the doctrine of double effect, suggesting that nuclear war threatens civilians with massive *collateral* damage. While no one intends to target civilians directly, they nonetheless face annihilation due to the indiscriminate nature of nuclear weapons. An alternative approach delves into the nature of the threat itself, suggesting that the intent to use nuclear weapons is sufficiently improbable that it sheds much of its moral repugnance. By this reasoning, successful deterrence does not require any firm intention to ever use nuclear weapons. Instead, policymakers may get by with vague, unformed intentions about what they will do in the future, or may bluff with no intention whatsoever to use nuclear weapons against civilian populations. Unfortunately, by appealing to the subjective aspect of intentionality, these claims invoke empirical arguments difficult to test: an experienced bluffer would be hard to ferret out, while half-formed intentions would be difficult to define, much less ascertain, with any precision (Walzer 1977, 269–283; Blake and Pole 1984; "Symposium on Ethics and Nuclear Deterrence," 1985; Coady 1988; McMahan 1988).

Nevertheless, there are theoretical teeth to this argument. While some suggest that a viable policy of deterrence absolutely requires the firm intention to use atomic, biological, or chemical weapons on the assumption that any equivocation shatters the credible threat that successful deterrence must project, one might consider many cases where firm intentions are not necessary. Given the utter destructiveness of nuclear weapons—that is, the overwhelming magnitude of the threat—it is sensible to suppose that the reasonable or even relatively weak prospect that one's opponent will deploy weapons of mass destruction is sufficient to maintain a deterrent capability. In other words, when a potential response is sufficiently devastating, the likelihood it will occur need not be great to sustain a rational decision to desist from a first strike. This clearly applies to nuclear deterrence; whether it applies to chemical and biological deterrence remains a matter of speculation. Although casualties from CBW can be staggering, there remain relatively effective measures to protect military personnel and civilian populations (Stockholm International Peace Research Institute, 1971–1975, vol. 3, 139). Nevertheless, casualties are sufficiently catastrophic to keep opponents at bay. Under these circumstances, a policy of successful deterrence does not necessarily require the firm intentions that deontologists attribute to actors.

Apart from deontological arguments, of course, one can evaluate deterrence on utilitarian grounds. Some utilitarians take note of the deontological quandary that actors face but simply set it aside as the lesser of two evils. Agents of deterrence may harbor immoral intentions but act to avoid a greater calamity. At the end of the day, targeting civilians enforces the ban on nuclear weapons. This forces a tragic choice to be sure, but a choice that nonetheless offers a superior alternative to unconventional war. Nevertheless, the same assessment of magnitude and probability that plagues deontological claims may also undermine consequentialist arguments. Deterrence is a morally superior doctrine because it works. Deterrence effectively prevents nuclear, chemical, and biological warfare at little cost, while the chances that it will fail are very small. But there is always some risk, and given the magnitude of the harm that failure will bring, the same combination of risk and magnitude that leads one adversary to deter another may also lead others, particularly those most risk aversive, to understand that any risk makes it too dangerous to play around with nuclear weapons. Although deterrence has worked, it remains an excessive risk—not because the probability of failure is high, but because any chance of failure, however slight, has catastrophic consequences. Deterrence, therefore, may be a very bad way to prevent nuclear war. Its pitfalls demand that rational actors seek other avenues to forestall nuclear conflict.

Finally, one may justify deterrence conditionally, aware that it is sometimes necessary to pursue a path one ultimately hopes to abandon. Advocates of "extrication" or "disentanglement" readily acknowledge the immorality of threatening civilians but likewise recognize that unilateral disarmament is fraught with overwhelming logistical complexities that may imperil a nation's security. One answer speaks to a policy of "finite" deterrence that demands progressively deeper cuts in unconventional arsenals while maintaining a limited deterrent capability that may continue to target civilian populations. Finite deterrence aims to slowly extricate adversaries from the quagmire of deterrence and proliferation. While force reductions remain the order of the day, adversaries may find it necessary to produce increasingly sophisticated or specialized weapons to maintain the deterrent capability they are not yet ready to renounce (Coady 1989).

CB Weapons and the Laws of Humanity: An Assessment
While the laws of humanity unequivocally condemn unconventional *warfare*, they do not offer an airtight defense against the development

of chemical or biological *weapons*. Weapons of mass destruction that include not only chemical and biological weapons in nations that have not ratified the Biological and Chemical Weapons Conventions, but also nuclear weapons currently on hand in some nations, are legitimate deterrent capabilities that do not violate the laws of humanity. Nor are less destructive weapons similarly proscribed simply because they "target a specific part of the human anatomy, physiology or biochemistry." Instead, these weapons—along with any others—must stand the test of humanitarian law and the laws of armed conflict that prohibit weapons that cause indiscriminate harm, unnecessary suffering, and superfluous injury. Nonlethal weapons, including those that employ chemical compounds (which I will consider shortly), do not necessarily violate these injunctions. Prompted by changing modes of warfare that place battles in close proximity to civilian populations, military planners recognize how conventional weapons may easily inflict disproportionate harm on noncombatants. Whether nonlethal weapons provide an answer for reducing the devastation of modern war remains at the center of a debate that cannot help but draw the medical community into the process of weapons development.

Physicians and other medical personnel who find themselves called on to contribute to the development of nonlethal weapons or of an unconventional deterrent capability cannot refuse, as the WMA strongly suggests, because these weapons violate the laws of humanity. This argument is too weak. The laws of humanity do not support a position, like the WMA's, that demands that medical workers unconditionally refuse to support arms development. Nevertheless, members of the medical community may certainly invoke their professional obligation to do no harm and so preclude participation in the development of unconventional weapons regardless of their military value. Here, as in many other cases, they run up against their civic obligations to support a just war. This raises two distinct questions. First, does weapons development necessarily violate a physician's obligation to do no harm? This question arises in the context of deterrence. Second, do doctors' professional obligations override their civic obligations? This question dogs the development of nonlethal weaponry and raises the specter of pacifism, a discussion that will carry through to the next chapter.

Bioethics and Unconventional Deterrence

Arguments supporting and opposing nuclear deterrence also bear on the ethics of chemical and biological deterrence. For now, the Chemical and Biological Weapons Conventions render the question of deterrence largely moot. The threat to many nations comes from attacks by terrorists or other nonstate actors, for whom the threat of retaliation deters no one. In the Mideast, however, the story is different. Here deterrence works precisely because it threatens civilians. Egypt and Syria maintain chemical and biological weapons to offset Israel's nuclear threat. Israel maintains a nuclear capability to forestall the threat of genocide it fears from the Arab nations. A concerned citizen in any of these nations will weigh an argument supporting deterrence against other moral principles that he or she holds dear. In many cases, the arguments noted above will persuade most individuals that an effective policy of deterrence based on the intention to harm innocent civilians is justified to prevent a greater catastrophe. Some individuals may find that the moral gravity of threatening harm to civilians pales beside the prospect of a chemical or biological attack. Others will remain unsettled by the sheer injustice of threatening innocents but will back down in the face of a greater evil. Still others may accept the argument that deterrence, however morally objectionable, ultimately paves the way for disarmament.

Individuals accepting any of these arguments will support a policy of CB deterrence and lend a hand when they possess the expertise to do so. Others will oppose deterrence that threatens civilians with weapons of mass destruction. They will recoil at the thought of intending to harm tens of thousands of innocent civilians. Instead, they may formulate a policy of nuclear deterrence aimed at military targets to deter chemical warfare or do their best to convince their governments that disarmament is the only moral route open to a progressive nation. Adopting any or all of these arguments, they will distance themselves from the development of CB weapons and/or engage in acts of civil disobedience if ordered to participate.

The moral principles that may motivate an individual to oppose chemical and biological deterrence reflect respect for international law and/or humanitarian norms of noncombatant immunity. These principles, however, have little to do with the principles of medical ethics described in chapter 2. Bioethics does not offer any *unique* reason for those practicing medicine to oppose CB weapons development, apart from the humanitarian reasons and general philosophical arguments just described. Why, then, do some organizations, such as the WMA, suggest that there are *special* obligations for health-care professionals to avoid chemical and biological weapons research? The WMA specifically cites humanitarian reasons for its prohibition. Yet if there are good reasons to claim, as proponents of deterrence often do, that deterrence does not violate humanitarian norms, then much of the WMA's argument collapses. Engaging in unconventional weapons research to produce a credible deterrent capability does not necessarily violate the laws of humanity.

At this juncture, one must ask whether bioethics offers physicians an argument to oppose CB weapons unrelated to humanitarian law. Here, one might look to the principle of nonmaleficence and demand that physicians, who may support deterrence on other grounds, should nevertheless shun unconventional weapons development because it violates their professional commitment to do no harm. The imperative to do no harm clearly seems to place health-care professionals in a quandary, creating an overwhelming dilemma for those who may reasonably support a policy in which they can take no part. To work through this dilemma, it is first important to understand what the argument from nonmaleficence looks like and, second, why it fails.

Deterrence and the Principle of Nonmaleficence

Nonmaleficence, the principle to do no harm, is one of the oldest norms of medical ethics. Clear to many as a principle that forbids physicians to harm their patients when this harm serves no therapeutic benefit, the norm of nonmaleficence is inherent in the meaning of health care and incumbent on any health-care provider. This makes it easy for the WMA to argue from a premise stipulating the physician's "mission to provide health care" to the conclusion that "it is unethical to participate in the research and development of chemical and biological weapons." But the argument is not so straightforward. The principle of nonmaleficence retains sufficient nuance so that it does not unequivocally prohibit physicians from participating in the development of a chemical and biological *deterrent*.

Nonmaleficence is distinct from negligence. While the latter often describes accidental—in other words, unintentional—harm, nonmaleficence forbids health-care professionals to intentionally harm their patients on balance, that is, without any offsetting greater good. A physician harming a patient, through painful surgery or other medical intervention, does so in the hope that the long-term benefits of better health dwarf the short-term pain and discomfort a patient suffers. Because the benefits are so overwhelming, it might seem incongruous to call routine surgery, for example, a harm at all. These harms merely entail temporary discomforts a patient must endure to recover good health. Harder cases of nonmaleficence ask whether physicians harm their patients by refusing to provide life-sustaining care or, alternatively, by insisting on painful, aggressive care in the face of deteriorating quality of life. I will not address these questions here but only emphasize that medical maleficence requires at least three conditions: intentionality, harm, and a patient. For health-care professionals to violate the principle of nonmaleficence, they must intentionally harm their patients. None of these conditions is necessarily part of a rational deterrence policy. Chemical and biological deterrence, like its nuclear cousin, is built on a credible threat to harm civilians under specified conditions. A credible threat, as noted above, does not require firm intention; it does not require, indeed must eschew, actual harm, otherwise it has failed; and it does not target patients in any meaningful sense but aims instead at enemy civilians and other noncombatants.

Nonmaleficence and "Patienthood"

It is important to remember that the duty of physicians to do no harm only extends to their patients. It is a professional duty, incurred in the context of a specific relationship between health-care professionals and patients. Physicians will violate the principle of nonmaleficence if their care brings more harm on balance than alternative forms of treatment do. More harm on balance is sometimes difficult to evaluate, because conflicting harms, such as death or poor quality of life, are often incommensurable. Nevertheless, medical maleficence can only take note of the harm physicians' own patients suffer. Physicians do not violate the principle of nonmaleficence if they harm individuals who are not their patients. They may violate the law by killing or harming other people, but they violate no bioethical norm. That is, under circumstances that do not involve their patients, health-care professionals have no greater obligation to avoid harming others than anyone else has. Whether deterrence, chemical, biological, or nuclear, harms anyone is a question I will consider in a moment. However, what seems clear is that deterrence harms no physician's patient. It might be harming others, sufficient cause for moral reflection for any person, but there is no room to indict physicians for maleficence if their behavior does not affect their patients.

Might it be possible, however, to define *patient* more broadly to not only include those a physician treats directly but anyone affected by the practice of medicine? Would it be sensible, in other words, to consider every child ever receiving a polio vaccination as the *patient* of Dr. Jonas Salk or Dr. Albert Sabin, developers of the vaccine? In one sense, perhaps, this makes sense. Salk and Sabin intended to treat every vulnerable child, just as a physician working on CB weapons intends to maltreat every vulnerable enemy soldier or civilian. Nevertheless, the extension of the argument is troubling. Salk and Sabin are not attending or treating physicians; they only make a particular product that is conceptually no different from the syringe used to deliver it. Salk and Sabin have no patient before them, nor do they evaluate their patient's medical needs, determine dosage, track and treat side effects, or administer booster shots. Similarly, the physician developing a biological weapon is divorced from its actual use and application.

It is important to note that the upshot of the argument is not to deny responsibility for outcomes—Salk and Sabin are just as responsible for the benefits of inoculation as physician–weapons experts are responsible for the harm their weapons cause—but to only deny that a doctor-patient relationship exists between researchers and those who suffer or enjoy the effects of their end products. This in no way mitigates the moral or legal responsibility for the product each develops, but is only to say that a physician harming or helping another through the development of a weapon or vaccine is in a position no different from anyone else who may cause harm to others through his or her intentional actions. Participating in the development of CB weapons may violate the general prohibition against harming others, but it does not speak to any violation of nonmaleficence if no doctor-patient relationship exists between the physician–weapons experts and those affected by the technology they develop. Nor do physicians developing CB weapons necessarily violate the principle of nonmaleficence by causing harm. Deterrence, in principle, harms no one, patient or otherwise.

Nonmaleficence, Deterrence, and Intentional Harm

Harm raises many issues, not the least of which is the idea of permissible harm. Some harms are permissible if they bring greater benefits on balance, while other harms are impermissible regardless of the good they bring. Generally, one cannot kill an innocent person to save other innocent people. War, however, upends this thinking for many people. While bioethics holds to a strict interpretation of nonmaleficence to protect a patient's interests, it is not self-evident that this obligation prevents a physician from contributing his or her expertise to weapons development for deterrent purposes. I will return to the question of permissible harms when I discuss nonlethal weapons. In the context of chemical and biological deterrence, however, I will preempt the question with another: Do weapons developed for deterrence actually harm anyone?

When deterrence works, no one suffers harm. Although some might suggest that individuals living under the specter of a nuclear or chemical attack might develop more than their share of anxiety, Walzer (1977, 271) has rightly described how the mutual deterrence—here he describes nuclear deterrence, but it could easily include chemical and biological deterrence as well—affects people's lives very little. The threat of catastrophic harm that comes with deterrence is rarely intrusive, and deterrence itself may even offer some measure of comfort if citizens know they can do little about where their adversaries point their weapons. The moral difficulty with deterrence lies with intent, not the actual harm it causes. If, however, one's intentions are sufficiently convincing and/or the destruction one intends to cause is sufficiently severe, then deterrence may successfully avert harm entirely. Where does this leave nonmaleficence and physicians who engage in CB weapons research?

Nonmaleficence entails intentional harm to patients. Putting aside the problem of identifying the patient, it is important to see how successful deterrence harms no one and, in fact, may protect many, many more. The moral difficulty of deterrence lies in the threat: if it is wrong to kill noncombatants intentionally, it is wrong to threaten to kill them. Whether one considers this threat immoral depends on how one construes the deontological relationship between causing harm and threatening harm, and on how one weighs the successful outcome of deterrence against the probability that the threat will fail. Assuming one can overcome these difficulties, as many people do, then deterrence is not maleficent. The threat overhanging targeted populations does not cause much harm. Nor do the weapons themselves. Nor is there necessarily any firm intention to harm anyone. Deliberate ambiguity and poker-faced bluffs often underlie believable threats. When President Ronald Reagan allowed the United States to manufacture binary chemical weapons (those that combine ingredients in flight to produce nerve gas) as nothing more than a bargaining chip to induce the Soviets to end their own CW program, intentional harm was conspicuously absent. The president harmed no one, soon destroyed the weapons, enhanced national security, and no one really knew if Reagan intended to begin bombing in five minutes. Any physician accepting these arguments may participate in the development of a chemical deterrent capability without violating the principle of nonmaleficence prohibiting intentional harm.

Medical Deterrence   To place these arguments in a different perspective, consider the case of *medical* deterrence. It is not inconceivable that a health-care professional might threaten a patient with harm to prevent dangerous behavior. Would this be wrong? Think about a patient trying to commit suicide who shows up in his doctor's office for treatment after trying to cut his wrists. Could a physician threaten this patient with nontreatment in the future, telling him that he will let him bleed to death the next time? Does the *threat* of harm violate nonmaleficence in the same way as causing harm? Here, as with deterrence, one may look to both the actor's intention, and the magnitude and probability of harm should deterrence fail.

If intent is a necessary condition of maleficence, one can easily imagine the physician thinking (to himself) that he is bluffing or, like our deterrence-minded policymakers, that he has not quite made up his mind how to act. In either case, he can effectively state his threat without holding a firm intention to carry it through. Intent, however, is a difficult state of mind to ascertain. Perhaps our threatening physician might lodge a letter with the local medical association stating that he has no intent to withhold treatment. He is only trying a novel way to force compliance. We might certainly excuse him from maleficent intent, assuming that his threat does not itself harm the patient. What then about the prospect of harm?

It is difficult to estimate the probability that medical deterrence will fail and the patient will suffer harm. The patient may find the threat believable and avoid harming himself. Or the physician may back down and bind his patient's wounds should he try suicide again. But these outcomes are no worse and, indeed, may be substantially better than the consequences of failing to ever make any credible threat. In the event the threats fail to deter, the suicidal patient may sooner or later kill himself— sooner should the physician do nothing at all. Were he to withhold treatment and let his patient die the outcome, too, is no worse than before. One could make this claim for deterrence as well. The outcomes of pursuing a credible deterrent are often better, and certainly no worse, than alternative courses of action. The most compelling problem arises when deterrence fails. Few would doubt that withholding life-saving treatment in these circumstances violates the principle of nonmaleficence. And if withholding life-saving treatment is maleficent, then unleashing unconventional warfare is nearly always condemnable. "Nearly always" because it is sometimes possible to raise the argument of supreme emergency.

Supreme Emergency   In contrast to the relatively benign nature of deterrence, the prospect of intentional harm emphatically informs the idea of "supreme emergency," those unique circumstances that permit a political community to violate the principles of just war by inflicting horrific injury to combatants and noncombatant alike if faced with utter destruction (see chapter 2). Supreme emergencies demand rigid criteria, and there are few compelling examples. To egregiously violate the principle of noncombatant immunity, a community must face a grave threat that only extreme means can avert. Neither the indignity or hardship of surrender nor the potential for significant military casualties allows a belligerent to obliterate an enemy's civilian population. Because the gravity of a threat is often in the eyes of the beholder and the effectiveness of indiscriminately bombing civilian populations is often questionable, the criteria of supreme emergency are difficult to apply in practice. This leaves its detractors to shun any sweeping breach of noncombatant immunity based on broad calculations of utility. But whether the extreme means necessitated by a supreme emergency are morally justified or simply a tragic choice between two evils, one must consider the possibility that physicians may face the call to arms. Just as one may seriously ponder the obligation of a Jewish scientist to manufacture a weapon of mass destruction to end the Holocaust, one cannot avoid asking about the duty of a Kurdish doctor, for example, to use his medical expertise to help build a chemical weapon to harm Iraqi civilians if it might have forestalled the same threat to his own people when Saddam Hussein attacked the Kurds with poison gas in 1988.

While much has been made of supreme emergency and the scenario it depicts, the argument repudiates rather than endorses the *use* of weapons of mass destruction while, at the same time, strengthening the need for a credible deterrent. Germany and Iraq embarked on genocide; they did not act in response to failed deterrence. In fact, one might reasonably argue that had Kurds or Jews commanded the wherewithal to manufacture and deliver a credible weapon, they would not have faced genocidal threats. Nations commit genocide precisely because they can exterminate their enemies at little cost. Avoiding genocide and with it, the prospect of unleashing a nuclear, chemical, or biological attack, is precisely the goal of deterrence. In a roundabout way, supreme emergency returns us to the necessity of unconventional deterrence and the contributions physicians can make to weapons development.

In the final analysis, there is sympathy for the claim that chemical and biological deterrence can work, that weapons of deterrence do not harm anyone, and that less-than-firm intentions can maintain a credible threat. If medicine wishes to invoke medical ethics to condemn deterrence, it must identify the principles of bioethics with the same arguments that belie the cogency of deterrence, namely, a deontology that identifies cause and intent, and a consequentialism that is highly risk aversive. This, however, may push medicine uncomfortably into the corner of pacifism, where many practitioners may not wish to be. Arguing otherwise, though, suggests that bioethics and medicine could live with a policy that sometimes justifies chemical and biological deterrence. Many may find this conclusion equally unpalatable. Those that do, however, must carefully distinguish between general philosophical arguments and the principles peculiar to bioethics. While there might be sound deontological arguments for decrying chemical and biological deterrence, the principle of nonmaleficence is essentially a consequentialist argument that is difficult to sustain in the face of the strong utilitarian merits of deterrence.

If the principle of nonmaleficence fails to deliver convincing grounds to oppose the development of chemical and biological weapons for building a credible deterrent in a hostile environment, it may fare better against other forms of CB weapons. While chemical, biological, or medical deterrence does not violate the bioethical principle of maleficence by intentionally harming others, nonlethal weapons are more difficult for this very reason. Nonlethal weapons intentionally cause harm. Yet these weapons are neither unlawful nor aim at unlawful targets. Do these weapons violate the principle of nonmaleficence or any other significant bioethical principle that would lead medical personnel to shun them regardless of any benefit they might bring?

Nonlethal Chemical and Biological Weapons

Military contractors design and build nonlethal weapons to inflict harm. Although the harm is transitory in most cases, it nonetheless can bring intense pain and suffering as adversaries fight to incapacitate one another. Unlike weapons developed for their deterrent potential, nonlethal weapons cannot distance the physician–weapons developer from maleficence by highlighting ambiguous intentions and the absence of real harm. While one may appeal to the argument that those suffering harm are no one's patients, I do not think this argument alone is sufficient to set a health-care professional's mind fully at ease.

In many respects, nonlethal weapons differ little from conventional weapons. Generally, both target combatants who are legitimately at risk for various degrees of bodily harm. Combatants are not controversial targets, nor is the harm they face from many nonlethal weapons beyond the limits of unnecessary suffering or superfluous injury. Just as they utilize conventional arms, armed forces may deploy nonlethal weapons during conventional warfare as a tactical measure subordinate to the dictates of military necessity and with the intention of preventing casualties to one's own forces as they secure a strategic goal. The morality of nonlethal weapons depends entirely on necessity and effectiveness, and in this respect they are similar to any other kinds of weapons. What grounds exist, if any, for physicians to spurn nonlethal weapons?

Coupland (1997b, 72; emphasis added) frames the moral issue succinctly:

There is a fundamental ethical dilemma for doctors. The development of this new generation of ["nonlethal"] weapons incorporates knowledge from the remarkable advances made in medical science; two examples are calmatives [compounds that depress or inhibit the function of the central nervous system] and eye attack lasers. . . . *The medical community must guard against use of its knowledge for the purposes of weapon development.*

The reference to medical knowledge is reminiscent of the WMA's prohibition that bans physicians from using their "personal or scientific knowledge" to develop chemical and biological weapons. Medical knowledge, however, is exceptionally difficult to define with precision. Is it restricted to the expertise associated with the medical profession, or does it comprise all forms of knowledge relevant to human health and well-being? Even in its narrowest sense, this would include medicine, microbiology, bacteriology, and molecular biology, thereby encompassing many more scientists than medicine would. Should nonlethal-weapons development be spurned by all scientists, or only by medical personnel, or is there an imperative for everyone to object to the development of these weapons? Before addressing this question, it is important to describe the nature of nonlethal weaponry and its place in armed conflict and international law.

The Nature of Nonlethal Weaponry

World War I first raised the possibility of deploying chemical weapons to incapacitate rather than kill enemy soldiers. Since then researchers have proposed and developed an astonishing array of nonlethal weapons. These include chemical and biological agents, low-energy lasers, and acoustic weapons. Nonlethal weapons may target personnel, or destroy or disable material and equipment. Those temporarily incapacitating personnel and dependent on medical expertise are described in table 8.1. I will not consider chemical and biological agents affecting material and equipment, or herbicides and defoliants that destroy nonhuman organisms. Medical personnel or medical knowledge are not an integral part of all nonlethal weaponry. Rubber bullets or land mines, which may

Table 8.1
Nonlethal Antipersonnel Weapons

Category	Type	Description/effects
Acoustical	Audible sound	Low-level noise to disperse crowds
	Infrasound	Low-frequency, high-intensity sound induces incapacitation, temporary nausea, vomiting, and bowel spasms
Optical	Low-energy laser	Temporary blindness*
	Optical munitions	Flash-bang grenades cause disorientation
	Strobe lights	Disorientation
Biological	Viruses and toxins	Respiratory and gastrointestinal disease
Chemical	Neural inhibitors	Paralyze synaptic pathways, causing incapacitation and loss of neurological control
	Calmatives	Inhibit central nervous system, causing incapacitation
	Neuroblockers	Tranquilizer darts and anesthetic bullets, causing incapacitation
	Irritants	Tear gas and pepper spray, causing tearing, coughing, choking, and intense and debilitating pain
	Psychotropic drugs	Hallucinations, disorientation, and incapacitation
	Gastroconvulsives	Nausea, vomiting, incapacitation

*In contrast to blinding lasers, which are outlawed by the Protocol on Blinding Laser Weapons (Protocol IV to the 1980 convention), October 13, 1995.
Source: Adapted from Nando 1996; Lewer and Schofield 1997; Sautenet 2000; Lewer and Davison 2005.

cause permanent disability, do not require medical expertise, but as military planners search for alternative methods to cripple an adversary's armed forces, it is necessary to accurately gauge the outer limit of human endurance below which one is incapacitated and beyond which one is irreversibly harmed or killed. It is not difficult to see how answering this question requires medical expertise.

While the early impetus for developing nonlethal weaponry came from a keen desire to limit the horrendous casualties of modern warfare and, perhaps naively, to wage war without death, the changing nature of contemporary armed conflict has presented an abiding challenge to weapons designers to develop alternative forms of weaponry (Coppernoll 1999; Alexander 2001; Lewer and Feakin 2001; Lewer and Davison 2005). Fighting in built-up areas against forces intermingled with noncombatants, large conventional armies find it impossible to bring their enormous firepower to bear. On the one hand, it has proved difficult to use massive, high-explosive munitions without causing extensive civilian casualties. On the other hand, conventional armies would find it just as difficult to use less powerful weapons against un-uniformed and therefore unidentifiable insurgents and guerrillas without risking harm to civilians. Therefore, "chemicals," writes the National Research Council (2003), "offer the theoretical possibility of peacefully incapacitating combatants/agitators, reducing the need for the violence that is frequently associated with many of the current methods." The need to avoid excessive noncombatant deaths arises not only in CAR conflicts—that is, the struggles against "colonial, alien and racist" regimes described by Protocol I—but in wars that very few envisioned until recently. These include wars of humanitarian intervention and wars against international terrorism, the latter a form of international law enforcement that often assumes the guise of conventional warfare in such places as Afghanistan and Iraq.

To address the hard tactical problems of waging these wars effectively and without undue civilian casualties, military planners turn to high-tech weaponry that would effectively allow them to shoot first and ask questions later, and to quell an uprising, rout an insurgency, or combat guerrillas without inflicting heavy civilian casualties. In contrast to previous approaches, nations waging nonlethal war might choose to be indiscriminate, and intentionally target combatants and noncombatants alike in an effort to ferret out and disable the former without causing permanent harm to the latter. It is not difficult to see, however, that this violates a fundamental and long-standing tenet of just war that prohibits intentionally targeting noncombatants.

Proponents insist that nonlethal weapons meet the challenge of changing modes of contemporary warfare by offering military planners a "force continuum" with which to respond to various levels of threats without causing indiscriminate or excessive civilian casualties. If conventional warfare only offers military planners one of two options—responding with overwhelming military force or doing nothing at all—nonlethal weapons significantly augment military strategy. There are very few scenarios, however, where nonlethal weapons are not accompanied or backed up with lethal force, a juxtaposition that has led critics to charge that nonlethal weapons may *increase* casualties.

Drawing on the American experience in Vietnam, critics describe how the U.S. military used irritants, harassing agents, and psychotropic drugs to exacerbate casualties by driving North Vietnamese soldiers from cover during artillery barrages (Stockholm International Peace Research Institute, 1971–1975, vol. 1, 185–210; vol. 5, 124–137). At the same time, high concentrations of tear gas killed Vietnamese civilians during tunnel-flushing operations to rout out North Vietnamese soldiers. In neither case did U.S. forces use nonlethal weapons to *minimize* casualties. On the contrary, they joined the arsenal of lethal weaponry designed to disable an enemy and attain military victory. Experiences such as these have led opponents to charge that nonlethal weapons compromise noncombatant immunity, exacerbate fighting, increase combatant casualties, and, in general, undermine the international community's efforts to do away with chemical and biological weapons (Dando 1996, 191–205; Lewer and Schofield 1997, 127–134). Establishing two categories of chemical and biological weapons only erodes the force of the Chemical and Biological Weapons Conventions, and provokes military escalation as one army suffering from nonlethal chemical and biological weapons responds with similar weapons of the lethal variety.

The jury is still out on these charges, and it remains unclear how effective nonlethal weapons will prove in future conflicts. Military planners rarely envision using nonlethal weapons to fight a bloodless war, but invariably back them up with lethal force. No advocate of nonlethal warfare advocates deploying troops without recourse to conventional arms, raising fears of inevitable combatant and noncombatant deaths. While supporters of nonlethal weaponry point to successes in Somalia's 1994 civil war or the growing need to think seriously about deploying nonlethal force in regional conflicts around the world, others are increasingly concerned with the misuse of nonlethal weapons—rubber-coated bullets, stun guns, pepper gas, and truncheons—by conventional police forces trying to quell domestic unrest (Wright 2001).

There is no doubt, however, that changing modes of warfare are forcing military officials to consider radically different forms of weaponry than they had in the past. The development of nonlethal weaponry takes into account changes along three fronts. Geopolitically, members of the international community face increasing challenges to wage limited kinds of war whether they intervene for humanitarian purposes or fight a global war on terror. Here, weapons designers will test existing forms of nonlethal weapons relative to criteria of effectiveness, discrimination, proportionality, and unnecessary suffering. Technologically, rapid scientific advances will offer the possibility of an array of weapons hitherto unimaginable. Finally, legal and ethical considerations will constantly come into play when individual nations and the international community gauge the legality of nonlethal weapons as they emerge from the assembly line and reach the battlefield. Medical personnel must evaluate these debates, consider their professional obligations, and weigh their civic duty. The development of biological and chemical nonlethal weapons highlights some of these dilemmas.

Nonlethal Weapons, Armed Conflict, and International Law

Nonlethal biological weapons include those that cause incapacitating rather than life-threatening illness. Although anthrax, plague, and botulinum carry very high mortality rates, some bacteria and toxins are considerably less lethal. These include brucellosis, Q-Fever, and Venezuelan equine encephalitis (VEE). VEE, for example, is particularly debilitating, afflicting nearly 100 percent of those infected with headaches, high fever, and several weeks of fatigue (World Health Organization, 2004,

229–276). Because mortality is less than 1 percent, it was a particularly attractive virus, and both the United States and the Soviet Union successfully weaponized VEE as an incapacitating agent before ending their biological-weapons programs (Croddy 2002, 208–211). Q-Fever and brucellosis cause similar symptoms and were also candidates for incapacitating biological weapons. Considering the casualties of a biological attack on a civilian population of 500,000, the World Health Organization estimated that Q-Fever would leave 150 dead and 125,000 incapacitated, while brucellosis would leave 500 dead and over 100,000 incapacitated. In contrast, a similar attack with weaponized anthrax would kill up to 95,000 people (World Health Organization, 1970).

Although they carry a low mortality rate, biological weapons armed with VEE or Q-Fever face the same shortcomings as lethal biological weapons. Both are subject to the same atmospheric conditions that make biological weapons unpredictable and difficult to deploy. Both suffer from the lack of any coherent strategic doctrine. Tactically, they create logistical nightmares for military planners, hamstring troops in action, and invite reprisals in kind, or worse, against civilian populations. Moreover, none of the agents described are entirely nonlethal, and while one may consider using them against combatants, one must realize that deploying any nonlethal biological weapon against a civilian or mixed population entails intentionally harming noncombatants, a considerable problem for anyone concerned with the morality of nonlethal weaponry. In any event, the Biological Weapons Convention (1972, Article I) makes no distinction between lethal and nonlethal biological antipersonnel weapons, obligating nations ratifying the convention to destroy both types of weapons.

In contrast to biological weapons, chemical weapons are not the subject of an absolute ban. While the Chemical Weapons Convention prohibits nations from developing, producing, otherwise acquiring, stockpiling, retaining, or using chemical weapons, including incapacitating agents, it does allow nations to use and develop "riot control agents" for the purposes of "law enforcement" (Article II, paragraph 9d). "Riot control agent" refers to "any chemical not listed in a [CWC] Schedule, which can produce rapidly in humans sensory irritation or disabling physical effects which disappear within a short time following termination of exposure" (Chemical Weapons Convention, 1993, Article II, paragraph 7).

Needless to say, this definition is less than airtight. While riot control agents traditionally include tear gas and other "harassing" agents, they permit other agents "not listed" and not yet developed or conceived and may include chemical agents (although not biological agents) such as "calmatives" that depress or inhibit the central nervous system.

"Law enforcement" is equally ambiguous. Including something more than "domestic riot control," many observers broadly interpret law enforcement to include "military operations other than war": international law enforcement, the fight against terror, peacekeeping, and humanitarian intervention (Coppernoll 1999; Fidler 2001). Commenting on the initial use of chemical irritants in Vietnam, for example, U.S. Secretary of State Dean Rusk introduced the idea of "situations analogous to riot control" when he stated:

We do not expect that gas will be used in ordinary military operations. Police-type weapons were used in riot control in South Vietnam . . . and in situations analogous to riot control, where the Viet Cong, for example, were using civilians as screens for their own operations. . . . The anticipation is, of course, that these weapons will be used only in those situations involving riot control or situations analogous to riot control. (Stockholm International Peace Research Institute, 1971–1975, vol. 1, 187)

Although the analogy is far from clear, the CWC leaves open a number of avenues for the development of nonlethal chemical weapons that may eventually find use in any number of conflicts around the globe.

Nations have developed many nonlethal agents for law-enforcement purposes, including various kinds of tear gases, irritants, and harassing agents. A harassing agent "disables exposed people for as long as they remain exposed. They are acutely aware of discomfort caused by the agent, but usually remain capable of removing themselves from exposure to it unless they are temporarily blinded or otherwise constrained. They will usually recover fully in a short time after exposure ends, and no medical treatment will be required" (World Health Organization, 2004, 44). Except in very high doses, harassing agents are generally not lethal and are the principal compound that the phrase "riot control agent" brings to mind. Agents such as CS (2-chlorobenzalmalononitrile) and CN (2-chloroacetophenone) are irritants causing coughing, choking, severe headaches, nausea, vomiting, and pain. In the best cases, law-enforcement agencies will use harassing agents to control crowds that threaten public safety. In other circumstances, CS and CN enjoy military use. After the U.S. army brought CN and CS to Vietnam as incapacitating agents, American forces often used them in conjunction with lethal weaponry, a turn of events that led critics to charge that irritants aggravated casualties when troops would use the irritants to flush out the Vietcong and then attack them with conventional weapons.

Vietnam also saw the Americans deploying the psychotropic agent BZ against North Vietnamese troops in 1968 (Stockholm International Peace Research Institute, 1971–1975, vol. 1, 189). BZ (3-quinuclidinyl benzilate) is an incapacitating agent rather than an irritant. Like an irritant, an incapacitating agent disables, but "people exposed to it may not be aware of their predicament, as with opioids and certain other psychotropic agents, or may be rendered unable to function or move away from the exposed environment. The effect may be prolonged, but recovery may be possible without specialized medical aid" (World Health Organization, 2004, 44). Exposure to BZ causes dizziness, confusion, hallucinations, and unpredictable behavior and renders troops unfit for combat almost immediately and for as long as seventy-two hours. Although BZ is a scheduled chemical agent banned by the CWC, the search continues for incapacitating agents that weapons designers can shoehorn into the CWC exceptions that allow riot control agents in the course of law-enforcement or military operations other than war.

Developing and Approving Nonlethal CB Weapons

Rather than pushing for changes in international law, some nations retain the right to interpret existing guidelines to allow weapons designers to develop viable chemical antipersonnel weapons. For members of the National Research Council (2003, 106–107), malodorants and calmatives are a top priority (see also Lakoski, Murray, and Kenny 2000). The approval process for chemical and other nonlethal weapons follows a two-stage process in the United States. The first evaluates emerging technologies for research-and-development potential and the second sets the stage to approve or reject the final proposal for a nonlethal weapon (NLW). The Judge Advocate General of the Navy, for example, has recently approved a number of emerging technologies for R&D—including gastrointestinal convulsives and calmative agents—that may lead to the development of viable nonlethal-weapons. Only when a weapon is technologically feasible will the navy evaluate its legal status. The criteria are by no means unequivocal, because military authorities retain considerable discretion when they approve a new weapon:

Such nonlethal weapons as neural inhibitors, gastrointestinal convulsives, neuropharmacological agents, calmative agents, disassociative hallucinogens and sedatives may be considered "temporary incapacitants" and therefore toxic chemicals and prohibited by the Chemical Weapons Convention for any purpose. . . . If Pentagon lawyers interpret "toxic chemicals" to include incapacitating NLW's, like calmative agents, their utility in combat will be questionable; the sole operations use of NLW's would be in operations other than war. (Coppernoll 1999, 122)

This is a big "if." Although a signatory of the Chemical Weapons Convention, the United States maintains that the ban on incapacitating weapons "does not apply to nonlethal technology that temporarily disables but does not cause permanent injury" (Fidler 1999, 69). As a result, the line between harassing chemicals, riot control agents, and incapacitating compounds is sufficiently ambiguous to allow military authorities considerable leeway. Nor do international treaties yet exclude acoustic or electromagnetic antipersonnel weapons (Fidler 1999, 75). Military and political leaders retain similar latitude in defining their nation's conflicts, particularly as "military operations other than war" take center stage across the globe and now comprise nearly every category of contemporary armed conflict.

I do not intend to resolve these ambiguities and discrepancies here, but only to point out, as I did in the previous chapter, that where ambiguities stymie legal scholars and jurists, it would be very difficult for medical personnel in the field to ferret them out. As with lethal CB weapons developed for deterrent purposes, medical personnel may raise their voices against nonlethal weapons with arguments that have nothing to do with medical ethics. In light of changing circumstances and the emerging demands of contemporary warfare, some may advocate revising international norms to accommodate NLWs, while others remain convinced that the same circumstances preclude nonlethal weapons (Alexander 2001). In opposition to the continued development and deployment of nonlethal weapons, some health-care professionals may object to classifying various chemical agents as riot control agents, dispute their government's insistence that a particular conflict is a "military operation other than war," or vehemently oppose using any weapon, however nonlethal or sublethal it may be, against unarmed civilians. Alternatively, medical personnel may place their faith with those charged with interpreting their nation's obligations under international law, entirely content with a procedurally proper ruling on the status of one weapons system or another, be it chemical, acoustic, or optical. A concerned, conscientious citizen could cogently pursue any of these arguments.

Yet each alternative course of action departs from the WMA and ICRC platforms. Both the World Medical Association and the Red Cross insist on the medical community's unique professional obligation to avoid weapons development however lawful it may be. These bodies raise another question: May medical personnel contribute their expertise and professional knowledge to the development of any weapon, nonlethal or otherwise, which by its very nature harms others?

Weapons Development and the Medical Community

Nonlethal weapons pose special problems for medical professionals. The WMA demands that physicians renounce any type of chemical or biological weapon, while some ICRC officials insist that no medical knowledge whatsoever finds its way into the development of weapons of any sort. Nevertheless, the medical community remains ambivalent. When physicians convened under the auspices of the ICRC in 1996 to consider their profession's role in the development of weaponry, it is noteworthy that they could not agree: "The working group wished to make a statement about members of the medical profession being involved knowingly in research which relates to the design and development of weapons. Whilst it was felt that the spirit of the desired statement was obvious, the wording has not been finalized despite correspondence since the Symposium" (International Committee of the Red Cross, 1996).

Nor has it been finalized to date; perhaps the spirit of the desired statement was not so obvious after all. No one could say unequivocally that the medical profession must entirely wash its hands of weapons development. Concern for military necessity seems to lurk in the background. Nevertheless, some of the working groups were able to offer suggestions for definitive guidelines:

1. The medical community has an obligation to monitor the deployment of weapons subject to the criterion of unnecessary suffering,
2. The medical community has an obligation to monitor weapons research, particularly research associated with utilizing biological and genetic technology,
3. Medical professionals may contribute to defensive research. (International Committee of the Red Cross, 1996)

As important as some of these suggestions are, none addresses the problem at hand, namely, medicine's role in the development of weapons. Medical personnel must monitor deployment and research. They may contribute their knowledge to developing defensive measures. Does their involvement end here or may they also contribute to weapons research and development? The question remains, perhaps intentionally, unanswered.

Two problems impede a clear understanding of medicine's role in weapons development. First, the distinction between offensive- and defensive-weapons research creates the impression that there are distinct ethical categories that permit medical personnel to participate in one but not the other. This distinction, though, is intensely problematic. Second, the principle of nonmaleficence suggests a professional duty to refrain from all kinds of weapons research. This is a more pressing issue, leading one to ask whether medicine is a pacifist vocation.

Offensive- and Defensive-Weapons Development

Although the delegates to ICRC symposium could not agree whether physicians should participate in weapons development, one working group recommended that "while doctors should not knowingly participate in the design of an offensive weapon, they could contribute to the development of a defensive capability without compromising their medical integrity" (International Committee of the Red Cross 1996).

Similar attitudes surface repeatedly throughout the history of chemical- and biological-weapons development:

The only similarities between defensive and offensive research are that common laboratory techniques are used in each at the outset but . . . the experimental hypotheses are diametrically opposed. . . . An offensive program would include a research program on mass producing or storing large quantities of microorganisms, on stabilization in an aerosol, on improving virulence or persistence, or on methods for dissemination and weapon development. In contrast, defensive research comprises development of biological agent detection methods, treatment and protection, and decontamination capability. (Huxsoll, Parrott, and Patrick 1989, 678–679)

How clear is this distinction? Commenting on postwar weapons development, Theodor Rosebury, director of American biological-weapons research at Fort Detrick during World War II, suggests that any attempt to draw a clear distinction between offensive- and defensive-weapons development is mired in practical and, more importantly, conceptual difficulties: "At Detrick, a certain delicacy concentrated most of the physicians into principally or primarily defensive operations—*principally* or *primarily*: the modifiers are needed because military operations can never be exclusively defensive" (Rosebury 1963, 514). In a similar vein, national security advisor Henry Kissinger wrote in 1969: "The United States bacteriological/biological programs will be confined to research and development for defensive purposes (immunization, safety measures, etc.). This does not preclude research into those offensive aspects of bacteriological/biological agents necessary to determine what defensive measures are required" (quoted in Tucker 1984–1985, 68).

Rosebury and Kissinger are pointing to the practical difficulties of drawing clear distinctions as the United States and other nations develop chemical and biological weapons. As nations pursued biological-weapons research in an era prior to the Biological Weapons Convention, it is not hard to imagine spheres of overlapping research when scientists engaged in different types of investigation. Following the ratification of the Convention, some observers claim that the international community drew a distinction between offensive and defensive biological research, prohibiting the former while permitting the latter (Frisina 1990). This is not quite right. The Biological Weapons Convention (Article 1) prohibits nations from "developing, producing, and stockpiling microbial or other biological agents, or toxins that have no justification for prophylactic, protective or other *peaceful* purposes." I emphasize the word *peaceful*, for opponents of biological-weapons research claim that its purpose, which may be prophylactic or protective, is intimately connected to war and far from peaceful, while its fruits inevitably find their way into contexts that harm others or may easily lend themselves to harm. Biological-weapons research, claim critics, draws off funds from public health and other peaceful pursuits of medicine and, at the same time, has the unintended effect of deluding nations into thinking they can wage and win an unconventional war (Frisina 2003). As such, biological-weapons research is no business of physicians. In response, medical researchers from the U.S. army's Biological Defense Research Program try to draw a firm distinction between offensive and defensive research, justifying the latter while condemning the former (Huxsoll, Parrott, and Patrick 1989).

Physicians who engage in weapons research may be looking for a distinction that does not exist. The distinction that medicine is after—that offensive weapons harm a person and defensive weapons protect a person—is difficult to maintain. What weapons fit this description? Gas masks and antidotes are necessary so soldiers can carry on. They may not carry on with chemical warfare, but they will certainly wage war by other means. Once one lends a hand to warfare, the line between offensive and defensive rapidly blurs, a situation analogous to trying to distinguish between the armor encasing a tank and its cannon. A defensive measure only enhances the efficacy of warfare.

But the problem goes much deeper than this. Conceptually, military operations can never be exclusively *offensive* insofar as one takes the tenets of just war seriously. Moreover, defensive measures nearly always entail inflicting harm. What exactly do offensive and defensive mean? In chapter 2, I describe the underlying intuitions of self-defense that allow an individual to use lethal force when facing a material and morally non-innocent threat and how bystanders who can intervene at relatively little cost to themselves often incur an obligation to aid victims of aggression. The laws of war largely adopt this domestic analogy. A nation unjustly attacked by another is a victim and may respond with armed force to forestall harm. While, traditionally, there is no international analogy to the domestic bystander who must render aid to victims if the cost is minimal, there is now growing support for wars of humanitarian intervention. These are justifiable uses of armed force.

A war of self-defense renders any moral distinction between offensive and defensive measures difficult to discern. In fact, one is hard-pressed to find the moral distinction medical workers sometimes try to impute. Instead, the distinction is merely strategic or tactical. Defensive measures are those designed to hold or protect a position; offensive measures aim to overpower and seize an enemy position. The moral distinction that perhaps one is looking for falls between "aggressive" and "law-abiding" behavior. An "offensive" nuclear strategy is aggressive and in defiance of international norms, while a deterrent capability strives to keep the peace. A war for territorial aggrandizement is aggressive; defense in its face is law-abiding—that is, an attempt to preserve and restore the norms of acceptable international behavior. From that standpoint, a nation fighting a war of self-defense can coherently categorize any of its operations as defensive. Recourse to any moral and practical distinction between offensive and defensive warfare is not very compelling, leaving medical professionals to search for other distinctions to govern their role in nonlethal-weapons development. Most likely, it lies in the nature of the harm they cause.

Building Weapons and Causing Harm

Weapons cause harm and while weapons research places medical workers in a difficult position, it is no more vexing, perhaps, than violating confidentiality or salvaging fit soldiers at the expense of those in greater need. These dilemmas force physicians to consider the limits of medical involvement in war. On the one hand, there remains a deep and visceral reluctance to involve medical workers directly in the business of war. "Medical professionals," instructs the U.S. Army's textbook on military medical ethics, "ought to stay in the business of healing and not hurting, which includes not participating in or contributing to weapons research and development" (Frisina 2003, 545). In this view, it seems obvious that the canons of medical ethics necessarily distance medicine from war and, perhaps, place medicine and its practitioners in a unique moral category. On the other hand, it is equally compelling to suggest that members of the medical profession occupy the same moral universe as every other person who must weigh his or her reluctance to harm others against reason of state or the common good. Commenting on the health-care professional's role in the development of CB weapons, Rosebury (1963, 296; 1949, 182) insists that

> There are no special moral standards for physicians or scientists. What is good for other men is also good for them. Scientists and physicians alike could lend their special talents to the destruction of man only in the hope that they are serving the more general preservation. . . . If it is right for a scientist to engage in war research whose purpose is the destruction of human life, it is equally right for a physician to do so.

Rosebury's categorical declarations are at the heart of some of the most pressing issues of bioethics and armed conflict. Medicine, it seems, faces a choice. Either it accepts Rosebury's claim and wages war without reservation when wars are just and balks when they are not, or the medical community rejects his claim and embraces pacifism, spurning weapons research and renouncing the practice of war.

9

Bioethics and the End of Armed Conflict

Pacifism, Peace, Medicine, and War

Is medicine a pacifist vocation? When American Quakers faced conscription in 1917, their first thought was to establish an ambulance unit modeled on the Friends Ambulance Unit that their pacifist brethren had operated with great success in Britain since the beginning of World War I. Warming rapidly to the idea, Adventist pacifists launched the Cadet Medical Corps prior to America's entry into World War II to allow young Adventists to fulfill their civic duty without violating the biblical precept that absolutely forbids killing. Nor was the idea lost on policymakers. Making room for conscripts who cannot, by reason of conscience, bear arms and serve in any capacity that might compel them to kill or harm others, military officials are prepared to offer conscientious objectors "service in the medical department of any of the Armed Forces, wherever performed" (U.S. Department of Defense, 2003a, paragraph 3.3).

Why does pacifism find such ready refuge in medicine? And, if many pacifists find medicine so accommodating, does it follow that medicine has a natural affinity for pacifism? Is medicine a pacifist vocation that should respond to the questions raised at the close of the previous chapter with the firm conviction that physicians should not build weapons because making war is no business for doctors and an affront to medicine? After all, if medicine satisfies the rigorous conditions that pacifism imposes on its adherents, then medicine's duty to "do no harm" is little different from the pacifist's duty to avoid killing or harming other human beings.

Like pacifism, however, medicine's relationship to war is multifaceted and nuanced. Just as relatively few pacifists unconditionally oppose war, few medical practitioners repudiate armed conflict absolutely. Many pacifists, for example, serve in noncombatant, military roles. They are not absolute pacifists, but like most physicians I imagine, accept the necessity of war under certain circumstances. They object instead to assuming a role that requires them to kill or harm others. While this form of pacifism is not without ambiguity and traces of self-contradiction, it comes close to characterizing the outlook of medical personnel during armed conflict. Otherwise, physicians could not so easily reject the call to arms when asked to contribute their expertise to the development of modern weapons systems that require medical knowledge.

There are many forms of pacifism, three of which bear on bioethics during armed conflict. One form is often religious and raises a similar aversion to bearing arms and causing harm that characterizes medicine. This is *"vocational" pacifism*, which reflects the unwillingness of members of certain communities or specific vocations to bear arms and kill during armed conflict. Instead, convinced that pacifism and medicine are fundamentally compatible, they accept noncombatant medical positions in regular armies.

A second form of pacifism is conditional or selective. This is *political pacifism*, a term that more accurately describes civil disobedience in the face of unjust war. As opponents object to specific wars, their purpose is not to "bear witness" to a religious creed or higher calling that eschews violence, but to act vigorously, and sometimes violently, to change public policy and end an unjust war. If vocational pacifists seek accommodation with the state, civil disobedients are confrontational; their actions are inimical to military and civilian authorities. Among civil disobedients are those willing to violate the law, undertake collective action, and suffer punishment. Others are more circumspect and engage in "evasive noncompliance" to evade the draft and avoid fighting in a war they feel is unjust. Physicians assume a uniquely important role when they engage in civil disobedience or aid those avoiding conscription.

Finally, it is important to consider the role medical professionals play in another form of pacifism—namely, *pacificism*, the idea "that war, though sometimes necessary, is always an irrational and inhumane way to resolve disputes, and that its prevention should always be an overriding political priority" (Ceadel 1980, 3). In this context, it is imperative to look at the special relationship between medicine and the peace movement.

Vocational Pacifism

There are two variants of vocational pacifism, communal and professional, and each raises difficult issues for the medical profession. Communal vocational pacifism illustrates the worldview of certain communities sworn to uphold principles that forbid them to participate in the practice of war in any form and for any purpose. While some members of these communities distance themselves from war entirely, many of these committed pacifists seek, and ultimately find, an ideologically safe haven in the medical profession that allows them to fulfill their humanitarian, religious, and civic obligations. Professional vocational pacifism, unlike its communal counterpart, addresses the pacifism of a particular vocation—medicine or the clergy—as its practitioners struggle with *professional* obligations that prohibit harm to others. While professional vocational pacifists grapple with the outer limits of their professional duties, their communal counterparts find refuge in medicine, firm in their conviction that its outer limits are secure.

Communal Vocational Pacifism: Turning to Medicine during War
During the two world wars, members of the historic peace churches—Quakers, Mennonites, and Brethren—struggled ceaselessly with the challenge that conscription in a war in defense of vital national interests and world peace posed for their pacifist beliefs (Keim 1979; Kohrman 1986; Bush 1998). Two core beliefs characterize their pacifism:

Antiwarism The belief that war is wrong and entirely incompatible with the spirit, example, and teachings of their religion.

Nonmaleficence The belief that one "cannot conscientiously engage in any activity or perform any function contributing to the destruction of human life" (Bowman 1944, 181).

These are two distinct principles. The first espouses an unconditional opposition to war in any form, the second to the role one must play during armed conflict. Individuals weigh these principles differently.

Refusing to compromise on either principle, some pacifists suffer imprisonment, while the vast majority of "absolute" pacifists during World War II, for example, chose alternative public service. They worked in civilian agricultural camps and performed essential national service without joining and supporting the military. Others, however, were willing to compromise in the face of German aggression and sought ways to fulfill their military and moral duties simultaneously. They would support war but practice nonmaleficence. In doing so, they chose *noncombatant* military service, and in nearly every case this translated into medical service in the U.S. army's Medical Department, the Royal Army Medical Corps, or the Friends Ambulance Unit.

Medicine as Noncombatant Military Service   Inasmuch as the Geneva Conventions define noncombatants as "persons taking no active part in the hostilities," the entire idea of "noncombatant military service" is something of an oxymoron. It is noteworthy, however, that the only noncombatant military service mutually agreeable to pacifists and the military is medical service. Nor is it a grudging compromise. On the contrary, pacifists find in medical service a happy union of their spiritual, humanitarian, civic, and antimilitarist beliefs, while military officials are only too pleased to co-opt conscientious objectors into their armed forces.

Within a year of introducing conscription in 1863, Union officials made provisions for accommodating those "conscientiously opposed to the bearing of arms" who, if drafted, could be declared noncombatants and "assigned by the Secretary of War to duty in the hospitals, or to the care of freedman (ex-slaves)" (Knight 1997, 164). Over the years this changed very little. Reintroducing conscription in World War I, the British offered conscientious objectors (COs) alternative service in the noncombatant corps (NCC), the Royal Army Medical Corps (RAMC), or the Friends Ambulance Unit (FAU). While the NCC directed COs toward agricultural or construction work, the RAMC and FAU trained COs as medics, stretcher-bearers, and ambulance drivers. The United States made no provisions for alternative service but permitted COs to train without weapons and serve in noncombatant positions in the engineering, quartermaster, and medical corps of the army. By World War II, the United States created two classes of COs, class 1-O, who "sincerely object to participation in war in any form," and class 1-A-O, who "sincerely object to participation in war in any form but whose convictions are such as to permit a Military Service in a non-combatant status" (U.S. Department of Defense, 2003a, 3.1.1, 3.1.2).

During World War II, the army offered COs classified as 1-O public service in nonmilitary, civilian camps that the peace churches organized and funded under the supervision the Selective Service System. COs classified 1-A-O, however, were inducted and by January 1942, assigned exclusively to the medical department. By the Korean War, the army no longer assigned so-called absolutists (1-O COs) to camps but allowed them to find alternative service in the public sector. Eighty percent made their way into health-related fields, so that by the Vietnam War, the only avenue available to COs of either stripe was service in a medically related field. For all intents and purposes, all noncombatant military roles were medical.

Although the number of COs was never very large, they tested the tolerance of Anglo-American democracy during wartime and assumed an importance far in excess of their numbers. During the American Civil War, most pacifists were content to purchase a substitute and avoid the dilemma of service altogether. World War I conscription made this impossible, leaving the peace churches to negotiate with the authorities. The British recognized 16,000 COs, while American authorities granted certificates of exemption from combat service to 21,000 men, of whom only 4,000 actually used them (Brock and Young 1999, 51). In World War II, the United Kingdom directed 16,000 men to noncombatant duties including the NCC and medical positions, and 23,000 men to civilian public service. In the United States, 25,000 of the nearly 10 million men under arms served in noncombatant military positions, while 12,000 found their way to civilian public service (Sibley and Jacob 1952; Flynn 1989, 35–55).

The Logic of Noncombatant Military Medical Service   What makes military medical duties so eminently suitable for pacifists? The obvious appeal lies in the symmetry between the nonmaleficence of pacifism and the nonmaleficence of medicine. Yet pacifists interpret this differently.

Quakers serving in the FAU, for example, hoped to offer humanitarian care in the tradition of those nonmilitary medical personnel who provided voluntary care to wounded soldiers in the wake of Dunant's successful effort to found the Red Cross. Neutral and above the fray, they refused to triage based on salvage utility and demanded the right to provide medical care to any wounded individual regardless of nationality (Smith 1999, 243–255). Other pacifists decidedly set aside their antiwarism and considered themselves "conscientious supporters" of war. They would back their nation's war effort but refuse to bear arms. It is a strange and marginal worldview but astonishingly close to one typically associated with the practice of medicine during armed conflict. Consider the following testimony: "He will participate in any service, in the military service or out of it, which will contribute to the saving of human life . . . [but is prevented] from engaging in any act which contributes to destroying or injuring human life, in the military service or out of it, in war or in peace" (Haynes 1943).

"He" sounds like a physician but is, in fact, an Adventist pacifist. Adventists did not embrace antiwarism but did adhere to the principle of nonmaleficence following their literal and absolute belief in the sixth Commandment. This belief led them to seek noncombatant military positions, and during World War II, nearly half of the 25,000 noncombatant medics were Adventists. Their numbers were not trivial but their perspective is decidedly idiosyncratic, and it would be disconcerting if medicine could not articulate its own version of nonmaleficence and general support for war in less than universally acceptable terms. But this is not easy. Can anyone coherently embrace the principle of nonmaleficence but reject antiwarism? Most pacifists, whether secular or religious, cannot. They find the entire idea of "noncombatant military service" disingenuous and make no room for any cogent argument that might reconcile support for war and the duty to do no harm.

Their argument is straightforward. Addressing the question "Can a nonresistant nurse serve in the Army?" H. S. Bender, chair of the Peace Problems Committee for the Mennonites during World War II, states categorically that she cannot. "The army nurse," writes Bender (1944, 7), "is a regular member of the army, . . . identifies herself with the organization which prosecutes the war, and takes her share of moral responsibility for the military operations of the army of which she is part. . . . The army nurse is essential to the operations of the army. Without nurses, the army could not continue to fight." The same is true, of course, for medics, physicians, and other male military medical personnel.

Handbooks advising secular conscientious objectors are no less circumspect:

Some men are actually inducted into the medical service thinking that medics are instruments of mercy apart from the Army and its primary objectives. This erroneous conclusion can lead to serious personal difficulties. True, the medics save lives and ease suffering, sometimes in a manner which takes real heroism. But the medic is a soldier, and the ultimate objective of medics is to win battles. (Tatum 1970, 87–88; also see Seeley 1998, 36)

The argument of each critic is the same: any military role, combatant or noncombatant, inevitably violates the principle of nonmaleficence when the military operations of which medical personnel are an integral part harm others. Medical personnel are not in any way neutral or above the fray. Quite the contrary, medical care is an adjunct of war; it does not speak to easing the pain and suffering of individual soldiers as an end in itself, but of conserving manpower, maintaining military capabilities, and preventing, as one military manual put it, "adverse effects of unevacuated casualties on combat efficiency by . . . providing adequate medical care and rapid evacuation" (*Army Field Manual*, FM 8–10, 1951, 195).

If those conscientiously committed to the principle of nonmaleficence cannot square their duty to avoid harming others with support for war, can medicine manage it? If it can, military medical personnel must ask themselves how they should support the business of war; if it cannot, they must either embrace pacifism and eschew war, or reject nonmaleficence and consider answering the call to arms by contributing their expertise to the development of modern weaponry. A difficult question, but one which an appeal to the pacifism of their profession may answer.

Professional Vocational Pacifism

Perhaps *professional* vocational pacifism best characterizes the practice of medicine during war. Historically, the idea is associated with the clergy: "Clerics and bishops are forbidden to take up arms, not as though it were a sin, but because such an action is incompatible with their state. . . . Certain occupations are so inconsistent with one another that they cannot be fittingly exercised at the same time" (Aquinas [1947] 1995). Substitute *physicians* for *clerics and bishops* and few would quarrel with paraphrasing Aquinas to describe the vocational pacifism of the medical profession. If this view is consistent with what we expect of ethical medical conduct, it means that medical personnel may not assume the professional, combatant duties of soldiers. This is not because they must oppose war or because harming others during war is wrong, but because harming others is wrong *for doctors*. In a modern army, this does not necessarily preclude military service, but it does prevent physicians from "taking up arms" in their professional capacity, and to return to Coupland's (1997b) plea in the previous chapter, from using medical knowledge "for the purposes of weapon development." While neither clerics nor doctors oppose war, their vocations are the only two that successfully resist the state's call to arms with an appeal to nonmaleficence while, at the same time, rejecting antiwarism. How can they defend war *and* profess to do no harm?

Their argument proceeds in three steps, each articulating a distinct principle.

The Principle of Just War   Nations have an obligation to their citizens to resist aggression by force of arms insofar as armed violence is necessary, does not bring more harm than good, takes reasonable care to protect the welfare of noncombatants, and avoids causing unnecessary suffering to combatants. These are the familiar principles of just war and humanitarian law explored throughout this book. By this argument, just war repudiates antiwarism and allows most individuals, including physicians, to support war under certain circumstances.

The Principle of Collective Responsibility   The state's obligation to defend its citizens is a collective undertaking. While a political community may incur an obligation to wage a just war, this obligation does not extend to each and every member of the community. Some are exempt if their participation undermines collective action (old men and children, perhaps) or if they can better contribute to the war effort without taking up arms. It is therefore neither presumptuous nor hypocritical that clerics and physicians eschew combatant duty while encouraging or aiding their compatriots to kill during a just war.

The Principle of Medical Necessity   The practice of medicine is necessary to wage war successfully. Some observers suggest that clerics may abstain from combat during war because they are "uniquely situated to help victims of violence" (Kemp 1995, 36). The same is true for physicians: they stand relieved of their duty to engage actively in armed violence because they pursue a profession that both aids the injured and conserves a nation's fighting strength and, therefore, brings greater good than any combat role they could pursue. At the same time, the practice of medicine is necessary to successfully secure peace, and any deviation from the principle of nonmaleficence irreparably undermines the integrity of medicine and the great good it brings to humankind.

The first two principles pose no difficulties. Once satisfied that a war is just and that certain vocations may have more important tasks to perform than to bear arms, one moves to weigh the necessity of medicine during war. Although the principle of medical necessity is sound, it is important to see that actions satisfying medical necessity are contingent. Its implications, therefore, are neither straightforward nor obvious.

One reason for allowing clerics, bishops, and religious pacifists to refuse to bear arms is that their participation in armed conflict *as combatants* is not necessary. Pacifists, in particular, pose a thorny problem for a democratic polity that finds itself compelled by its very principles to show tolerance for diverse ethical and religious viewpoints that would, if significant numbers were to espouse the same view, otherwise undermine the state. Military officials are less perturbed precisely because the numbers of pacifists are small and manpower is fungible. Drafting conscientious objectors into medical service releases others for combat duty. There were never too many pacifists that officials could not afford to be magnanimous and avoid forcing pacifists to test their commitment to nonmaleficence by obligating them to bear arms.

Physicians, however, face a different problem because their duty *as combatants* is sometimes necessary. Ordinarily, practicing medicine with an eye toward never doing harm is of inestimable value to a nation waging war. In the overwhelming majority of cases, there is no reason to question the necessary role that medical nonmaleficence plays in just war. The goal of military medicine is to conserve a nation's military capability. Sound medical practice accomplishes this by protecting soldiers from disease, supervising proper hygiene, and evacuating and treating the wounded. However, one can also imagine a different set of circumstances when medical expertise is, in fact, necessary for the development of essential weapons systems, whether for deterrence or nonlethal warfare. If the principle of just war allows nations to defend themselves by force of arms and the successful deployment of arms requires medical knowledge, then the principle of nonmaleficence may not serve medical necessity if it impairs the development of the means necessary to wage a just war.

At this juncture, medical professionals face a stark choice: nonmaleficence or just war. Choosing the former will, in those hard cases under consideration, inevitably affect the latter. Here, as is often the case during war, they must consider the relationship between medicine and the welfare of the community. Unlike religious pacifism, medicine is not a vocational calling that transcends the welfare of the community within which it is embedded. Rather, medicine is a professional calling subordinate to the interests of the community that bestows on its practitioners their obligations and privileges. When David Thomasma and Edmund Pellegrino refer to medicine's "sacred trust" or "covenant," they do not mean, I hope, a covenant akin to the one binding God and the ancient Hebrews, but one that binds physicians and the community. Most often, the medical interests of the community translate into the interests of its individual patients, and here medicine finds its vocation and imperative to do no harm. But not always; during war the interests of the community may move from individual health care to collective welfare. Communities have interests of their own that sometimes complement but sometimes conflict with those of their members and reflect the shared ethos or way of life that nations and their citizens fight for during war. During war, collective welfare shapes the duties of medical practitioners, just as it shapes the duties of other members of the community within which doctors live. In fact, it is precisely because the community sanctions the medical community's privileged access to medical knowledge that physicians must use their knowledge in the service of their community. Ordinarily this demands overriding attention to beneficence and scrupulous attention to their duty to do no harm. However, during armed conflict communal interests change. The health-related interests of individual patients give way to the welfare of the political community. Non-maleficence may then yield to active participation in a just war and bring physicians to contribute their expertise to the development of weapons. Unjust war, on the other hand, elicits a different response as medical professionals consider the merits of civil disobedience.

Physician-Assisted Draft Evasion

From the early days of conscription, physicians have declared their opposition to unjust wars and used their good offices to aid draft evaders:

William McCanless, a [Confederate] physician arrested in 1863 for giving resisters false medical deferments and for harboring deserters, justified his anti-draft activity by declaring that 'it was a shame to take men off to this army to be slaughtered; and that it would be considered a dishonor in future years to have been in favor of the rebellion'. (Honey 1986)

One hundred years later the situation was much the same:

Many men were obtaining medical deferments because their personal physicians were writing letters claiming ailments that would qualify them for exemptions. A favorite ailment was manic depression. The *New York Times* reported that one New York psychiatrist was writing about seventy-five letters a week for a fee of $200 each, all to be paid "cash in advance." With the help of physicians, whether for financial gain or opposition to the war, the failure rate for Vietnam War–era inductees was triple what it had been during World War II. (Dickerson 1999, 71)

Although anecdotal tales abound, it is impossible to estimate the number of physicians who have conscientiously aided draft evaders (Baskir and Strauss 1978; Gottlieb 1991, 139–172). The cases above demonstrate how physicians defy both the law of the land and the canons of medical ethics when they lie and write fraudulent medical reports. In response, we surmise that physicians who abet draft evasion are answering to a higher moral principle that transcends both the law *and* bioethics. This is unusual, for in those rare instances when physicians exercise civil disobedience, they usually violate the law precisely so they may *uphold* a fundamental principle of medical ethics that serves their patient's best interests. Draft evasion, however, invokes the specter of just war and places the relationship between medicine and civil disobedience in a different light.

The Idea of Civil Disobedience

Delivering an impromptu lecure to Crito when he came to rescue Socrates from execution, Socrates admonishes his students to obey the law. Knowing that the people of Athens unjustly condemned him to death, Socrates nonetheless does not see their lapse as sufficient reason to turn his back on the law, the state, and his fellow citizens. Although condemned to die, Socrates remains convinced that he continues to owe the state a debt of gratitude for all the benefits it provided him throughout his life and, moreover, is too important an institution to undermine by a poor example of disgruntled citizenship. Refusing exile, he stays and accepts his fate.

Plato's dilemma focuses squarely on a citizen's obligation to obey the law. Socrates was not unsympathetic to Crito's plea, but his view of the state as the organism that gives life and meaning to the individual precluded him from placing his interests, however wronged, or his own sense of justice, however right, above the welfare of the polis. We have come a long way since Athenian democracy. Turning the polis on its head, the modern state trumpets individual welfare as the state serves as the vehicle for personal self-development. Safeguarding human rights and civil liberties is at the heart of the state's fiduciary responsibility toward its citizens. Good riddance to the state that violates its sacred trust.

Civil disobedience, however, is not a theory for dismantling the modern democratic state. Instead, as Rawls (1971, 365–366) suggests, civil disobedients work *within* the framework of a well-ordered state and defy certain laws to convince an errant majority that it has swayed from its own sense of justice:

In justifying civil disobedience, one invokes the commonly shared conception of justice that underlies the political order. . . . The persistent and deliberate violation of the basic principles of this conception over any extended period of time, especially the infringement of the fundamental equal liberties, invites either submission or resistance. By engaging in civil disobedience a minority forces the majority to consider whether it wishes to have its action construed in this way, or whether, in view of the common sense of justice, it wishes to acknowledge the legitimate claims of the minority.

As they consider resistance, civil disobedients do not have an easy time. Unlike conscientious objection, civil disobedience is inimical to the state. Guided by magnanimity and tolerance for religious freedom, many states will make room, either by alternative service or deferment, for those who sincerely espouse the principles of antiwarism and nonmaleficence. The state cannot show similar tolerance for those who believe a particular war is unjust and who challenge, rather than respect, the authority of the state. If a democratic state can accommodate pacifists who cannot conscientiously obey a law committing them to armed violence, the same state must repudiate and diligently prosecute those who defy the law, censure the government, and make a concerted effort to rally others to their cause.

Civil Disobedience and the Principles of Just War   While COs anchor their beliefs in an idiosyncratic and private worldview, civil disobedients draw on a shared sense of justice that appeals to the Western tradition of human rights and humanitarian law. Underlying this sense of justice is the conviction that states that violate fundamental equal liberties, whether at home or abroad, during peace or war, are open to rebuke. Nevertheless, states do not often face civil disobedience during war. Ordinarily they command the legal and moral authority to conscript citizens in the interest of legitimate national defense. And, most often, the vast majority of citizens comply. Those that do not, face arrest and imprisonment, while their compatriots look on with few misgivings and indeed a sense of just desert. Unjust wars, on the other hand, merit a different response. Traditionally, the just ends of war (*jus ad bellum*) exclude any war that is not a last-resort measure necessary to stave off an armed attack against a nation-state or recognized political community. More recently, however, the legitimate ends of war are expanding to embrace wars of humanitarian intervention and international law enforcement. Nor are the just means of war (*jus in bello*) stable. At the very least, just war demands that belligerents respect human rights, refrain from using weapons that cause unnecessary suffering, make a concerted effort to protect noncombatants from unnecessary harm, and cease hostilities once they have disabled their enemy. Just wars do not indiscriminately target civilians, forever displace indigenous populations, or seek to annihilate an enemy. Yet difficulties arise when some belligerents turn to terror, when civilians aid and abet militants and guerrillas, and when military planners consider nonlethal weapons.

In spite of ever-shifting conditions, the principles of just war continue to invoke the same shared principles of justice that justify any form of civil disobedience when they are persistently and deliberately violated by the state. Armed conflict, by its very nature, abridges, curtails, and often denies combatants and noncombatants fundamental *civil* rights by restricting freedom of movement and assembly, the right to a free press, and political representation. Generally, these measures are a temporary expedient, necessary to maintain order but subject to restoration at the cessation of hostilities and end of occupation. Abridged or unequal civil rights do not usually serve as cause for civil disobedience during war unless they remain unrestored for unnecessarily long periods of time. Human rights, on the other hand, deserve special consideration and save anyone, but particularly noncombatants, from cruelty, enslavement, wanton death and suffering, indignity and humiliation, indigence, and political impotence. Blatant wars of aggression, unnecessary wars that defend dubious interests, and wars prosecuted without regard for the welfare or human rights of noncombatants merit condemnation.

Although each principle of just war is conceptually distinct, a just war requires both legitimate ends and means. Many Americans objected to the Vietnam War because it did not serve the interests of self-defense, did not stave off an armed threat to the United States, brought unnecessary death and destruction upon the civilian population of Vietnam, and ignored the legitimate political interests of the Vietnamese by propping up a corrupt regime. In the postwar period, nations such as France found themselves locked in unpopular colonial wars that sparked similar moral outrage as the French tortured and abused Algerian insurgents. More recently, Israel's ongoing war with the Palestinians has elicited a similar response because Israel's attempt to generally preserve humanitarian law in the face of vicious terror attacks has done little to quiet claims that it continues to wage an unjust war of occupation. Wars like these invite civil disobedience.

Civil Disobedience and Evasive Noncompliance   There are many ways to defy the law. Some are public and confrontational as civil disobedients try to rouse and sometimes enrage their fellow citizens so they will overcome their acquiescence to injustice. For some observers, therefore, civil disobedience must be public, nonviolent, aim solely at laws civil disobedients believe are unjust (and no other), and obligates offenders to suffer punishment for their misdeeds. In this way, civil disobedients have the best chance to transform public policy without undermining the very regime whose policies they oppose. Nevertheless, it is easy to see how some of these conditions are difficult to fulfill in practice. When demonstrators fight civil rights abuses or protest an unjust war they invariably break laws unrelated to the injustice they oppose. Violence, too, is sometimes inevitable when protestors clash with police and inflame public passions.

Others, such as draft evaders, are less inclined to accept the punishment the state metes out and, therefore, act surreptitiously as they violate the law. Their actions, often described as "evasive noncompliance," are quieter and less confrontational than civil disobedience. While these actions are perhaps tinged with self-interest, one assumes that most draft evaders would not hesitate to serve in a just war (otherwise they would be conscientious objectors and gain the forbearance of the state). At worst, their motives combine self-interest with a commitment to a moral principle that appeals to the justice of war. Moreover, potential draftees, unlike student demonstrators who publicly declare their opposition to the war and their willingness to take on the authorities, face much higher costs for their opposition. Stiff prison terms and/or conscription are the norm. Given these costs, it is reasonable for draft evaders to stay out of the public eye. Nevertheless, there is no reason to assume that many evaders do not feel a passionate and conscientious opposition to a particular war and hope that through their evasion they may weaken public support for the government.

Draft evasion presents an intriguing challenge to physicians who oppose unjust war and wish to aid draft evaders. While physicians may engage in civil disobedience like anyone else, they do not often violate the law in their *professional* capacity. When they do, it is to uphold and defend the canons of medical ethics. Draft evasion, however, is considerably more problematic, for as physicians aid draft evaders, they violate the law and the most basic principles of medical ethics.

Medical Civil Disobedience

"Dissent," writes James Childress (1985, 63), "is not common in health care." Significant examples are as tightly defined as Rawls demands. Fighting abortion, resisting laws that restrict the withdrawal of life support, and similar causes have brought doctors and nurses to publicly defy the law, treat their patients as they feel their professional integrity demands, and go public and bear the consequences. Championing abortion rights or the right to die with dignity, doctors who defy the law ultimately appeal to the welfare and/or rights of their patients, as they demand that certain policies are unjust and must be changed. The abortion argument turns on both the benefit of safe and legal abortions for pregnant women who might otherwise resort to dangerous, back-alley procedures and the deontological force of a woman's right to self-determination and privacy. In these circumstances, conscientious physicians place their professional obligations as healers against their prima facie obligation to obey the law. As the former gain strength and the latter weaken in the face of a law that infringes on fundamental liberties, disobedience becomes a legitimate moral option. Physicians can appeal to beneficence or respect for autonomy to justify their actions when they endorse contraception, perform abortions, withdraw life support, or help critically ill patients die (Madden and Hare 1978; Childress 1985; Wicclair 2000). In these cases medical civil disobedients operate within the paradigm of medical ethics and invoke its moral norms to override the law when the two conflict.

Support for draft evasion is significantly different, because disobedient physicians are appealing to the principles of just war to override both medical ethics—that is, the injunction against lying—and the law of the land that forbids draft evasion. Physicians can justify their actions only by arguing that both the law *and* professional medical ethics are subordinate to higher moral principles of justice. For this argument to work, civil disobedients must assert a greater good or greater deontological principle that overrides their other duties. This has brought antiwar activists—protesters, draft evaders, and sympathetic physicians alike—to support *selective* antiwarism, the belief that war is wrong when it violates the principles of just war. This has in turn led the most conscientious to violate the law and, in some cases, their professional duties as well.

Selective antiwarism is not vocational pacifism. Unlike vocational pacifists, selective pacifists are not at all convinced that war is wrong or unnecessary but only that certain wars violate the conditions of just war and therefore merit denunciation. When wars are unjust, some individuals will refuse to fight, either because they cannot in good conscience take part in an unjust war and/or because they hope their refusal will sufficiently impair manpower or influence public opinion to force a change in policy. In these circumstances, physicians can play a crucial role if they choose to aid and abet draft evasion. Because conscription is subject to good health, physicians find themselves uniquely situated to certify draft evaders as unfit for duty.

Physician-Assisted Draft Evasion and the Demands of Beneficence

Before appraising a decision to abet draft evasion, consider first the obligation to obey the law and respect the principle of truth telling. Asked to abet draft evasion, a physician might reasonably respond with the following arguments:

- It is against medicine's professional code of ethics to lie.
- Draft evasion is against the law.
- Draft evasion may harm others:
  By undermining a nation's ability to defend itself.
  By reducing the pool of eligible young men and women and thereby placing a greater burden on others.
- Every citizen must do his or her duty, and I cannot assist those who shirk theirs.

Physicians now contemplating requests to aid draft evaders face the prospect of violating their duty to tell the truth and to obey the law.

To justify either violation requires an argument grounded in utility, substantiating that in some instances lying and blatantly violating the law bring a greater good than truth telling and obedience, or that the duty to tell the truth and obey the law of the land falls before some higher moral principle that overrides both. Consider the first obstacle: must a physician always tell the truth? Sometimes the answer is no; one may appeal to beneficence to override the imperative to respect autonomy and always tell the truth. This is true of therapeutic lies:

The Therapeutic Lie   In a hypothetical case, White and Gampel (1996) describe how a woman critically injured in a car wreck is not told that her children also died in the accident. When asked directly, her caregivers lie, convinced that the truth might cause her irreversible harm.

This is not yet an act of civil disobedience, for no law has been broken. In other instances, violating medical ethics may also violate the law. This happens in efforts to game the system.

Gaming the System   In Oregon, a certain illness, A, is uninsured and patients cannot obtain treatment. However, another illness, B, is ranked higher and guarantees the insured will receive treatment. By happy coincidence, treatment for A and B is identical although the diseases are different. To provide treatment, doctors game the system and lie about their patient's true condition so they may receive care (Jacobs, Marmor, and Oberlander 1999; Leichter 1999).

In each of these cases, beneficence—the duty to see to their patients' welfare—overrides physicians' obligation to tell the truth and obey the law. The therapeutic lie is, perhaps, less controversial. Here doctors lie to their patients with the understanding that divulging the true nature of their tragedy will harm their health and impair their chance of recovery. Here, too, the breach of autonomy is temporary. Once the patients sufficiently recover, they will learn the truth. Beneficence overrides respect for autonomy and the physicians' duty to tell the truth. The risk is minimal. Although lying may impair the integrity of physicians and jeopardize their patients' trust, these effects disappear once the patients recover, learn the learn for the deception, and trust is restored.

The second case is more complex. The physicians do not lie to their patients but to a third-party provider, perhaps an employer. Their actions are illegal as well as unethical. Here, too, however, the patients' welfare motivates their doctors to lie and confirm an illness only because it guarantees the treatment patients need for their actual, but uninsured, condition. But the lie is not short-lived, nor does the truth ever emerge. Nor are the long-term consequences clear: gaming the system might easily undermine the provision of fair health care.

Evasive noncompliance accurately describes gaming because the physicians' actions are covert and nonconfrontational. Nevertheless, noncompliance, like civil disobedience, must meet several tests. To lie and meet the conditions for legitimate evasive noncompliance, physicians must demonstrate that illegal actions

• Constitute a last resort, without which it is impossible to avert harm

• Appeal to a higher or at least equally weighty moral principle

• Pass the test of utility, so that physicians' illegal acts bring greater benefit than harm

In this case physicians lie to uphold beneficence and/or protect their patients from what may be discrimination. They must ask themselves whether they might forestall harm to their patients by other means, whether beneficence and/or fair access to health care are sufficiently weighty principles to stand against the duty to tell the truth, and whether gaming the system does not do more harm to more people than abiding by the rules. One can also imagine another variant of gaming that allows physicians to lie by appealing to global beneficence—that is, the welfare of other patients. Convinced, perhaps, that the entire system is corrupt or discriminatory, caregivers go out of their way to help many patients game the system to both protect their welfare and, at the same time, change the structure of local health care. Civil disobedience here, too, must stand the test of last resort and utility.

Physician-Assisted Draft Evasion and the Demands of Justice

Gaming the system is close to abetting draft evasion with one significant difference. Physicians who game the system appeal to beneficence and act to prevent health-related harm to their patients that comes from a system that functions to their disadvantage. The justification for gaming the system lies within the paradigm of patient care and stems from an assessment of the health-related consequences that undermining the system may have for others. While physicians have an interest in their patients' welfare, they may not harm others as they pursue their patients' well-being. Convinced their actions harm no one else, they may decide to game the system to care for their patients.

Any decision to aid draft evaders, in contrast, cannot appeal to beneficence. If beneficence is an overriding norm and physicians are concerned solely about their patients' welfare, they must *always* refuse to certify the fitness of conscripts for military service, just as they should endeavor to prevent their wounded patients from returning to service (by doctoring their medical records, for example) whether the war is just or unjust. But they do not. Most physicians would not and should not give a second thought to aiding draft evaders during a just war. Abetting draft evasion only gains moral force when war is unjust—that is, violates a political conception of justice. It has nothing to do with beneficence or health-related norms of justice or narrow considerations of patients' welfare.

Disobedience to the law must meet the same conditions that drive any act of civil disobedience or evasive noncompliance. A decision to aid draft evaders must consider both the act of draft evading and the act of lying to avoid conscription. Each act poses a moral dilemma, for it places the obligation to oppose an unjust war against the duty to obey the law. For physicians, the dilemma is compounded by their professional obligation to tell the truth. The principle of beneficence is not at stake. Assuming that gross violations of the principles of just war offer sufficient grounds to temper one's prima facie obligation to obey the law, one must ask whether they also offer sufficient grounds to override the professional obligation of physicians to tell the truth. Ordinarily, this principle is fundamental, but I have already noted two cases where truth telling falls to beneficence and, more generally, to calculations of utility. Nevertheless, one can still imagine physicians responding that they must never lie. They would not tell therapeutic lies but would perhaps temporarily avoid telling the truth. They would refuse to game the system while perhaps referring their patients to other physicians. Under these circumstances, the dilemma does not get off the ground. In fact, there is no dilemma for the Kantian who refuses to lie under any circumstances.

Scratching the surface, however, one often finds a utilitarian argument: lying is wrong because it brings harm. To make a case, draft evasion must exemplify a last-resort means to avoid injustice and meet the test of utility. This is often difficult to ascertain. A draft evader may publicly disobey the law and accept punishment or evade the law and flee the country before asking a physician for a fraudulent medical report. Each of these options involves significantly higher costs. Evasion by means of a fraudulent medical deferment, on the other hand, adds the cost of a physician lying, the harm this brings to others, and the harm this may bring to the medical profession. Draft evasion by any means may save one person but endanger another who must take his or her place.

An assessment of these costs varies with the circumstances. When wars are very unpopular, physicians may argue that although medical civil disobedience violates the law and the principles of medical ethics, it enhances rather than undermines their professional integrity. The harm that evasion may bring to others is extraordinarily difficult to evaluate. It is impossible to know who, if anyone, will take one's place, what may befall him or her, and whether that person, too, may evade the draft. Moreover, harm to others might be precisely the point the draft evader wants to make. By forcing the government to triple its efforts to find recruits, draft evaders hope to hobble military capabilities and turn public opinion against the war. These are the costs and benefits any civil disobedient weighs in considering the benefits of violating the law and undermining public policy.

I will not attend to these utility calculations any further, but emphasize the point that the principles of just war may clash with and override fundamental principles of medical ethics. As physicians consider their duty to oppose unjust war, they move outside the paradigm of medicine and violate the law out of a commitment to justice that overrides the principles of medical ethics. This is a remarkable shift in priorities as medicine subordinates its professional duties to civic justice and the shared moral norms of the community. And, this is precisely what they are also asked to do when called on to develop weaponry.

Physician-assisted draft evasion reveals the asymmetry of professional and civic obligations, and demonstrates how the latter sometimes override the former, particularly during war.

In armed conflict, the principles of medical ethics may fall to collective interests that include reason of state or national self-defense. During war, physicians generally certify their patients for military duty knowing full well they may suffer death or injury. We attribute this to military medicine's commitment to building a nation's fighting force and conserving manpower at the expense of individual liberties and ordinary patient rights. As physicians serve the interests of the community, war tests many of medicine's fundamental principles. Patients, particularly soldiers, lose their autonomy, privacy, and right to die. To keep a unit fit, military personnel treat the wounded with an eye on salvage utility rather than on medical need. And, of course, medical doctors certify a person's fitness to fight and die. In each of these instances, it is tolerable and indeed necessary for physicians to place their professional services and their canon of ethics in the service of war when it is just.

When war is unjust, however, doctors must use their good offices to achieve other ends. Unjust wars signify a gross violation of justice that threatens to tear apart the moral fabric of the community. Physicians who understand that truth telling is not sacrosanct may be inclined to aid draft evaders if this, indeed, contributes to the end of an unjust war. The effects of lying may be difficult to ascertain. One must be careful to avoid the slide toward beneficence and the conviction that lying to avoid the draft is justified because it benefits a doctor's patient. While the individual patient invariably has the most to gain, his or her welfare does not and cannot justify draft evasion in the same way it justifies gaming the system or a therapeutic lie. Instead, one must be content to take the extreme steps of violating the law and violating a physician's duty to tell the truth in the hope that it will assuage one's conscience that he or she did everything possible to end an unjust war.

For all its merit, civil disobedience remains defensible in only extreme circumstances and under carefully defined conditions. Selective pacifism comes to the fore in those rare instances that nations unjustly choose armed conflict to meet threats from other countries. In many other situations, war may be imprudent, unnecessary, and tremendously costly, suggesting to many observers that there are better ways to resolve conflict between nations. This prompts us to think about world peace and the special role medicine may play as physicians demonstrate social responsibility.

Medicine and Pacifism: The Quest for World Peace

One need not espouse absolute pacifism or engage actively in civil disobedience to worry about the effects of war on the human race or believe that war is a poor method of settling disputes. Drawing on a more benevolent vision of human nature than that which prompted Hobbes to famously describe man's life as "nasty, brutish, and short," many Enlightenment thinkers were soon convinced that both domestic and international politics might run better in the spirit of cooperation than competition. The turn toward peace was neither quick nor inevitable but a rational preference fired by the belief, as Kant ([1784] 1991, 47) suggested, that ultimately humankind "will take the step that reason could have suggested without so many sad experiences—that of abandoning the lawless state of savagery and entering a federation of peoples." Sorely tested by the First and Second World Wars, this commitment to pacifism—that is, the belief that a rational, liberal, and enlightened world can eventually abandon war—gained force when it became clear that the world would not survive another world war. To the weighty claims of enlightened rationalism, health-care professionals add their professional commitment to nonmaleficence and beneficence. As it has done for pacifists and civil disobedients, the former lends weight to the opposition of war while the latter fosters a commitment to peace and the greater good it can bring humankind in terms of health and development:

Health care workers are especially sensitive to the issue of prevention of war, as both war itself and the preparation for war are highly destructive to health. Not only is it a natural motivation for health workers to improve health by preventing war but we are also inspired by the Hippocratic tenet "first do no harm" to prefer healing and preventative rather than forceful or military means to address conflict and war. (International Physicians for the Prevention of Nuclear War, 2001b, 309)

Although medical professionals have actively supported the peace movement for well over a century, medical organizations came to prominence following World War II as they sought ways to reduce the likelihood of nuclear war (Lewer 1992; Maddocks 1996). Most were not pacifist organizations; they did not oppose conventional war or the need to wage war in self-defense. Instead, they sometimes described themselves as internationalists, heirs to a tradition of international liberalism that emphasizes the importance of cooperative world bodies to maintain collective security, reduce conflict, and safeguard human rights. Inspired by their professional commitment to beneficence and the duty to do no harm, many physicians take to the optimistic vision that liberalism offers the international community. What, then, can medicine specifically bring to the end of conflict and the achievement of peace? The answer is twofold: medical research and political activism. The overwhelming need to document the medical effects of war, convince a reluctant public of war's futility, and promote alternative means of conflict resolution cuts across two fields—nuclear disarmament and human rights.

Nuclear Disarmament

Between the end of World War II and the collapse of the Soviet Union a half century later, the medical peace movement dedicated its efforts to nuclear disarmament and preventing nuclear war. While physicians were not the only activists to grasp the dangers of nuclear war, they roused considerable interest among many members of the profession by appealing to the principle of medical nonmaleficence and to the unique contributions medical professionals could make to the cause of peace. "We physicians who shepherd human life from birth to death," declared Bernard Lown (1985) as he accepted the Nobel Prize on behalf of the International Physicians for the Prevention of Nuclear War (IPPNW), "have a moral imperative to resist with all our being the drift toward the brink."

Together with the Medical Association for the Prevention of War (MAPW) and Physicians for Social Responsibility (PSR), the IPPNW embarked on a concerted campaign to rid the world of nuclear weapons. By carefully analyzing the human, material, and environmental costs of nuclear war, peace activists hoped to impress policymakers with the simple fact that no nation could ever fight and survive, much less win, a nuclear war (Cassel et al. 1980). Through persistent lobbying and well-funded educational campaigns, the physician's peace organizations labored to change policy by describing the catastrophic effects and calamitous impact of nuclear war. Just as infectious disease, urban decay, poor housing and sanitation, and inadequate health care threatened public health at the turn of the century, nuclear war posed the single greatest threat to human health and survival in the aftermath of World War II.

While the empirical data about the effects of nuclear war are clear and overwhelming, their implications are not. Should nations pursue disarmament or deterrence? Is civil defense a vital part of national security or a waste of resources that would bring greater benefit elsewhere? Strategic weapons aside, are there any military benefits to tactical—that is, battlefield—nuclear weapons? As these questions occupied policy-makers throughout the postwar period, most peace groups took exception to any policy short of disarmament. Medical peace groups were no exception.

As they struggled to convince the public of the merits of disarmament, antinuclear organizations confronted a number of issues. Weighing the merits of nuclear deterrence, peace groups raised many of the concerns outlined in the previous chapter: deterrence, although obviously preferable to war, threatens the lives of innocent noncombatants in the best case and flirts with the obliteration of humankind in the worse. To forestall any justifiable claim of nuclear armament that deterrence might support, the physicians' peace organizations emphasized the futility of any reasonable medical response to strategic and tactical nuclear war, going so far as to wonder whether medical workers may need to euthanize large numbers of civilians that they could not effectively treat (Haines, de B. White, and Gleisner 1983). Deterrence moreover, even successful deterrence, was not without ancillary costs. The environmental costs of developing and testing any nuclear weapon were overwhelming and funds earmarked for nuclear weapons could, in their opinion, better improve education and fight disease. Each of these arguments—the high cost of medical treatment, the tragic effects on the environment, and alternative uses for the funds earmarked for nuclear weapons—also fueled arguments for eliminating tactical nuclear weapons.

On the subject of civil defense, the peace organizations found themselves divided. Civil defense measures—bunkers, public shelters, stockpiled medical supplies, and evacuation—obviously demanded funds for construction, and medical and nonmedical personnel for implementation. The question that plagued the peace movements, however, was military. Committed to disarmament and the end of nuclear war, many felt that civil defense might only encourage nations to fight a nuclear war in the hope that they could survive a retaliatory second strike. At best, widespread civil defense measures would lead arms manufacturers to develop increasingly powerful devices that could destroy reinforced bunkers. Either way, the scenario they painted remained dark: no nation could ever hope to wage or win a nuclear war. Physicians for Social Responsibility responded with similar arguments to American contingency plans to allocate existing medical facilities for care during a nuclear war. The issue did not turn on medical care but nuclear war: PSR activists feared that any preparation for war, including shelters or contingency medical care, allowed policymakers to reasonably contemplate the possibility of limited nuclear hostilities. War, they reasoned, might become a self-fulfilling prophecy (Bisgard 1982; Geiger 1982; Johnson 1982; Murray 1982; Day and Waitzkin 1985).

For the most part, the medical peace organizations were single-issue, special-interest groups. The IPPNW in particular was careful to emphasize a single goal—nuclear disarmament and the prevention of nuclear war—and pointedly ignored questions of human rights abuses or conventional war. Recipients of the Nobel Peace Prize, it is nonetheless difficult to evaluate their success independent of the geopolitics that brought the collapse of the Soviet Union. Although they pressed tirelessly for nuclear disarmament, mutual deterrence best describes the nuclear policy of the superpowers prior to the disintegration of the Soviet Union. Subsequently, the United States and Russia signed treaties—START I (1994) and SORT (Strategic Offensive Reductions Treaty, 2003)—that promised substantial reductions of American and Russian nuclear capabilities. At the same time, the international community continues to move slowly toward the Comprehensive Nuclear Test Ban Treaty (CNTBT).

In the best tradition of prominent and highly visible social movements, "success breeds failure," and with the decreasing danger of thermonuclear war as East-West relations realigned at the end of the twentieth century, many peace movements dedicated to ending nuclear war were suddenly on the verge of fulfilling their mission and disappearing. As the nuclear threat waned and the vast majority of nations accepted the conventions against chemical and biological warfare, the world moved slowly away from the danger of unconventional wars of mass destruction. In their place, however, low-intensity wars simmered among state and substate actors. Colonial wars of independence, vicious ethnic conflicts, wars of humanitarian intervention, and international terror presented a different kind of threat to world peace and eventually brought the *Bulletin of Atomic Scientists* (2002) to move its doomsday clock forward by two minutes. Sensing the urgency of these conflicts, peace movements like the IPPNW sought novel ways to end all conflicts and ensure human rights and civil liberties around the world.

Medical Humanitarianism

Medical humanitarianism and concern for human rights is steadily replacing concern for nuclear war among the physicians' peace organizations. Inasmuch as humanitarian aid has always been the watchword of medicine, it might seem redundant to describe the contribution that physicians' peace movements make to alleviate suffering during armed conflict. Medical humanitarianism, however, pushes beyond the provision of medical care during war and highlights the role physicians can play as neutral, independent actors who can make a special contribution to ending armed conflict and ensuring human rights. When it altered its mission statement in 1993 to accommodate a new agenda, the IPPNW (2005) transformed its organizational goals: "IPPNW is ... dedicated to research, education, and advocacy relevant to the prevention of nuclear war. To this end, IPPNW seeks to prevent all wars, to promote non-violent conflict resolution, and to minimize the effects of war and preparations for war on health, development, and the environment."

Relieved of the threat of nuclear war and consistent with its belief that war is the least desirable means of conflict resolution, the IPPNW

(2001a, 2001b) turned its attention to nonviolent means of conflict resolution. In doing so, it proposed to draw on the unique resources of the
medical community by formulating a program to defuse conflicts or
reduce their attendant violence. Drawing on their expertise in the arena
of nuclear war, advocates proposed a program of public education to
discredit the efficacy of armed conflict by forcefully bringing the tragic
effects of war to the public's attention. This was not a diffuse effort aimed
solely at the world community, but an "on-the-ground" approach that
would place medical workers in conflict-ridden areas to document
human rights abuses and establish a bridge of support with the local population and warring parties. Building on the prestige of physicians
together with traditional respect for physician neutrality, IPPNW officials hoped that physicians could serve as impartial observers and mediators between conflicting sides.

While the medical community continues to draw on its professional
expertise to provide humanitarian aid and relieve the physiological and
psychological suffering of war, the IPPNW broadens the role it envisions
for physicians. Among many physicians, there is a growing understanding that in the absence of human rights, it is impossible to provide adequate medical care. Physicians for Human Rights and Médecins Sans
Frontières (MSF) (Doctors Without Borders), for example, not only
provide humanitarian medical aid in war-torn areas but expend considerable resources monitoring, documenting, protesting and prosecuting
human rights abuses (Iacopino and Waldman 1999; Nolan 1999;
Bortolotti 2004 Weissman 2004). By moving toward mediation, these
organizations expand the role of the physician further still as aid
workers, apart from offering medical care, serve in a *political* role.
Medical and political efforts are mutually reinforcing; the underlying
idea is to remove physicians from contributing to the fighting in any way,
restore their traditional neutrality, reinstate the transcendence of bioethical principles, and indeed place physicians above the fray so they are in
a position to end armed conflict. Other groups of medical workers, often
locally based, strive for more modest goals, hoping to use medical cooperation to foster understanding, promote solidarity, and provide a forum
for free and open discussion between mistrustful and warring groups
(Skinner et al. 2005; MacQueen and Santa-Barbara 2000). These efforts

highlight medical humanitarianism in rogue regimes as well as in those the international community seeks to change by force of arms.

Medical Humanitarianism in Rogue Regimes   Unique moral problems arise when aid workers knowingly support despotic regimes. Markus Michael and Anthony Zwi (2002) report on Red Cross efforts to provide surgical care in Taliban-controlled Afghanistan (1996–2002) and ask an important question: "Does providing health care prop up a repressive regime?" "Propping up" can mean (1) allowing government officials to redirect scarce resources to its armed forces or other agencies of repression, knowing that international organizations are providing health care; (2) using health care to instill loyalty and win the people's support for a cruel and oppressive government; (3) exploiting an international organization to win legitimacy for the regime. In reviewing the Red Cross efforts in Afghanistan, Michael and Zwi conclude that these conditions were not met. "The Taliban," they write, "never attempted to politicize humanitarian aid or specifically capitalize on its provision" (p. 118).

But what if they had? Should medical workers continue to provide aid? If the ethical principle that medical care should not prop up despotic regimes is compelling, then humanitarian organizations should desist if their aid allows repressive regimes to divert funds or encourages support for the government. Complying with this principle, however, demands a definition of a *repressive* or *rogue* regime and the empirical means to determine whether humanitarian aid supports the government in any significant way. Taliban Afghanistan was certainly a rogue regime, if by this we mean a regime unrecognized by most nations. Assessing the effects of humanitarian aid is a more difficult task and, in this case, was only possible *after* the Red Cross went to work in Afghanistan. Aid workers will require considerable data to draw conclusions before intervening. Moreover, it is insufficient that humanitarian aid merely maintains a repressive regime. Rather, aid is only unwarranted if the harm it causes by supporting an oppressive regime outweighs the good it brings by providing medical care. This seems to be an exceedingly difficult conclusion to draw under any circumstances, leaving most aid organizations to ignore, and with good reason, the question that Michael and Zwi raise.

Nevertheless, it remains the obligation of the world community to address the question that relief workers can only set aside, and intervene militarily when it becomes clear that international aid organizations are fighting, and losing, an uphill battle as they provide medical care in a regime that is not only repressive but genocidal and massively abusive of human rights as well. This does not always happen. Although the UN had long imposed sanctions on the Taliban government while hoping for a peaceful regime change, the United State took notice only once its own interests were at risk. Nevertheless, many hope that in the future the world community will look beyond national interests and forcibly replace rogue regimes and so relieve aid workers of the dilemma of having to support corrupt regimes while they provide medical care to their beleaguered inhabitants. In such cases, humanitarian aid will join forces with armed intervention.

Medical Humanitarianism and Armed Intervention   Medical humanitarianism does not repudiate war. On the contrary, as medical observers mediate conflict and/or offer humanitarian aid they may find that nonviolent intervention goes hand in hand with armed intervention to prevent human rights abuse or genocide. While peace organizations prefer law enforcement and police forces to military operations and professional armies, this line is often blurred (International Physicians for the Prevention of Nuclear War, 2001b, 315). The United Nations provides for international law enforcement with forces that look much like military troops, while the entire concept of "military operations other than war" opens up possibilities for armed violence that may include some weapons, nonlethal arms for example, that are generally not a part of conventional war. As the international community considers the complexity of enforcing human rights, preventing terror, and expanding the practice of democracy, peace organizations face the possibility that armed intervention, at least in the short term, is necessary to curb the excesses of rogue regimes that harbor terrorists, illegally trade in nuclear material, or develop weapons of mass destruction in contravention of international treaties.

As the international community moves slowly toward humanitarian intervention, the relationship between medicine and war begins to change. Throughout this book, medicine is depicted in the service of war. When wars are necessary, effective, and justly waged, the role of medicine remains to serve reason of state and maintain the forces necessary for nations to pursue vital interests. Wars of humanitarian intervention, however, are not about vital interests but reflect the duty dictated by beneficence to end massive and egregious human rights violations in despotic regimes. These wars pose an enormous challenge for an international community that has hitherto conceptualized just war in terms of defense against armed aggression (Chatterjee and Scheid 2003; Holzgrefe and Keohane 2003). As the world community weighs the importance of human rights, there is growing agreement that nations should act in concert and at the behest of the United Nations to intervene when rights are abused, and when no other alternative can aid victims of injustice. Insofar as contemporary armed conflict holds to emerging principles of humanitarian intervention that include UN authorization, the amelioration of human rights abuses, the establishment of local democratic government, and a clear exit strategy, armed conflict will represent the moral force of the world community, not the parochial interests of nation-states. Now the tables are turned. Armed force serve humanitarian interests and with them the practice of medicine.

As nations undertake humanitarian intervention, medicine may find itself in the position of assuming the neutral—that is, impartial—role it originally enjoyed when volunteer medical forces first entered the battlefield. Proposals for a 15,000-member European Human Security Response Force mobilized to respond to "gross human rights violations" envision both military and civilian personnel. Among the latter are police, legal specialists, humanitarian aid workers, doctors, and medical personnel (*A Human Security Doctrine for Europe*, 2004). Both military and civilian forces serve humanitarian interests. As such, war does not serve national security or any nation's reason of state, but goes hand in hand with international legal, educational, and medical efforts. How well medical personnel will fare in this novel climate of humanitarian intervention under international military auspices remains to be seen. They will continue, no doubt, to face some of the problems confronting MEDCAP personnel described in chapter 6, particularly the inability to overcome linguistic and cultural differences inherent in humanitarian medical care. Yet multinational, humanitarian medical personnel should remain unencumbered by the suspicion that they provide medical care for ulterior purposes or that continued care is contingent on the donor nation's military interests. This recognition may alleviate some elements of distrust and ensure continuity of care and a long-term medical presence even as military troops depart. It may also open the door to relative peace and tranquility.

The Lure of Pacifism and Peace

Medicine is not a pacifist vocation, but it is certainly imbued with principles of pacifism. Medicine attracts pacifists because it can offer its practitioners an opportunity to do no harm and avoid killing. Medicine can permit pacifists to carve out a space within the sphere of military service where they can serve in noncombatant capacities. Assuming that they are not bothered by the apparent contradiction of "noncombatant military service," some pacifists will find refuge in medicine during armed conflict. But this requires noncombatant medical workers to bracket cardinal characteristics of military medicine and ignore that its primary aim is to treat sick and wounded soldiers so they may return to fight and kill. Others are cognizant of the role medicine plays during war and accept the necessity of armed conflict but are content that they themselves neither bear arms nor do harm. While this is sufficient for some, pacifists firm in their convictions do not find medicine a proper refuge because they understand that medicine's commitment to do no harm is conditional on the obligations of physicians to contribute to their nation's war effort. Medicine cannot escape this responsibility. At best, vocational pacifism is coherent only insofar as the practice of medicine cannot make alternative contributions to war. Often it cannot; the care of the sick and wounded is its only effective function. More recently, however, medicine may also provide the expertise necessary to forestall armed aggression in other ways, namely, by contributing to the development of weaponry. Absolute pacifists, whether physicians or laypeople, will resist weapons development as they will resist any noncombatant military position. But medicine, solely based on vocational pacifism and its commitment to do no harm, cannot nor should not avoid an active role in war. Doctors must sometimes help build bombs.

What physicians should also do is scrutinize war and use their singular and often socially privileged vantage point to obstruct the prosecution of unjust wars. The obligation to oppose war selectively is one that everyone faces; there is little room to claim that it is the exclusive purview of the medical profession. Its members are, however, in a unique position to prevent the induction of conscripts by exaggerating medical maladies and doctoring medical records. Evidence is admittedly anecdotal, but there are few accounts of physicians facing criminal prosecution for assisting others to avoid the draft. Perhaps it is difficult to prove or perhaps medicine has sufficient wiggle room when certain illnesses are at issue. The important point is that medical civil disobedience during war positions medical ethics opposite and subordinate to civic duty. Physicians who believe a war is unjust will knowingly subvert the principles of medical ethics, lie about a patient's health, and use their patients to further a political agenda. The justification comes from above. When war is just, civic duty reaches beyond the principles of biomedical ethics to obligate physicians and other medical workers to support their nation's war effort. When wars are unjust, civic duty, subject as always to the common weal, requires citizens to disobey.

The obligation to disobey is anchored in strong political morality and the general duty of ethical activism (Gross 1997). While some forms of classical political morality do not require citizens to take interest in the affairs of others beyond those that impinge on their own welfare, strong political morality demands more. Strong political morality assumes that most citizens command the requisite sense of justice to evaluate public policy relative to underlying principles of liberal justice, and maintain the capacity to take appropriate action to restore moral equanimity to a functioning democracy. Ethical activism embraces a cognitive capacity for well-developed and objective moral judgment together with the capability to act when an otherwise fair and generally well-ordered society is beset by intolerance, discrimination, and an absence of basic human rights. This may occur in war or peace, at home or abroad. Ethical activism, however, does not necessarily entail civil disobedience. On the contrary, while Rawls and others writing during the Vietnam and civil rights years often agreed that civil disobedience was the most effective means to fight political injustice, civil disobedience remains the avenue of last resort when public policy undermines principles of social justice and just war. In less contentious times, voting may be sufficient to maintain a society's moral integrity, assuming, as John Stuart Mill ([1861] 1950, 304) demanded, that the voter is ever cognizant of his [or her] "absolute moral obligation to consider the interest of the public [and] not his private advantage." In a more complex political environment, reforming social movements are indispensable for integrating moral interests into public policy as activists vigorously confront their governments on basic social issues such as peace, nuclear arms, and civil liberties.

Many social movements that serve the ends of peace take a broad view of what a peaceful world should look like. In contrast to realism, peace does not rest solely on an absence of armed conflict and on the stable alignment of states in an anarchic community that pays scant attention to the domestic affairs of member nations. Instead, social movements often embrace the idea of a liberal peace based on international cooperation, collective security, and a vision of human good that the world community should actively pursue. This is an aggressive peace that takes a keen interest in the internal affairs of sovereign states and envisions a world not only characterized by expansive civil liberties and human rights but also by the means necessary to achieve these ends: education, housing, social welfare, and medical care.

With these goals in mind, medical workers may find themselves in one or more of several new roles. In some cases, they may serve as part of the military or civilian medical staff accompanying intervention forces. The current model for humanitarian intervention remains in a state of flux. In some cases, medical personnel served and continue to serve as military medical offices in intervening forces, be they national (the United States in Iraq, for example), multinational (NATO forces in the Balkans), or international (UN peacekeeping forces in Rwanda, Somalia, or Cambodia). Alternatively, they may join the staff of NGOs that work solely to provide medical and humanitarian aid. Often military forces and NGOs work hand in hand as the former provide the security necessary for relief operations. Finally, one must take note of the NGOs that embrace medical *and* political goals such as the IPPNW, PHR, MSF, or a myriad of local projects that hope to use medicine to achieve peace through mediation, the protection of human rights, or cross-border cooperation.

Each kind of medical activism replaces MEDCAP-type programs that place medical personnel in the service of individual nations pursuing parochial state interests. While this may go part of the way toward restoring some measure of neutrality that armed conflict normally denies the practice of medicine, these various forms of medical humanitarianism are often no less politically charged. The moral, legal, and political justification of humanitarian intervention remains a source of contention in world politics. Not everyone accepts the necessity or the justice of war to suppress regimes guilty of human rights abuses. Medical personnel may not be immune to antagonism or distrust as they ply Western medicine in nations with profoundly different views of human dignity, personal autonomy, family relations, and sexual norms. Nor will medical workers remain exempt from charges of hubris. "Thinking they have an answer for every ill," some medical NGOs, charge critics, pursue unrealistic political goals in the absence of hard evidence that medicine can serve peace (Vass 2001, 1020). What some see as an extension of medical beneficence, others fear may politicize medicine, jeopardize neutrality and impartiality, and, ultimately, undermine medical care (Jabbour 2005).

In spite of these obstacles, the longtime relationship of medicine, war, and reason of state may change dramatically as nations aggressively pursue liberal peace and seriously consider the merits of humanitarian intervention. When states must fight wars to protect their vital interests, medical care and expertise serve these interests as well. However, when states fight wars to protect the welfare of those beyond their borders, war no longer serves reason of state and medicine is released from its subordinate role. While this may resolve some of the hard choices that medical professionals must make during war, and eventually allow physicians to work above the fray, it should not obscure the fact that armed conflict continues to pose hard moral dilemmas for the practice of medicine.

10
The Moral Dilemmas of Medicine and War

"Nouns always trump adjectives," some writers like to remind their readers, and as we consider the phrase "military medical ethics" it is always important to ask which of these words is which. Are *military* and *medical* the adjectives that modify the noun *ethics*? Or is *medical ethics* the noun at the center of our discussion, convincingly trumping its modifying adjective *military*?

Many, I believe, are tempted to understand *military* as the sole adjective modifying *medical ethics* and assert that medical ethics is unaffected by war, in much the same way that it remains unswayed by other modifying adjectives, be they *acute-care, ambulatory, pediatric,* or *geriatric.* While these varieties of medical ethics may differ in complexity or subject matter, they remain intimately connected by common principles and decision-making strategies. The noun, *medical ethics* remains upright and constant. The opening reminder, however, cautions us to beware of such a hasty conclusion. *Ethics* is our proper subject matter. *Medical* ethics applies general moral principles to the practice of medicine. *Military* medical ethics reflects the state of medical ethics during war. Contrary to the position of the World Medical Association, medical ethics in times of armed conflict is *not* identical to medical ethics in times of peace. One reason is that ethics in times of war is not identical to ethics in times of peace.

The Transformation of Ethics during War

From a moral perspective, realists sometimes think they have an easy time of it. War does not transform or affect ethics in any meaningful way. Rather, it sets ethics aside entirely. For realists, the nation-state assumes a unique position in the human community. Nations are the arbiters of laws and morality and, as such, beyond their reach. If ethics cannot reach beyond the nation-state, then it cannot bind their behavior; moral categories of right and wrong do not apply to nations adrift in an anarchic state of nature. Nations, therefore, know only one law—the imperative of their own survival—and so will covenant or fight with one another with that sole end in mind. This does not mean that nations will not agree to limit the destructiveness of war, refrain from harming noncombatants, or repatriate prisoners of war. But it does mean that they will set these aside if compliance threatens reason of state, for the conventions of war carry no independent moral weight that one must take seriously.

Moral philosophers alarmed by the ascendancy of state over reason were quick to point out that the state, together with the interests it protects, are not beyond the reach of morality, but serve as an important vehicle for achieving an ethical life. Ethics embraces the rules and maxims that help us to understand and lead us to act on what is good. *Good* may mean many things, but without pursuing this point any further, it is clear that many versions of ethics hope to offer some universal vision of the good, one that is incumbent on all individuals endowed with reason. Under ideal circumstances, we posit ideas of the good—utilitarian norms of happiness and well-being or deontological visions of self-determination and inviolable human rights—together with the maxims of behavior necessary to achieve them. The state, in turn, at least the liberal state, is charged with the responsibility of ensuring the conditions necessary for liberty and human happiness. Fundamental among these are the preservation of human life and the prevention of gratuitous harm.

During war, we set aside many of the principles that prohibit intentional harm to others and accept the need to take life and wreak destruction, either to save ourselves, save others, protect cultural artifacts and traditions, or avenge a wounded sense of pride and honor. Each of these—our lives, our states, our traditions, and our self-esteem—reflect, we think, the conditions necessary for human existence and for making our lives worth living. To protect all or some leads nations to wage war of many types. One is cataclysmic: the war of national self-defense that nations wage to protect or free themselves from foreign domination. Another is beneficent: wars of humanitarian intervention that some nations undertake to prevent genocide or massive human rights abuses in lawless or authoritarian nations. The former are at the core of traditional just-war theory, while the same theory currently struggles with justifying armed violence on behalf of the unfortunate citizens of rogue regimes. In between are those conflicts that constitute perhaps the majority of wars nations fight: the wars of honor, glory, and power that Hobbes and Thucydides remind us of so well.

During these armed struggles, a nation's war effort—that is, its collective undertaking to safeguard personal safety and shared, communal interests—often takes center stage and leapfrogs over a number of important ethical principles as lives are placed at risk in an effort to secure what many think to be a greater good. "Reason of state" and "the war effort" are by no means above common morality, but direct our attention to moral goods that are generally not at stake during peacetime and emphasize the necessity of war when other means fail. Once war emerges as the only viable option to protect the moral goods that armed aggression or despotic rulers endanger, we make do with limiting war to the attainment of political aims, with protecting innocents who fall into harm's way, and, in general, with trying to accomplish more good than the harm war inevitably brings. These efforts are of overriding concern for ethics during armed conflict. Medical ethics is no exception.

The Transformation of Medical Ethics during War

In light of the changes that ethics undergoes during wartime, it is not surprising that medical moral decision making changes substantially in wartime and that many of the dilemmas the medical community must resolve are entirely novel. But this alone is not enough; other branches of medical ethics also present new and challenging dilemmas. During war, however, the everyday principles of biomedical ethics, like those of ethics itself, must compete with equally weighty and conflicting principles anchored in military necessity and national security. There is no doubt that the principle of military necessity colors many of the arguments throughout this book and impinges on moral decision making as military necessity, reason of state, and the war effort compete with and sometimes overwhelm the axioms that animate medical ethics during peace. While the outcome of this fierce competition is by no means self-evident, it cannot but affect the practice of medical ethics in times of armed conflict.

As nations wage wars of all types, they conscript or enlist young men and women and place them in harm's way with little or no compunction. As they do, military forces mobilize medical resources and personnel for a single express purpose: to maintain combat readiness and facilitate the ends the military finds itself authorized to achieve. The patient, at first glance, is nowhere to be seen. "Vital" interests, the touchstone of just war and of the medical corps war mobilizes, have far less to do with the welfare of any individual patient and far more to do with the welfare of the state and the political community the state protects. Searching for the patient amid the detritus of war, we encounter two remarkable phenomena. First, the very idea of patient—that is, an individual in need of medical care—is no longer monolithic. Instead of one "patient" there are several, each with a different identity and attendant rights and duties. Second, we see that the effect of military necessity is to substantially overturn the traditional hierarchy of bio-medical principles. Under normal, peacetime circumstances the principles of bioethics form a pantheon of multiple first principles that exists in an uneasy but stable coexistence. Whatever philosophical reservations we have about *multiple* first principles are cast aside during war as military necessity, in an equally uneasy manner, often trumps the right to life, self-determination, and patient welfare. Those threads of uneasiness form the tension that runs throughout this entire book and are unique to war.

Consider first the range of moral questions that arise during war. While some are similar to those medicine faces during peace—Why should medical personnel treat the sick and injured? What patient rights must caregivers respect? How best to distribute scarce resources?—the actors at the center of these vital questions have changed. While each question poses a challenge to caregivers, there is no longer a single, paradigmatic patient but several recipients of medical care: soldiers, enemy and friendly, and civilians, also enemy and friendly. Each type of patient holds different rights and, therefore, demands different duties from caregivers. During war, claim rights vary from patient to patient as a function of medical need *and* identity. The questions just posed, therefore, are always augmented by another, namely, who is the patient? Is he or she a combatant or noncombatant, soldier or civilian, friend or enemy?

Physicians care for sick and wounded soldiers for reasons that are different from those they invoke to treat other patients. While medical workers care for ordinary patients with an end to restoring their health, they treat soldiers to preserve manpower and to protect the vitality of a collective, fighting force. During war, medicine cannot ignore the instrumental value placed on the lives of its patients or its duty to preserve their lives for the purpose of waging war. Patients' rights, too, vary with their identity. These difficulties arise because different classes of patients, particularly friendly and enemy soldiers, find that military service in general and war in particular greatly impinge on basic human rights that are transformed during war. One of these rights is self-determination; another is the right to life.

While in peacetime we grant overwhelming, if not decisive, weight to an individual's right of self-determination, the free range that we normally extend to personal decision making shrinks within the confines of a tightly layered hierarchy like the military. In fact, the entire structure of moral decision making changes in light of both the military's vertical organization and the exigencies of war. Ordinarily, medical decision making together with the resolution of moral dilemmas that may arise in its wake are often deliberative and nonhierarchical: patient, family, nurses, doctors, and other caregivers and advisors generally remain on equal footing. Even under the best conditions, the decision-making process can be extraordinarily difficult, particularly as information about the effects of outcomes is not always clear, and disagreement about the priority of conflicting principles, and principals, remains. Nevertheless, resolution is often collective and deliberative. Families confer, professionals consult, and committees reach majority if not consensual decisions. In other, less common cases, decision making becomes adversarial and acrimonious. Here the courts or other authoritative institutions may deliver decisions.

Wartime medical decision making is entirely different. Many medical decisions, as Larrey first noted, belong to military commanders, not medical officers. Families are not present or necessarily a part of decision making, there may be no recourse to the courts, decisions are made without informed consent, and emergency conditions often prevail. Many questions, common in peacetime, do not arise because military personnel do not command the right to refuse medical treatment that will keep them fit to perform the jobs for which they trained. Their "job"—that is, effective soldiering—assumes primary importance and is ever more crucial during war. Effectively fulfilling a military role has little to do with personal welfare, and everything to do with the collective good. Here again, collective interests overwhelm individual welfare, and the tension between self-determination and utility is palpable.

Working through these tensions is a constant challenge for military medical ethics precisely because the peacetime decision-making paradigms are not always relevant or entirely helpful. The debate over the use of investigational drugs illustrates this point vividly. Peacetime standards of medical ethics demand informed consent when anyone receives investigational drugs. When military officials needed to protect American soldiers against botulinum toxoid and later airborne anthrax, they sought either investigational compounds or drugs previously approved for different applications. In each case, officials invoked military necessity and feasibility, arguing that the drug was necessary to preserve military capability and that obtaining informed consent under prevailing conditions was impractical. In chapter 4, I then pushed this argument one step further, suggesting that medical risk, an important criterion for obtaining informed consent in peacetime, is replaced by military risk during war. Only when the risk of an investigational drug approaches the very high risk that combat personnel encounter in war might one consider invoking the rules of informed consent. At issue is not simply higher risk, but a different kind of risk that comes from the "military," not the "medical," side of military medical ethics.

Military necessity similarly affects the right to life of all the actors party to armed conflict. Human life is among the first casualties of war, and in its defense nations and their citizens resort to armed violence and invoke the right to kill. Civilians remain vulnerable to "collateral" damage in the course of necessary military operations, while soldiers lose their right to life vis-à-vis their enemy the moment they are in uniform, regain it when they are wounded, and lose it again once they recover. While medicine struggles to save life, war offers a legitimate framework for taking it. If medicine serves the aims of war, its duty to safeguard human life at all costs will suffer. Triage is a prime example. Peacetime triage is largely a matter of efficiency and how best to ensure that all those in need obtain necessary care given constraints of time and available personnel. Wartime triage pushes further when casualties overwhelm medical facilities. The question is not *when* a patient is treated, but *who* is treated. Mass-casualty triage favors salvage over medical need, strives to restore health to those fit to return to duty, and places greater value on the lives of friendly soldiers over enemy soldiers and over civilians of either stripe. Medical care is no longer a function of medical need but guided instead by military necessity, a nation's war effort, and, generally speaking, by the collective good, a principle that is generally foreign, if not antithetical, to peacetime medical ethics. This reverses the burden of proof that generally governs the practice of medical ethics. As I noted in chapter 4, in peacetime, those *violating* patient rights must justify their action; during war, those *upholding* patient rights and interests usually bear the burden of proof and must defend their decisions to respect informed consent, protect confidentiality, honor a patient's right to die, treat the sick and wounded on the basis of medical need, and refrain from controlling the flow of scientific information.

The full weight of *military* medical ethics comes to the fore in the entirely new dilemmas that armed conflict poses. Neutrality, interrogational torture, and weapons development are very real dilemmas. They cannot be set aside by fiat independently of the ethical arguments that justify or condemn each practice. Neutrality means both immunity and impartiality. But medical facilities retain their immunity only insofar as parties to an armed conflict agree that they remain inviolable. Once one side violates immunity, the other may have reason to reconsider the convention. Medical facilities are not inherently immune from attack, although it generally serves everyone's interests to protect these facilities from harm. Unconventional war, however, challenges this convention, just as it affects other practices and protections that, for example, turn on a clear distinction between combatants and noncombatants. As this distinction fades, the conventions that preserve neutrality or seek to protect the welfare of noncombatants are increasingly difficult to maintain.

Medical stability operations, although sometimes benign, set the stage for the harder dilemmas that follow by starkly asking which master medicine serves during war: the patient or the war effort. Many critics object vociferously to any program that uses medical care to stabilize fragile regimes by fostering loyalty to the government and thereby providing a bulwark against insurgent forces. Here, however, we must remember that nouns still trump adjectives; medicine is but another form of military operation. This problem has not, and will not, go away. As the nature of warfare shifts from wars of self-defense to those of humanitarian intervention, medicine may eventually relinquish the constraints that military necessity imposes. In a war of intervention, armed conflict serves humanitarian and, by extension, medical interests. The relationship between war and medicine is reversed insofar as nations do not conflate national interests and humanitarian concerns. The world is still a long way from this state of affairs, preferring self-defense to justify recourse to armed conflict. As intervention becomes an international rather than unilateral undertaking and as security forces incorporate medical personnel in a nonmilitary capacity, it may be possible to restore medical ethics to its more comfortable peacetime paradigm.

The same cannot be said, however, for those dilemmas that are clearly noncaregiving and antithetical to the principle of "do no patient harm." Peacetime medical ethics offers no paradigm for resolving these dilemmas because it recognizes no moral difficulty. Torture and weapons development are simply forbidden; no physician may share a role. However, the force of the medical community's prohibition leans heavily on condemning interrogational torture and weapons development regardless of who participates and for what end. In spite of the tremendous moral difficulties one may encounter as one considers both harsh interrogation and weapons research, neither is resistant to defense or justification.

The difference between *defense* and *justification* is significant. Interrogational torture remains legally proscribed but may be morally defensible under conditions that offer the possibility of preventing egregious harm to others. This is the upshot of Shue's (1978, 143) argument when he demands that anyone who "sincerely believes an act of torture to be the least available evil is placed in the position of needing to justify his or her act morally in order to defend himself or herself legally." Physicians and other medical personnel find themselves in a similar position should they also believe that an act of interrogational torture is the least available evil necessary to preserve a "supremely important moral goal." Given the importance of human dignity and its subsidiary rights of self-esteem and human life, this goal can only be the preservation of innocent human life. Whether these human lives are so threatened to make torture defensible remains a decision for those who authorize and undertake interrogational torture and for the political community that must judge them. Medical personnel, however, are not immune to these arguments solely on the basis of their professional duties. If one can substantiate a *supremely* important moral goal then, by definition, the same goal must direct the behavior of medical professionals.

Unlike interrogational torture, weapons and the purpose for which they are developed, namely the destruction of human life during war, remain lawful. To avoid participating in weapons research medical workers must move beyond a claim of illegality and invoke a conflict of moral interest. But unless medicine is a pacifist vocation—that is, opposed to the taking of life in any circumstances—the argument is tenuous at best. The practice of medicine is not committed to doing no harm under any and all conditions; rather it is committed to avoiding harm *on balance*. "On balance" reflects the welfare of those affected by medical care, which, during war, expands beyond patients of various combatant and noncombatant statuses to embrace the collective well-being and the good of the political community. Subject to the dictates of humanitarian law, the same interests that justify war also justify the means to wage it. The medical community, therefore, cannot pursue business as usual during armed conflict and ignore the need to help build weapons that require medical expertise. Like everyone else, its members can only direct their best efforts to prevent wars before they break out and bring to an end those that already threaten the world community.

These two dilemmas, interrogational torture and weapons development, are unique dilemmas of military medical ethics. They are not only unique in the sense that they bring a novel convergence of bioethical principles in a new environment (as some new scientific discovery might), but because they bend time-honored principles to the breaking point. This not only tests the practice of medicine but assails any individual bound by the duty not to kill or harm others. War puts these moral principles to the test in the same way it tests the principles of biomedical ethics. Medical professionals have perhaps struggled with this challenge more than others, particularly as they very often believe that their professional obligations supercede all others.

Armed Conflict and Professional Obligation

Throughout their textbook on military medical ethics, Thomas Beam, Edmund Howe, and their colleagues return to the tension between medicine and war, between the professional obligations of a physician and those of a soldier. Is the physician-soldier a physician first or a soldier first? As they think about this question, they consider the possibility that the two are mutually exclusive professions and confront Victor Sidel and Barry Levy's (2003) pointed argument that military medical service inevitably and irretrievably undercuts the practice of medicine by subordinating the best interests of the patient, undermining patient rights, discriminating against enemy soldiers and civilians, and failing to provide proper medical care. Sidel and Levy react to the exigencies of war by backing medicine away from armed conflict and placing medical care in the hands of neutral nonmilitary personnel who can provide care with the same neutrality and fairness of Dunant's volunteer doctors and nurses. It is a bold move that embraces vocational pacifism, effectively strips medical workers of their national identity, and builds them into cosmopolitan citizens of the world. Only then can they fulfill their medical obligations and distance themselves from war making. At the same time, they can also assume the duties of conflict mediators that organizations like the IPPNW envision.

There is much to be said for depicting the role of medical professionals during armed conflict in this way. It is particularly suited to the type of "human security response forces" that some envision as the best tool for humanitarian intervention (chapter 9). Here, medical personnel together with other aid workers, teachers, and legal specialists form the vanguard of humanitarian relief. Doctors working in this capacity will, to be sure, face fewer dilemmas than their colleagues in uniform and, under ideal conditions, may not face any of the dilemmas that face military medical personnel who husband their resources for entirely different purposes.

It is difficult to see, however, that the anarchy inherent in the international order will ever allow any nation to completely demilitarize medicine. International efforts at humanitarian intervention may bring about the slow democratization of authoritarian states, and these fledging democracies may show the same reticence about fighting one another that the older liberal nations maintain. In the meantime, however, nations will continue to field armies of their own. They will continue to maintain deterrent capabilities as well as the forces necessary to repel armed aggression. In all these efforts, medical personnel will continue to face dilemmas of treating the wounded, defining and ensuring patient rights, and distributing scarce resources. Questions about the reciprocity of neutrality, permissible interrogational torture, and unconventional deterrent capabilities will continue to plague the medical profession. Nor must it be forgotten that wars of humanitarian intervention will very likely demand an increasing array of nonlethal weapons that will require medical expertise.

As a result, many military medical professionals will respond to Sidel and Levy with the conviction of any concerned citizen-soldier: while it is imperative to curtail abuse, prevent poor care, and check discrimination, reason of state remains paramount during armed conflict. Circumscribed patient rights, limited autonomy, and salvage-based triage are sometimes necessary to conserve manpower and aid the common good (Howe 2003). Physician-soldiers cannot escape the demands of military necessity. They may question its reach, but when convinced that their state's interests are at risk, professional medical obligations emphasizing the priority of the patient fall to collective survival: "The survival of society" insist Beam and Howe (2003, 856), "is the ultimate goal of the military profession. Because this goal is absolute, the needs of individuals must be considered secondary and ethically can be overridden by military necessity."

Unfortunately, this conviction does little to resolve the tension between professional and military obligations. While some are prepared to simply live with this tension as best they can, it is important to realize that this is one we must all live with. Any citizen must question the reach of military necessity and the demands of reason of state during war. At issue is not whether one is a physician or any other professional first and a soldier second, but whether one is a citizen first and a soldier second. Sidel and Levy resolve the friction by doing away with citizens and soldiers and, perhaps in time, this will come to pass. In the meantime, the challenges of armed conflict are overwhelming.

This is not a simple-minded struggle. If we take military necessity and reason of state seriously, and concede that they may override other professional obligations, then why exclude anyone from answering the call to arms? If professional medical obligations emphasizing the priority of a patient's interests sometimes fall to military necessity, then why should the obligation to do no harm or, for example, the duty to avoid weapons development remain sacrosanct? These are precisely the questions that pacifists ask when they consider any form of military medical service, and they highlight the charge that military service cannot but destroy the basis of medicine. The questions are not, however, novel, but the logical outcome of any attempt to resolve conflicting roles and duties during war. To answer them only demands that physicians reason through the dilemmas of war like other concerned citizens. In the end, it means that physicians, together with their fellow citizens, bear the responsibility to support their community and participate in wars that are just and oppose those that defy humanitarian and international law. Despite its commitment to nonmaleficence and beneficence, medical ethics is not a pacifist doctrine, if by that we mean the absolute and unconditional repudiation of war. Nor is peace, if by that we mean a state of nonwar, an axiomatic principle of bioethics.

In spite of what I think is a clear symmetry between the moral conflicts ordinary citizens face and those that confront medical workers as they weigh their professional and civic duties in time of war, physicians face historical and conceptual hurdles that sometimes impede a clear grasp of their conflicting obligations. The first stems from the shameful history of Nazi medicine, while the second, ironically enough, stems from medicine's appeal to a higher calling.

The Nazi Doctors

When doctors are called on to serve the political community by taking up arms in their professional capacity, it is impossible to ignore the legacy of Nazi Germany. While Nazi barbarity shocked the human race, the behavior of German physicians was beyond comprehension. While one might somehow grasp the psychological dynamics that allow one group of human beings to systematically exterminate another as the result of authoritarian personalities (Adorno 1950), or repressed hatred for an abusive parent figure (Cohn 1981), or imperceptible banalities that mask the horror of their deeds (Arendt 1963; Hilberg 1985), we are unable to extend the same understanding to members of the medical profession. Like Elie Wiesel, we are apt to believe that a medical degree ought to "shield" doctors from evil (Annas and Grodin 1992).

Yet German physicians committed unspeakable horrors in the service of the state (Lifton 1986; Proctor 1988). How then are subsequent generations of physicians going to avoid a similar fate when called on to violate confidentiality, ignore medical need during triage, or develop weapons to protect the state or the common good? The answer must be: they will avoid it just as we all will, not by appealing to parochial professional obligations or a "minority" morality but to the common principles of humanity. There is nothing inherently evil or misguided about granting inordinate weight to the principle of military necessity or reason of state during war. Neither principle, however, stands alone; each will readily bring evil when citizens ignore the imperatives of just war. Nazi doctors trumpeted medical necessity or the "medicalization" of war without ever examining the justice of the war they were fighting. The abject failure to consider the ends and means of German aggression was not only a problem for Nazi doctors but for anyone who gladly took up the Nazi cause.

Nevertheless, we are often perturbed by the behavior of physicians because we expect their professional duties to come to the fore and temper, if not override, their duty to the state in time of war. We expect the professional obligations of the physician, and the clergy, to stand as a bulwark against wartime inhumanity. In this sense, members of both professions serve witness to their pacifist and humanitarian principles. While one might not expect an individual's professional obligations to assume overriding importance when one contemplates the dilemmas of war, physicians must necessarily pause before they deny combatants patient rights, violate neutrality, or help build weapons. At the same time, the medical profession demands vocational pacifism and convincingly recommends pacificism to its members because physicians are "shepherds" of life. Ignoring the fact that we all, and parents in particular, shepherd life no less than physicians do, it is difficult to escape the impression that medicine imposes *special* obligations on its practitioners and places them above the practice of war. The WMA certainly believes this to be true, and for this reason alone can conclude that medical ethics in times of war is identical to medical ethics in times of peace. They are not identical, however, precisely because medicine does not answer to a calling any higher than that of any other profession. On the contrary, faced with unjust war, many physicians gladly surrender their professional obligation to tell the truth so they may undermine a war that violates fundamental principles of justice.

Medicine is not a pacifist vocation, nor do its principles necessarily override a physician's commitment to his or her community during times of armed conflict. As citizens evaluate the arguments surrounding patient rights, neutrality, and unconventional warfare, and, more generally, assess the moral implications of going to war, they are easily confronted with conflicting duties. Familial duties, small-group loyalties, and professional obligations are all thrown off track when states go to war, impose military service, and partake in armed violence. Generally, individuals identify with their country's reasons for going to war and subordinate their conflicting obligations to their civic duties. When states pursue war to preserve or enlarge their territory or protect national honor, many men seem willing to risk their own lives in order to take those of others. They will desist, if at all, only when higher moral principles compel them to pursue conscientious objection or civil disobedience when wars are unjust. But this is not a higher calling; nor is it unique to medicine.

Medicine's Higher Calling

Commenting on medicine's higher calling, Solomon Benatar (1993, 142) distinguishes among three kinds of duties: those we acquire "by virtue of our common humanity," those we undertake in the context of our "institutionalized duties" as we participate in civil society, and "another class of moral obligations—those acquired or voluntarily self-imposed by the exercise of free will." The latter, in Benatar's view, champion "supererogatory caring actions" during armed conflict and take precedence over the other obligations a health-care professional may have. Beyond the pale of ordinary civic and moral duties, supererogatory actions infuse the practice of medicine. "It is this 'higher calling' response within medical practice," writes Benatar, "which many consider to be the true moral essence of a health professional's work." However one looks at it, medical practitioners have placed themselves beyond ordinary moral obligations. They are, indeed, flirting with a different moral universe that, in a way I admittedly do not quite understand, supercedes the norms of our common humanity.

But a higher calling need not reach to a novel moral universe inaccessible to most individuals and dangerously conferring moral authority on those who claim entrance. Instead, any idea of a higher calling need only reach to the same universal moral principles that bring ordinary individuals to sometimes act as their conscience dictates. Recall the WMA's declaration prohibiting physicians from contributing to the development of lethal or nonlethal chemical and biological weapons: "It is the privilege of the medical doctor to practice medicine in the service of humanity, to preserve and restore bodily and mental health without distinction as to persons, to comfort and ease the suffering of his or her patients. The utmost respect for human life is to be maintained even under threat, and no use made of any medical knowledge contrary to the laws of humanity" (World Medical Association 1990).

The WMA uses the word *humanity* in two distinct senses here, and this perhaps sums up the ambiguity inherent in the idea of a "higher calling" and the strain of competing roles and obligations. In the first sentence, the "service of humanity" refers to beneficence—that is, the imperative to preserve and restore human health. This is a professional obligation and, in principle, no different from those duties that obligate other professions that serve different human needs and that may fall before reason of state during just war. Professional obligations gain their force from the community that confers privileges and duties upon each vocation. These are supererogatory commitments only in the sense that they are moral obligations that one freely chooses within the context of a specific profession; it is not that they supercede any other. The "laws of humanity," in contrast, invoke humanitarian law and respect for the human rights on which communities themselves are based. These norms and rights are inviolable insofar as they do not conflict with one another, and in spite of the tendency to sometimes conflate the laws of humanity and medicine's professional duty of beneficence, the two are not synonymous. Preserving this distinction is important. While one would not expect a physician or anyone else to use his or her knowledge contrary to the laws of humanity, there is sometimes room to ask whether any individual, physicians included, may violate another person's "bodily and mental health." This, in the end, is the question we all face in the shadow of armed conflict.

Notes

Chapter 1

1. Of engaged forces in American wars since the Civil War, 18 percent were killed in action and 42 percent were wounded. Engaged strength refers only to those engaged in battle and excludes staff and logistics support (Gabriel and Metz 1992, vol. 1, 23).

Chapter 2

1. Notable among the nations not ratifying the Protocols are the United States and Israel.

2. The idea of "illegal" combatants remains murky. Neither the Geneva Conventions nor the Protocols recognize the term *illegal combatant.* One is either a legal combatant or a civilian. War criminals are a subset of the former, ordinary criminals a subset of the latter. See Human Rights Watch, 2002.

3. But Hobbes was less clear about the obligation to die for the state. See chapter 3.

4. Rawls, too, equivocates, calling self-esteem *"perhaps* the most important primary good" (Rawls 1971, 440; emphasis added). For a critique of Rawls's position see Massey 1983.

Chapter 3

1. Figures are extrapolated from Dupuy (1995, 50–54). If 20 percent of those hit are killed, then some 335,000 Union soldiers suffered hits during the Civil War. Using Dupuy's figures, 15 percent or roughly 50,000 of these suffered serious wounds and only 34 percent or 17,000 survived. While Dupuy does not clearly define "seriously" wounded in action, one can assume that many of those requiring amputation were seriously wounded. The Union Army reported 20,559 amputations of the forearm, upper arm, and leg (whole or part). Of these, 13,555

survived, leaving only approximately 3,500 of the 17,000 seriously wounded to survive with other disabilities and relatively few to return to duty after suffering serious wounds (amputation figures from *Official Records, Medical and Surgical History of the War of the Rebellion* (Washington, DC: Government Printing House, 1870), cited in Gabriel and Metz, 1992, vol. 2, 183).

2. The figure of 30,000 is an estimate for illustrative purposes only. Total American casualties (killed and wounded) in World War II were 625,000. Saving an additional 57 soldiers per thousand could have saved approximately 30,000 more lives. For casualty figures see Dupuy 1995, 141.

3. Rawls does not refer to medical care as a "primary" good, although there are compelling arguments that contracting, rational agents would include it as a primary good, for without health care, individuals will be hard-pressed to take advantage of their other basic liberties. See Daniels 1988.

4. Troop strength in Vietnam was about 500,000 in 1968. In 1968, there were 2,252 inpatient care neurosurgeons practicing in the United States, or 1.1 per 100,000 people. This was about half the ratio of the neurosurgeons present in Vietnam (Haug et al. 1970, 39).

Chapter 4

1. American service personnel refusing treatment that will keep them "fit" (i.e., "able to reasonably perform the duties of his or her office, grade, rank or rating") are subject to charges of "willful neglect" (Secretary of the Navy, 2002, Instruction 1850.4E, paragraph 3413, p. 3–28).

2. Casualties as a percent of soldiers mobilized were 13 percent in the Civil War, 6 percent in World War I, 7 percent in World War II, and 3.4 percent in Korea (Dupuy 1995, 141).

3. See, for example, 21 Army Group, 1945; U.S. Office of War Information, 1944. Most of these studies are retrospective, and analyze data collected from the records of soldiers previously treated with penicillin and sulfanilamides during the war. However, investigators also built controlled experiments using two different surgical clearing stations, so that patients from one received only penicillin and patients from the other received penicillin and sulfanilamides. In most of these cases, many of the wounds were not so severe as to prevent communication, but informed consent was never reported.

Chapter 5

1. While it is not clear whether Howard is referring to one patient or many, the same criteria apply when treating many patients. The priorities are: correction of defects that immediately endanger life, then defects that ultimately endanger life, then defects that immediately endanger limb or organ, and finally defects that ultimately endanger limb or organ (see also Beam 2003).

Chapter 6

1. The early Geneva Conventions of 1864 (Article 1) and 1868 (Article 7) as well as *The Laws of War on Land*, Oxford, September 9, 1880 (Article 13), refer to ambulances, military hospitals, hospital ships, and their staff as "neutral" and "as such protected and respected by the belligerents as long as they accommodate the sick and wounded." Later conventions no longer designate medical personnel and facilities as neutral but as "protected."

2. Rogers (1996) is right to point out that the provision allowing combatants to fight without uniforms is the exception rather than the rule (personal communication, May 3, 2005). However, its implications are far-reaching; see Green 2000, 234.

3. Terror, as a recent UN report defines it, is "any action intended to cause death or serious bodily harm to civilians or noncombatants, when the purpose of such an act, by its nature or context, is to intimidate a population or to compel a government or international organization to do or abstain from doing any act" (United Nations, 2004, paragraph 164d).

4. Whether American bombing of medical facilities was deliberate remains debatable (Lewy 1980).

5. Physicians for Human Rights (2005), however, describes how security forces sometimes demand collaboration from patients as a condition for receiving health care.

6. For illegal combatants, see chapter 2, note 2.

Chapter 7

1. The Tokyo Declaration (World Medical Association, 1975) defines torture as "the deliberate, systematic or wanton infliction of physical or mental suffering by one or more persons acting alone or on the orders of any authority, to force another person to yield information, to make a confession or for any other reason."

2. Whether a new manual will leave less room for similar exceptions remains unclear (Schmitt 2005).

3. For a possible exception, see Dershowitz 2002, 131–164.

4. I make a similar argument in Gross 2004. There are several weaknesses in this deontological argument that I raise in the next paragraph of the text. My thanks to Danny Statman and Saul Smilansky for highlighting these flaws.

5. Commenting on the 1949 Geneva Conventions (Conventions I, II, Article 12) that forbid leaving the wounded without medical care, Draper (1958, 76–77) describes how German interrogators found that "wounded aircrew suffering from shock, burns and wounds tend to be profitable subjects for interrogation purposes . . . and frequently delayed treatment until after interrogation."

6. In a personal communication from Amnesty International and B'tselem in April 2005, neither organization reported any evidence of investigators using psychotropic drugs during interrogations.

7. The 1975 Tokyo Declaration (World Medical Association, 1975) forbids artificial feeding when a prisoner refuses nourishment. In 1991 the WMA decided that "when the hunger striker has become confused . . . or lapsed into a coma the doctor shall be free to make the decision for his patient as to further treatment which he considers to be in the best interest of that patient."

Chapter 8

1. Of America's 70,000 gas casualties, 3 percent died. Among the 190,000 wounded by high explosives, 26 percent died (Dupuy 1995, 141; Croddy 2002).

2. Thanks to Saul Gross for this insightful comment.

3. Grade 3 wounds are those causing skin wounds of 10 cm and a large (two-finger) cavity or comminuted fracture (crushed and splintered bone).

4. The World Health Organization (1970) estimates 95,000 dead and 125,000 incapacitated following an attack with anthrax on a city of 500,000. A defended military installation would sustain fewer casualties, as would an attack using typhus, brucellosis, and tularemia.

References

Adams, D. P. 1989. "Wartime Bureaucracy and Penicillin Allocation: The Committee on Chemotherapeutic and Other Agents, 1942–44." *Journal of the History of Medicine and Allied Sciences* 44: 196–217.

Adams, D. P. 1991. *The Greatest Good to the Greatest Number: Penicillin Rationing on the American Home Front, 1940–1945*. New York: P. Lang.

Adorno, T. W., Frenkel-Brunswik, E., Levinson, D. J., and Sanford, R. N. 1950. *The Authoritarian Personality*. New York: Harper & Row.

Alexander, J. P. 1999. *Future War: Non-Lethal Weapons in the Twenty First Century*. New York: Thomas Dunn Books.

Alexander, J. P. 2001. "An Overview of the Future of Non-Lethal Weapons." *Medicine, Conflict and Survival* 17: 180–193.

Allen, T., and Gordon, S. 1971. *The Scalpel, the Sword: The Story of Doctor Norman Bethune*. Toronto: McClelland and Stewart.

Amnesty International. 2004. "Iraq: Amnesty International Reveals a Pattern of Torture and Ill-Treatment." http://web.amnesty.org/pages/irq-torture-eng

Annas, G. J. 1978. "Patient Rights Movements." In W. T. Reich, ed., *Encyclopedia of Bioethics*, vol. 3. New York: Free Press.

Annas, G. J. 1998. "Protecting Soldiers from Friendly Fire: The Consent Requirement for Using Investigational Drugs and Vaccines in Combat." *American Journal of Law and Medicine* 24 (2, 3): 245–260.

Annas, G. J., and Grodin, M. A. 1992. *The Nazi Doctors and the Nuremberg Code*. Oxford: Oxford University Press.

Aquinas. [1947] 1995. *Summa Theologiae* 2-2, q. 40, a 2. Trans. Fathers of the English Dominican Province. New York: Benziger.

Arendt, H. 1963. *Eichmann in Jerusalem: A Report on the Banality of Evil*. London: Faber and Faber.

Army Field Manual, FM 8-10, Medical Service Theater of Operations, March, 1951. Washington, D.C.: Department of the Army.

Bailey, B., and Farber, D. 1992. "Hotel Street: Prostitution and the Politics of War." *Radical History Review* 52: 54–77.

Baker, M. S., and Ryals, P. 1999. "The Medical Department in Military Operations Other Than War. Part II: Medical Civic Assistance Program in Southeast Asia." *Military Medicine* 164 (9): 619–625.

Baker, R., and Strosberg, M. 1992. "Triage and Equality: An Historical Reassessment of Utilitarian Analyses of Triage." *Kennedy Institute of Ethics Journal* 2 (2): 103–123.

Balmer, B. 2002. "Biological Warfare: The Threat in Historical Perspective." *Medicine, Conflict and Survival* 18: 120–137.

Barak, E. 2003. "Where Do We Go From Here? Implementation of the Chemical Weapons Convention in the Middle East in the Post-Saddam Era." *Security Studies* 13 (1): 106–155.

Baskir, L. M., and Strauss, W. 1978. *Chance and Circumstance: The Draft, the War, and the Vietnam Generation.* New York: Knopf.

Baumgold, D. 1983. "Subjects and Soldiers: Hobbes on Military Service." *History of Political Thought* 4 (1): 43–64.

Beam, T. E. 2003. "Medical Ethics on the Battlefield: The Crucible of Military Medical Ethics." In T. E. Beam and L. R. Sparacino, eds., *Military Medical Ethics*, vol. 2, 369–402. Textbooks of Military Medicine. Washington, DC: Office of the Surgeon General, Borden Institute.

Beam, T. E., and Howe, E. G. 2003 "A Proposed Ethic for Military Medicine." In T. E. Beam and L. R. Sparacino, eds., *Military Medical Ethics*, vol. 2, 851–865. Textbooks of Military Medicine. Washington, DC: Office of the Surgeon General, Borden Institute.

Beam, T. E., and Sparacino, L. R., eds. 2003. *Military Medical Ethics.* Textbooks of Military Medicine. 2 vols. Washington, DC: Office of the Surgeon General, Borden Institute.

Beauchamp, T. L., and Childress, J. F. 1994. *The Principles of Biomedical Ethics.* 4th ed. Oxford: Oxford University Press.

Bedau, H. A. 1971. "Military Service and Moral Obligation." *Inquiry* 14: 244–270.

Beecher, H. 1971. *Research and the Individual.* Boston: Little, Brown.

Bellamy, R. F. 1985. "Contrasts in Combat Casualty Care." *Military Medicine* 150 (5): 405–410.

Benatar, S. R. 1993. "Medical Ethics in Times of War and Insurrection: Rights and Duties." *Journal of Medical Humanities* 14 (3): 137–147.

Bender, H. S. 1944. "Can a Nonresistant Nurse Serve in the Army?" *Mennonursing* 1 (1): 7.

Benn, A. 2001. "Mounting Pressure on the Rule of Law." Ha'aretz, February, 15.

Berlin, F. S., Malin, H. M., and Dean, S. 1991. "Effects of Statutes Requiring Psychiatrists to Report Suspected Child Abuse of Children." *American Journal of Psychiatry* 148 (4): 449–453.

Best, G. 1980. *Humanity in Warfare*. New York: Columbia University Press.

Bickel, L. 1972. *Rise Up to Life: A Biography of Howard Walter Florey Who Gave Penicillin to the World*. New York: Scribner.

Biological Weapons Convention. 1972. *Convention on the Prohibition of the Development, Production and Stockpiling of Bacteriological (Biological) and Toxin Weapons and on Their Destruction*. www.state.gov/t/ac/trt/4718.htm

Bisgard, J. C. 1982. "The Obligation to Care for Casualties." *Hastings Center Report* 12 (2): 15–17.

Bishop, R. 1969. "Medical Support of Stability Operations: A Vietnam Case Study." Carlisle, PA: U.S. Army War College.

Blachar, Y. 1997. "The Truth about Israeli Medical Ethics." *The Lancet* 35 (9096): 1247.

Blachar, Y. 1999. "Unpressured Physicians." *Ha'aretz*, November 15, (In Hebrew.)

Blake, N., and Pole, K., eds. 1984. *Objections to Nuclear Defence: Philosophers on Deterrence*. London: Routledge and Kegan Paul.

Bloche, M. G., and Marks, J. H. 2005. "When Doctors Go to War." *New England Journal of Medicine* 352 (1): 3–6.

Bok, S. 1989. *Secrets: On the Ethics of Concealment and Revelation*. New York: Vintage.

Bok, S., and Kottow, C. 1986. "Medical Confidentiality: An Intransigent and Absolute Obligation." *Journal of Medical Ethics* 12: 117–122.

Bonner, R., Natta, D., Jr., and Waldman, A. 2003. "Questioning Terror Suspects In a Dark and Surreal World" *New York Times,* March 9, p. 1. http://lists.stir.ac.uk/pipermail/media-watch/2003-July/000719.html

Bortolotti, D. 2004. *Hope in Hell: Inside the World of Doctors Without Borders*. Buffalo: Firefly.

Bowman, R. D. 1944. *The Church of the Brethren and War 1708–1941*. Elgin, IL: Brethren Publishing House.

British Medical Association. 1992. *Medicine Betrayed: The Participation of Doctors in Human Rights Abuses*. London: Zed Books.

Brock, P., and Young, N. 1999. *Pacifism in the Twentieth Century*. Syracuse: Syracuse University Press.

B'tselem (Israeli Information Center for Human Rights in the Occupied Territories). 2000. *Position Paper, Legislation Permitting Physical and Psychological Pressure in the Investigation of the General Security Services*. Jerusalem: B'tselem.

B'tselem. 2001a. *No Way Out: Medical Implications of Israel's Siege Policy.* Jerusalem: B'tselem.

B'tselem. 2001b. *Torture of Palestinian Minors in the Gush Etzion Police Station.* Jerusalem: B'tselem.

B'tselem. 2002. *Impeding Medical Treatment and Firing at Ambulances by IDF Soldiers in the Occupied Territories.* Jerusalem: B'tselem.

B'tselem. 2002–2004. "Testimonies, Medical Treatment." http://www.btselem .org/english/Testimonies/index.asp?TF=21.

B'tselem and Physicians for Human Rights. 2003. *Harm to Medical Personnel: The Delay, Abuse and Humiliation of Medical Personnel by the Israel Security Forces.* Jerusalem: B'tselem and Physicians for Human Rights.

Buck, P. 1986. *The Enemy.* Mankato, MN: Creative Education.

Bulletin of Atomic Scientists. 2002. "From the Board of Directors: It's Seven Minutes to midnight." February 27. http://www.bulletin.org/media/ current_print.html.

Bush, P. 1998. *Two Kingdoms, Two Loyalties: Mennonite Pacifism in Modern America.* Baltimore: Johns Hopkins University Press.

Callahan, D. 1988. *Setting Limits: Medical Goals in an Aging Society.* New York: Simon and Schuster.

Callahan, D. 1990. *What Kind of Life: The Limits of Medical Progress.* Washington, DC: Georgetown University Press.

Carter, G. B., and Pearson, G. S. 1999. "British Biological Warfare and Defense, 1925–45." In E. Geissler and J. E. van Courtland Moon, eds., *Biological and Toxin Weapons: Research, Development and Use from the Middle Ages to 1945,* 168–189. SIPRI Chemical and Biological Warfare Studies 18. Oxford: Oxford University Press.

Cassel, C. K., Jameton, A. L., Sidel, V. W., and Storey, P. B. 1985. "The Physician's Oath and the Prevention of Nuclear War." *Journal of the American Medical Association* 254 (5): 652–654.

CAT. 1984. *Convention against Torture and Other Cruel, Inhuman or Degrading Treatment or Punishment.* www.unhchr.ch/html/menu3/b/h_cat39.htm

Ceadel, M. 1980. *Pacifism in Britain 1914–1945: The Defining of a Faith.* Oxford: Clarendon Press.

Chatterjee, D. K., and Scheid, D. E. 2003. *Ethics and Foreign Intervention.* Cambridge: Cambridge University Press.

Chemical Weapons Convention. 1993. *Convention on the Prohibition of the Development, Production, Stockpiling and Use of Chemical Weapons and on Their Destruction.* www.cwc.gov/treaty/cwcIndex_html

Childress, J. F. 1985. "Civil Disobedience, Conscientious Objection, and Evasive Noncompliance: A Framework for the Analysis and Assessment of Illegal Actions in Health Care." *Journal of Philosophy and Medicine* 10: 63–84.

Childress, J. F. 1990. "The Place of Autonomy in Bioethics." *Hastings Center Report* 20: 12–16.

Chisholm, J. J. 1861. *A Manual of Military Surgery for the Use of Surgeons in the Confederate Army*. Richmond, VA: West and Johnston.

Chodoff, E. P. 1983. "Ideology and Small Groups." *Armed Forces and Society* 9 (4): 569–593.

Christopher, G. W., Cieslak, T. S., Pavlin, J. A., Eitzen, E. H., Jr. 1999. "Biological Warfare: A Historical Perspective." In J. Lederberg, ed., *Biological Weapons: Limiting the Threat*, 17–35. Cambridge, MA: MIT Press.

Coady, C. A. J. 1988. "Deterrent Intentions Revisited." *Ethics* 99: 98–108.

Coady, C. A. J. 1989. "Escaping from the Bomb: Immoral Deterrence and the Problem of Extrication." In H. Shue, ed., *Nuclear Deterrence and Moral Restraint: Critical Choices for American Strategy*, 163–225. Cambridge: Cambridge University Press.

Coates, A. J. 1997. *The Ethics of War*. Manchester: Manchester University Press.

Cohen, D. 1987/8. "The Development of the Modern Doctrine of Necessity: A Comparative Critique." In A. Eser, and G. Fletcher, eds., *Justification and Excuse: Comparative Perspectives*, vol. 2, 991. Freiburg: Max Planck Institute.

Cohn, N. 1981. *Warrant for Genocide: The Myth of the Jewish World-Conspiracy and the Protocols of the Elders of Zion*. Chico, CA: Scholars Press.

Connell, F. J. 1967. "Double Effect, Principle of." *The New Catholic Encyclopedia*, vol. 4, 1021. New York: McGraw Hill.

Coppernoll, M. 1990. "The Non-Lethal Weapons Debate." *Naval War College Review* 52 (2): 112–131.

Costello, J. 1986. *Virtue under Fire: How World War II Changed Our Social and Sexual Attitudes*. Boston: Little, Brown.

Coupland, R. M. 1991. *The Red Cross Wound Classification*. 2nd ed. Geneva: International Committee of the Red Cross.

Coupland, R. M. 1996. "The Effect of Weapons: Defining Superfluous Injury and Unnecessary Suffering." *Medicine and Global Survival* 3: A1. http://www.ippnw.org/MGS/V3Coupland.html

Coupland, R. M. 1997a. "Abhorrent Weapons and 'Superfluous Injury or Unnecessary Suffering': from Field Surgery to Law." *British Medical Journal* 315: 1450–1452.

Coupland, R. M. 1997b. "'Non-Lethal Weapons': Precipitating a New Arms Race." *British Medical Journal* 315: 72.

Coupland, R. M. 1999. "The SIrUS Project: Progress Report on 'Superfluous Injury or Unnecessary Suffering' in Relation to the Legality of Weapons." *International Review of the Red Cross* 835: 583–592.

Crane, S. [1895] 2003. *The Red Badge of Courage*. New York: Barnes and Noble Classics.

Croddy, E. 2002. *Chemical and Biological Warfare: A Comprehensive Survey for the Concerned Citizen.* New York: Springer-Verlag.

Cummings, M. L. 2002. "Informed Consent and Investigational New Drug Abuses in the U. S. Military." *Accountability in Research* 9: 93–103.

Dai, L. C. 2004. *The Central Highlands: A North Vietnamese Journal of Life on the Ho Chi Minh Trail 1965–1973.* Annotated trans. by Lady Borton. Hanoi Vietnam: Gioi Publishers.

Dando, M. 1996. *A New Form of Warfare: The Rise of Non-Lethal Weapons.* London: Brassey's.

Daniels, N. 1988. *Just Health Care.* Cambridge: Cambridge University Press.

Daniels, N., and Sabin, J. 1997. "Limits to Health Care: Fair Procedure, Democratic Deliberation, and the Legitimacy Problem for Insurers." *Philosophy and Public Affairs* 26 (4): 303–350.

Danon, Y. L., Nili, E., and Dolev, E. 1984. "Primary Treatment of Battle Casualties in the Lebanon War, 1982." *Israel Journal of Medical Science* 20: 300–302.

Day, B., and Waitzkin, H. 1985. "The Medical Profession and Nuclear War: A Social History." *Journal of the American Medical Association* 254 (5): 644–651.

Dershowitz, A. M. 2002. *Why Terrorism Works.* New Haven, CT: Yale University Press.

Dickerson, J. 1999. *North to Canada: Men and Women against the Vietnam War.* Westport, CT: Praeger.

Dillon, R. S. 1995. "Introduction." In R. S. Dillon, ed., *Dignity, Character and Self-Respect.* New York: Routledge.

Dolev, E. 1996. "Ethical Issues in Military Medicine." *Israel Journal of Medical Science* 32: 785–788.

Dolman, J. E. 1995. "Obligation and the Citizen Soldier: Machivellian Virtu versus Hobbesian Order." *Journal of Political and Military Sociology* 23: 191–212.

Doswald-Beck, L. 1999. "Implementation of International Humanitarian Law in Future Wars." *Naval War College Review* 52 (1): 24–52.

Downie, R. S. 1993. "The Ethics of Physician Participation in Torture." *Journal of Medical Ethics* 19: 135–137.

Dunant, H. [1862] 1986. *A Memory of Solferino.* Geneva: International Committee of the Red Cross.

Dupuy, T. N. 1995. *Attrition: Forecasting Battle Casualties and Equipment Losses in Modern War.* Falls Church, VA: Nova Publications.

Emanuel, E. 1991. *The Ends of Human Life.* Cambridge, MA: Harvard University Press.

Feinberg, H. 1998. "North to Palestine: Napoleon Marches against the Turks." *Journal of Napoleonic Scholarship* 1 (2). Available at http://www.napoleonicso ciety.com/english/scholarship98/c_palestine.html

Fidler, D. P. 1999. "The International Legal Implications of 'Non-Lethal' Weapons." *Michigan Journal of International Law* 21 (1): 51–100.

Fidler, D. P. 2001. "Non-Lethal Weapons and International Law." *Medicine, Conflict and Survival* 17: 194–206.

FitzPatrick, W. J., and Zwangziger, L. L. 2003. "Defending against Biological Warfare: Ethical Issues Involving the Coercive Use of Investigational Drugs and Biologics in the Military." *Journal of Philosophy, Science and Law* 3: 1–16.

Flynn, G. Q. 1989. "Selective Service and the Conscientious Objector." In M. F. Noone, ed., *Selective Conscientious Objection: Accommodating Conscience and Security*, 35–55. Boulder, CO: Westview.

Foot, P. [1975] 1994. "Killing and Letting Die." In B. Steinbock and A. Norcross, *Killing and Letting Die*, 2nd ed., 280–289. New York: Fordham University Press.

Four Feathers. 2002. Paramount Pictures. (Based on the novel by A. E. W. Mason. New York: MacMillan, [1902] 2000.)

Frisina, M. E. 1990. "The Offensive-Defensive Distinction in Military Biological Research." *Hastings Center Report* 20 (3): 19–22.

Frisina, M. E. 2003. "Medical Ethics in Military Biomedical Research." In T. E. Beam, and L. R. Sparacino, eds., *Military Medical Ethics*, vol. 2, 533–561. Textbooks of Military Medicine. Washington, DC: Office of the Surgeon General, Borden Institute.

Gabriel, R. A., and Metz, K. S. 1992. *A History of Military Medicine.* 2 vols. New York: Greenwood Press.

Gal, J. 2001. "The Perils of Compensation in Social Welfare Policy: Disability Policy in Israel." *Social Service Review* 75 (2): 225–244.

Garrison, F. H. [1922] 1970. *Notes on the History of Military Medicine.* New York: Georg Olms Verlag.

Geiger, H. J. 1982. "Why Survival Plans Are Meaningless." *Hastings Center Report* 12 (2): 17–19.

Geissler, E., and van Courtland Moon, J. E., eds. 1999. *Biological and Toxin Weapons: Research, Development and Use from the Middle Ages to 1945.* SIPRI Chemical and Biological Warfare Studies 18. Oxford: Oxford University Press.

Geneva Conference. 1863. *Resolutions of the Geneva International Conference,* Geneva, October, 26–29. http://www.icrc.org/ihl.nsf

Geneva Convention 1864. *Convention for the Amelioration of the Condition of the Wounded in Armies in the Field.* Geneva, August 22. http://www.icrc.org/ihl.nsf

Geneva Convention. 1868. *Additional Articles Relating to the Condition of the Wounded in War*, Geneva, October 20. http://www.icrc.org/ihl.nsf

Geneva Convention. 1929. *Convention for the Amelioration of the Condition of the Wounded and Sick in Armies in the Field*, Geneva, July 27. http://www.icrc.org/ihl.nsf

Geneva Convention (I). 1949a. *Convention for the Amelioration of the Condition of the Wounded and Sick in Armed Forces in the Field, Geneva*, August 12. http://www.icrc.org/ihl.nsf

Geneva Convention (I). 1949b. *Commentary, Convention (I) for the Amelioration of the Condition of the Wounded and Sick in Armed Forces in the Field, Geneva*, August 12. http://www.icrc.org/ihl.nsf

Geneva Convention (II). 1949c. *Convention for the Amelioration of the Condition of the Wounded and Sick in Armed Forces at Sea, Geneva*, August 12. http://www.icrc.org/ihl.nsf

Geneva Convention (IV). 1949d. *Convention Relative to the Protection of Civilian Persons in Time of War, Geneva*, August 12. http://www.icrc.org/ihl.nsf

Ginn, R. V. N. 1977. *The History of the US Army Medical Service Corps.* Washington, DC: Office of the Surgeon General and Center for Military History of the United States Army.

Glick, S. 1997. "Unlimited Human Autonomy: A Cultural Bias?" *New England Journal of Medicine* 336 (13): 954–956.

Gonzales, A. R. 2002. *Memorandum for Alberto R. Gonzales, Counsel to the President re: Standards of Conduct for Interrogation under 18 U.S.C. 2340–2340A*, August 1, no. 1. http://www.gwu.edu/~nsarchiv/NSAEBB/NSAEBB127/02.08.01.pdf.

Gordon, H. 1995. "Political Evil: Legalized and Concealed Sadism." In N. Gordon, and R. Marton, eds., *Torture: Human Rights, Medical Ethics and the Case of Israel*, 11–19. London: Zed Books.

Gottlieb, S. 1991. *Hell No, We Won't Go! Resisting the Draft during the Vietnam War*. New York: Viking.

Graham, G. L. 1997. *Ethics and International Relations*. London: Blackwell.

Green, L. C. 1998. "Cicero and Clausewitz or Quincy Wright: The Interplay of Law and War." *United States Air Force Academy Journal of Legal Studies, Annual* 9: 59–98.

Green, L. C. 2000. *The Contemporary Law of Armed Conflict*. 2nd ed. Manchester: Manchester University Press.

Grissinger, J. W. 1927. "The Development of Military Medicine." *New York Academy of Medicine* 3 (5): 301–356.

Gross, M. L. 1997. *Ethics and Activism: The Theory and Practice of Political Morality*. Cambridge: Cambridge University Press.

Gross, M. L. 1999. "Autonomy and Paternalism in Communitarian Society: Patient Rights in Israel." *Hastings Center Report* 29 (4): 13–20.

Gross, M. L. 2003. "Fighting by Other Means in the Mideast: A Critical Analysis of Israel's Assassination Policy." *Political Studies* 51: 350–368.

Gross, M. L. 2004. "Doctors in the Decent Society: Medical Care, Torture and Ill-Treatment." *Bioethics*, 18 (2): 181–203.

Gross, M. L. 2005. "Treating Competent Patients by Force: The Limits and Lessons of Israel's Patient Rights Act." *Journal of Medical Ethics* 16 (1): 29–34.

Grotius, H. [1625] 1901. *The Rights of War and Peace*. Trans. A. C. Campbell. New York: M. Walter Dunne.

Hague Convention. 1899. *Convention (II) with Respect to the Laws and Customs of War on Land and Its Annex: Regulations Concerning the Laws and Customs of War on Land*, The Hague, July 29. http://www.icrc.org/ihl

Haines, A., de B. White, C., and Gleisner, J. 1983. "Nuclear Weapons and Medicine: Some Ethical Dilemmas." *Journal of Medical Ethics* 9: 200–206.

Haldane, J. J. 1987. "Ethics and Biological Weapons." *Arms Control* 8 (1): 24–35.

Hammond, P. M., and Carter, G. 2002. *From Biological Warfare to Healthcare: Porton Down 1940–2000*. Centre for Applied Microbiology Research. Houndmills, UK: Palgrave.

Handelman, S., and Alibek, K. 2000. *Biohazard: The Chilling Story of the Largest Covert Biological Weapons Program in the World, Told from the Inside by the Man Who Ran It*. New York: Delta.

Hardin, G. 1974. "Lifeboat Ethics: The Case against Helping the Poor." *Psychology Today* 8: 38–43.

Hardin, R. 1982. *Collective Action*. Baltimore: Johns Hopkins University Press.

Hare, R. M. 1993. "The Ethics of Physician Participation in Torture: Commentary." *Journal of Medical Ethics* 19: 138–141.

Harel, A. 2002. "Shin Bet Tested by Legal Restraints and a Growing Caseload." *Ha'aretz*, July 25.

Harel, A. 2001. "Suicide Bombing Averted in Haifa." *Ha'aretz*, July 23.

Harris, R., and Paxman, J. 2002. *A Higher Form of Killing: The Secret History of Chemical and Biological Warfare*. New York: Random House.

Harris, S. 1999. "The Japanese Biological Warfare Programme: An Overview." In E. Geissler and J. E. van Courtland Moon, eds., *Biological and Toxin Weapons: Research, Development and Use from the Middle Ages to 1945*, 127–152. SIPRI Chemical and Biological Warfare Studies 18. Oxford: Oxford University Press.

Haug, J. N., Roback, G. A., Theodore, C. N., and Balfe, B. E. 1970. *Distribution of Physicians, Hospitals, and Hospital Beds in the U.S., 1968*. Chicago: American Medical Association.

Haynes, C. B., ed. 1943. "Seventh Day Adventist, General Conference Committee, September 1940." In *Studies in Denominational Principles of Non-combatancy and Governmental Relations*, 22–24. Washington, DC: Seventh Day Adventist War Service Commission.

Haynes, W. J. 2002. *Action Memo, from William J. Haynes, General Counsel, to the Secretary of Defense, regarding "Counter-Resistance Techniques."* November 27. www.defenselink.mil/news/JUN2004/d20040622doc5.pdf

Heller, J. 1996. *Catch 22*. New York: Simon and Schuster.

Hilberg, R. 1985. *The Destruction of the European Jews*. New York: Holmes & Meier.

Hinds, S. 1976. "On the Relations of Medical Triage to World Famine: An Historical Survey." In G. Lucas, and T. Ogletree, eds., *Lifeboat Ethics*, 29–61. New York: Harper & Row.

Hobbes, T. [1651] 1996. *Leviathan*: Revised student edition (Cambridge Texts in the History of Political Thought). Ed. R. Tuck. Cambridge: Cambridge University Press.

Holmes, R. L. 1989. *On War and Morality*. Princeton, NJ: Princeton University Press.

Holzgrefe, J. L., and Keohane, R. O., eds. 2003. *Humanitarian Intervention: Ethical, Legal and Political Dilemmas*. Cambridge: Cambridge University Press.

Honey, M. K. 1986. "The War within the Confederacy: White Unionist of North Carolina." *Journal of the National Archives* 18 (2): 75–93. http://home-pages.rootsweb.com/~ncuv/honey1.htm.

Horne, A. 1977. *A Savage War of Peace: Algeria 1954–1962*. New York: Viking.

Howard, J. M. 1954. "Triage in the Korean Conflict." In *Recent Advances in Medicine and Surgery, 19–30 April 1954, Based on Professional Medical Experiences in Japan and Korea 1950–1953*, vol. 1. Medical Science Publication No. 4. Washington, DC: U.S. Army Medical Service Graduate School, Walter Reed Army Medical Center.

Howard, M., Andreopoulos, G. J., and Shulman, M. R. 1994. *The Laws of War: Constraints on Warfare in the Western World*. New Haven, CT: Yale University Press.

Howe, E. G. 2003 "Point/Counterpoint—A Response to Drs. Sidel and Levy in Victor W. Sidel and Barry S. Levy, "Physician-Soldier: A Moral Dilemma. In T. E. Beam and L. R. Sparacino, eds., *Military Medical Ethics*, vol. 2, 312–320. Textbooks of Military Medicine. Washington, DC: Office of the Surgeon General, Borden Institute.

Howe, E. G., and Martin, E. D. 1991. "Treating the Troops." *Hastings Center Report* 21 (2): 21–24.

Howie, J. 1979. "Gonorrhea: A Question of Tactics." *British Medical Journal* 2 (6205): 1631–1632.

Human Rights Watch. 2002. *Background Paper on the Geneva Conventions and Persons Held by US Forces*, January 29. http://www.hrw.org/backgrounder/usa/pow_bck.htm#P49_10180.

Human Rights Watch/Middle East. 1994. *Torture and Ill-Treatment: Israel's Interrogation of Palestinians from the Occupied Territories*. New York: Human Rights Watch.

A Human Security Doctrine for Europe. 2004. The Barcelona Report of the Study Group on Europe's Security Capabilities, Presented to EU High Representative for Common Foreign and Security Policy Javier Solana, Barcelona, September 15, 2004. http://www.lse.ac.uk/Depts/global/Human%20Security%20Report%20Full.pdf.

Humphreys, J. 1968. "The Aid Medical Mission in Vietnam." *Military Medicine* 133: 201–207.

Huxsoll, D. L., Parrott, C. D., and Patrick, W. C. III. 1989. "Medicine in Defense against Biological Warfare." *Journal of the American Medical Association* 262 (5): 677–680.

Iacopino, V., and Waldman, R. J. 1999. "War and Health from Solferino to Kosovo—The Evolving Role of Physicians." *Journal of the American Medical Association* 285 (5): 479–481.

International Committee of the Red Cross. 1996. *The Medical Profession and the Effects of Weapons*. ICRC Publication Ref. 0668. Geneva: International Committee of the Red Cross.

International Committee of the Red Cross. 1997. *The SIrUS Project: Towards a Determination of Which Weapons Cause "Superfluous Injury or Unnecessary Suffering*. Geneva: International Committee of the Red Cross.

International Committee of the Red Cross. 2004. *Report of the International Committee of The Red Cross (ICRC) on the Treatment by the Coalition Forces of Prisoners of War and Other Protected Persons by the Geneva Conventions in Iraq during Arrest, Internment and Interrogation*. http://www.globalsecurity.org/military/library/report/2004/icrc_report_iraq_feb2004.htm

International Covenant on Civil and Political Rights. 1976. www.unhchr.ch/html/menu3/b/A_opt.htm.

International Physicians for the Prevention of Nuclear War. 2001a. "Preventing War through Non-violent Direct Involvement in Conflict, I, Principles and Background." *Medicine, Conflict and Survival* 17: 309–322.

International Physicians for the Prevention of Nuclear War. 2001b. "Preventing War through Non-violent Direct Involvement in Conflict, II, Proposal for the Role of IPPNW." *Medicine, Conflict and Survival* 17: 323–336.

International Physicians for the Prevention of Nuclear War. 2005. Mission Statement. http://www.ippnw.org/IPPNWBackground.html.

Ireland v. the United Kingdom. 1976. In *Yearbook of the European Conventions on Human Rights* 19: 512–928.

Israeloff, J. 1985. "Medical Field Service in the US Army Medical Department and the Israel Defense Forces." *Military Medicine* 150 (8): 416–422.

Jabbour, S. 2005. "Healing and Peace Making in the Middle East: Challenges for Doctors." *The Lancet* 365: 1211–1212.

Jacobs, L., Marmor, T., and Oberlander, J. 1999. "The Oregon Health Plan and the Political Paradox of Rationing: What Advocates and Critics Have Claimed and What Oregon Did." *Journal of Health Politics, Policy and Law* 24 (1): 161–180.

Johnson, J. T. 1982. "The Moral Basis of Contingency Planning." *Hastings Center Report*, 12 (2): 19–20.

Jones, D. P. 1980. "American Chemists and the Geneva Protocol, *Isis* 71 (3): 426–440.

Jones, G. E. 1980. "On the Permissibility of Torture." *Journal of Medical Ethics* 6: 11–15.

Jonson, A. R. 1998. *The Birth of Bioethics.* Oxford: Oxford University Press.

Kadish, S. H. 1989. "Torture, the State, and the Individual." *Israel Law Review* 23 (2, 3): 345–356.

Kagen, D. 1995. *On the Origins of War and the Preservation of Peace.* New York: Anchor.

Kant [1784] 1991. "Idea for a Universal History with Cosmopolitan Intent." In *Kant: Political Writings* (Cambridge Texts in the History of Political Thought). Edited by H. S. Reiss. Translated by H. B. Nisbet. Cambridge: Cambridge University Press: 41–53.

Katz, R. D. 2000–2001. "Friendly Fire: The Mandatory Military Anthrax Vaccination Program." *Duke Law Journal* 50: 1835–1865.

Kegley, C. W., Jr. 1990. "The Characteristics of Contemporary International Terrorism." In C. W. Kegley Jr., ed., *International Terrorism: Characteristics, Causes, Controls*, 11–26. New York: St. Martin's Press.

Keim, A. N. 1979. "Service or Resistance? The Mennonite Response to Conscription in World War II." *Mennonite Quarterly Review* 52 (2): 141–155.

Kellet, A. 1982. *Combat Motivation: The Behavior of Men in Battle.* Dordrecht, The Netherlands: Kluwer.

Kellet, A. 1990. "The Soldier in Battle: Motivational and Behavioral Aspects of the Combat Experience." In G. Glad, ed., *The Psychological Dimensions of War*, 215–235. Newbury Park, CA: Sage.

Kemp, K. W. 1995. "Personal Pacifism." *Theological Studies* 56: 21–38.

Knight, G. K. 1997. "Adventism and Military Service." In T. F. Schlabach and R. T. Hughes, ed., *Proclaim Peace: Christian Pacifism from Unexpected Quarters*, 157–171. Chicago: University of Illinois Press.

Koehler, R. H., Smith, R. S., and Bacaner, T. 1994. "Triage of American Combat Casualties: The Need for Change." *Military Medicine* 159 (8): 541–547.

Kohrman, A. 1986. "Respectable Pacifists: Quaker Response to World War I." *Peace and Change* 75 (1): 35–53.

Lakoski, J. W., Murray, B., and Kenny, J. M. 2000. *The Advantages and Limitations of Calmatives for Use as a Non-Lethal Technique.* Hershey, PA: College of Medicine; Applied Research Laboratory, Pennsylvania State University.

Landau Commission. 1989a. "Commission of Inquiry into the Methods of Investigation of the General Security Service Regarding Hostile Terrorist Activity." *Israel Law Review* 23 (2, 3): 146–188.

Landau Commission. 1989b. "Landau Commission Report—Was the Security Service Subordinated to the Law, or the Law to the 'Needs' of the Security Service?" *Israel Law Review* 23 (2, 3): 216–279.

Larrey, D. J. [1814] 1987. *Memoirs of Military Surgery and Campaigns of the French Army.* Trans. from the French by Richard Willmott Hall. 2 vols. Baltimore: Joseph Cushing. (Reprint, Birmingham, AL: Classics of Modern Medicine, Gryphon Editions, 1987.)

Lazersfeld, P. F. 1949. "The American Soldier: An Expository View." *Public Opinion Quarterly* 13: 377–404.

Leichter, H. M. 1999. "Oregon's Bold Experiment: Whatever Happened to Rationing?" *Journal of Health Politics, Policy and Law*, 24 (1): 147–160.

Lewer, N. 1992. *Physicians and the Peace Movement.* London: Frank Cass.

Lewer, N., and Davison, N. 2005. "Non-Lethal Technologies—An Overview." *Disarmament* 1: 36–51.

Lewer, N., and Feakin T. 2001. "Perspectives and Implications for the Proliferation of Non-Lethal Weapons in the Context of Contemporary Conflict, Security Interests and Arms Control." *Medicine, Conflict and Survival* 17: 227–286.

Lewer, N., and Schofield, S. 1997. *Non-Lethal Weapons: A Fatal Attraction?* London: Zed Books.

Lewis, N. A. 2004. "Red Cross Finds Detainee Abuse at Guantánamo." *New York Times*, November 30. www.cis.ksu.edu/~schmidf/misc/30gitmo.html

Lewy, G. 1980. *America in Vietnam.* Oxford: Oxford University Press.

Lieber Code. 1863. Francis Lieber, *Instructions for the Government of Armies of the United States in the Field.* General Orders no. 100. Washington, DC: War Department.

Lifton, J. 1986. *The Nazi Doctors: Medical Killing and the Psychology of Genocide.* New York: Basic Books, 1986.

Lown, B. 1985. "Nobel Peace Prize." December 10. http://www.ippnw.org/Lown.html.

MacQueen, G., and Santa-Barbara, J. 2000. "Peace Building through Health Initiatives." *British Medical Journal* 321: 293–296.

Madden, E. H., and Hare, P. H. 1978. "Civil Disobedience in Health Services." In W. T. Reich, ed., *Encyclopedia of Bioethics*, vol. 1, 159–162. New York: Free Press.

Maddocks, I. 1996. "Evolution of the Physicians' Peace Movement: A Historical Perspective." *Health and Human Rights* 2 (1): 88–109.

Mallory, M., Jr. 1954. "Emergency Treatment and Resuscitation at the Battalion Level." Presented April 19, 1954, to the *Course on Recent Advances in Medicine and Surgery*, Army Medical Service Graduate School, Walter Reed Army Medical Center, Washington, DC.

Margalit, A. 1996. *The Decent Society*. Cambridge, MA: Harvard University Press.

Marsh, A. R. 1983. "A Short but Distant War—The Falklands Campaign." *Journal of the Royal Society of Medicine* 76 (11): 972–982.

Mason, J. K., and McCall Smith, R. A. 1999. *Law and Medical Ethics*. 5th ed. London: Butterworth.

Massey, S. J. 1983. "Is Self-Respect a Moral or Psychological Concept?" *Ethics* 93: 246–261.

McFarlane, G. 1998. "Howard Florey, Part Two, The Health Report with Norman Swan." Radio interview, Radio National (Australia). September 21. http://www.abc.net.au/rn/talks/8.30/helthrpt/stories/s12820.htm.

McMahan, J. 1988. "Deterrence and Deontology." *Ethics* 95 (3): 517–536.

McMahan, J. 1994a. "Innocence, Self-Defense and Killing in War." *Journal of Political Philosophy* 2: 193–221.

McMahan, J. 1994b. "Revising the Doctrine of Double Effect." *Journal of Applied Philosophy* 11 (2): 201–212.

Michael, M., and Zwi, A. B. 2002. "Oceans of Need in the Desert: Ethical Issues Identified While Researching Humanitarian Aid in Afghanistan." *Developing World Bioethics* 2 (2): 109–130.

Michalowski, S. 2001. "Medical Confidentiality for Violent Patients? A Comparison of the German and English Approach." *Medicine and Law* 20 (4): 569–577.

Miles, S. 2004. "Abu Ghraib: Its Legacy for Military Medicine." *The Lancet* 364: 725–729.

Mill, J. S. [1859] 1989. *On Liberty*. Cambridge: Cambridge University Press.

Mill, J. S. [1861] 1950. *Utilitarianism, Liberty and Representative Government*. New York: Dutton.

Miller, R. K. 2002. "Informed Consent in the Military: Fighting a Losing Battle against the Anthrax Vaccine." *American Journal of Law and Medicine* 28 (2, 3): 325–345.

Montague, P. 1981. "Self-Defense and Choosing between Lives." *Philosophical Studies* 40: 207–219.

Moore, M. S. 1989. "Torture and the Balance of Evils." *Israel Law Review* 23 (2, 3): 280–344.

Moreno, J. D. 2001. *Undue Risk: Secret State Experiments on Humans.* New York: Routledge.

Moreno, J. D., and Lederer, S. E. 1995. "Revising the History of Cold War Research Ethics." *Kennedy Institute of Ethics Journal* 6 (3): 223–237.

Moskop, J. C. 1998. "A Moral Analysis of Military Medicine." *Military Medicine*, 163 (2): 76–79.

Murray, T. H. 1982. "The Physician as Moral Leader." *Hastings Center Report* 12 (2): 20–21.

Nando, Malcolm. 1996. *A New Form of Warfare: The Rise of Non-Lethal Weapons.* London: Brassey's.

National Commission for the Protection of Human Subjects of Biomedical and Behavioral Research. 1979. *The Belmont Report: Ethical Principles and Guidelines for the Protection of Human Subjects of Research.* DHEW Publication No. OS 78-0012. Washington, DC: Government Printing Office.

National Research Council. 2003. *An Assessment of Non-Lethal Weapons Science and Technology.* Committee for an Assessment of Non-Lethal Weapons Science and Technology, Naval Studies Board Division on Engineering and Physical Sciences. Washington, DC: National Academies Press.

National Research Council. 2004. *Biotechnology Research in an Age of Terrorism: Confronting the Dual Use Dilemma.* Washington, D.C.: The National Academies Press.

Neel, S. 1967. "The Medical Role in Army Stability Operations." *Military Medicine* 132: 605–608.

Neel, S. 1991. *Medical Support of the U.S. Army in Vietnam 1965–1970.* Washington, DC: U.S. Department of the Army.

Nolan, H. 1999. "Learning to Express Dissent: Médecins Sans Frontières" *British Medical Journal* 319: 446–447.

Norman, R. 1995. *Ethics, Killing and War.* Cambridge: Cambridge University Press.

Nuremberg Code. 1947. http://www.hhs.gov/ohrp/irb/irb_appendices.htm#j5

Office of the Surgeon. 1944. *Circular Letter no 36.* Office of the Surgeon, Headquarters, North African Theatre of Operations, July 1. http://history.amedd.army.mil/booksdocs/wwii/Othromed/Appendix.html.

Orend, B. 2001. "Just and Lawful Conduct in War: Reflections on Michael Walzer." *Law and Philosophy* 20: 1–30.

Parker, G. 1994. "Early Modern Europe." In M. Howard, G. J. Andreopoulos, and M. R. Shulman, eds. *The Laws of War: Constraints on Warfare in the Western World,* 40–58. New Haven: Yale University Press.

Pacheco, A. 1999. *The Case against Torture in Israel.* Jerusalem: Public Committee against Torture in Israel.

Pagaard, S. A. 1986. "Disease and the British Army in South Africa, 1899–1900." *Military Affairs* 50 (2): 71–76.

Palmer, C. A., and Zwi, A. B. 1998. "Women, Health and Humanitarian Aid in Conflict." *Disasters* 22: 236–249.

Paré, A. 1968. *The Apologie and Treatise.* New York: Dover Publications.

Pellegrino, E. D., and Thomasma, D. C. 1993. *The Virtues in Medical Practice.* Oxford: Oxford University Press.

Peters, E. 1996. *Torture.* Rev. ed. Philadelphia: University of Pennsylvania Press.

Peterson, R. K. D. 1995. "Insects, Disease, and Military History: The Napoleonic Campaigns and Historical Perception." *American Entomologist* 41: 147–160.

Pfeffermann, R. et al. 1976. "Modern War Surgery Operations in an Evacuation Hospital during the October 1973 Arab Israeli War." *Journal of Trauma* 16: 694–703.

Physicians for Human Rights. 2002. *Medicine under Attack: Critical Damage Inflicted on Medical Services in the Occupied Territories: An Interim Report.* Jerusalem: Physicians for Human Rights–Israel.

Physicians for Human Rights. 2003. *Keep Medical Institutions out of the Conflict.* Jerusalem: Physicians for Human Rights–Israel.

Physicians for Human Rights. 2005. "Medical Treatment Conditional upon Collaboration." Press release, Physicians for Human Rights–Israel, May 1.

Porter, R. 1997. *The Greatest Benefit to Mankind: A Medical History of Humanity.* New York: Norton.

President's Commission for the Study of Ethical Problems in Medicine and Biomedical and Behavioral Research. 1983. *Deciding to Forego Life-Sustaining Treatment.* New York: Concern for Dying–An Educational Council.

Priest, D. 2004. "CIA Puts Harsh Tactics on Hold." *Washington Post*, June 27. http://www.washingtonpost.com/wp-dyn/articles/A8534-2004Jun26.html

Proctor, R. N. 1988. *Racial Hygiene: Medicine under the Nazis.* Cambridge, MA: Harvard University Press.

Protocol I. 1977a. *Protocol I to the Geneva Conventions of 12 August 1949, and Relating to the Protection of Victims of International Armed Conflict,* June 8. http://www.icrc.org/ihl.nsf

Protocol I. 1977b. *Commentary, Protocol Additional to the Geneva Conventions of 12 August 1949, and Relating to the Protection of Victims of International Armed Conflicts,* June 8. http://www.icrc.org/ihl.nsf

Protocol II. 1977. *Commentary, Protocol Additional to the Geneva Conventions of 12 August 1949, and Relating to the Protection of Victims of Non-International Armed Conflicts,* June 8. http://www.icrc.org/ihl.nsf

Protocol IV to the 1980 Convention. 1995. *Protocol on Blinding Laser Weapons,* October 13. http://www.icrc.org/ihl.nsf

Public Committee against Torture in Israel. 1993. *Dilemmas of Professional Ethics as a Result of the Involvement of Doctors and Psychologists in Interrogation and Torture.* Jerusalem: Public Committee against Torture in Israel.

Public Committee against Torture in Israel. 2001a. *Breaches in the Defense: Torture and Ill-Treatment during GSS [General Security Services] Investigations Following the Verdict of the High Court of Justice, 6 September 1999.* Jerusalem: Public Committee against Torture in Israel.

Public Committee against Torture in Israel. 2001b. *Racism, Violence and Humiliation, Findings, Conclusions and Recommendations of the Public Committee against Torture in Israel Concerning the Behavior of the Security Forces toward Persons Detained during the Events of September-October 2000.* Jerusalem: Public Committee against Torture in Israel.

Public Committee against Torture in Israel v. The State of Israel. 1999. HC 5100/94.

Quester, G. H. 1990. "The Psychological Effects of Bombing Civilian Populations: Wars of the Past." In B. Glad, ed., *The Psychological Dimensions of War,* 201–214. Newbury Park, CA: Sage.

Quinn, W. S. 1989. "Actions, Intentions and Consequences: The Doctrine of the Double Effect." *Philosophy and Public Affairs* 18: 334–351.

Rawls, J. 1971. *A Theory of Justice.* Cambridge, MA: Harvard University Press.

Reister, F. A. 1973. *Battle Casualties and Medical Statistics, U.S. Army Experience in the Korea War.* Washington, DC: Office of the Surgeon General.

Rettig, R. A. 1999. "Military Use of Drugs Not Yet Approved by FDA for CW/BW Defense: Lessons from the Gulf War." *Rand Report,* MR-1018/9 OSD. http://www.rand.org/cgi-bin/abstracts/e-getabbydoc.pl?MR-1018/9-OSD.

Richardson, F. M. 1985. "Wellington, Napoleon and the Medical Services." *Journal of the Royal Army Medical Corps* 131: 9–15.

Ritchie, E. C., and Mott, R. L. 2003. "Military Humanitarian Assistance: The Pitfalls and Promise of Good Intentions." In T. E. Beam and L. R. Sparacino, eds., *Military Medical Ethics,* vol. 2, 805–830. Textbooks of Military Medicine. Washington, DC: Office of the Surgeon General, Borden Institute.

Rodley, N. S. 1999. *The Treatment of Prisoners under International Law.* Oxford: Clarendon Press.

Rogers, A. P. V. 1996. *Law on the Battlefield.* Manchester: Manchester University Press.

Rosebury, T. 1949. *Peace or Pestilence: Biological Warfare and How to Avoid It.* New York: McGraw-Hill.

Rosebury, T. 1963. "Medical Ethics and Biological Warfare." *Perspectives in Biology and Medicine* 6: 512–523.

Rozin, R., Klausner, J. M., and Dolev, E. 1988. "New Concepts in Forward Combat Surgery." *Injury* 19: 193–197.

Rush, R. S. 2001. *Hell in the Hürtgen Forest: The Ordeal and Triumph of an American Infantry Regiment.* Lawrence: University of Kansas Press.

Ryan, J. M. 1984. "The Falklands War—Triage." *Annals of the Royal College of Surgeons of England* 66: 195–196.

Ryan, J. M., Sibson, J., and Howell, G. 1990. "Assessing Injury Severity during General War: Will the Military Triage System Meet Future Needs?" *Journal of the Royal Medical Corps* 136: 27–35.

Sautenet, V. 2000. "Legal Issues Concerning Military Use of Non-Lethal Weapons." *Murdoch University Electronic Journal of Law* 7 (2). http://www.murdoch.edu.au/elaw/issues/v7n2/sautenet72.html

Sayigh, Y. 2001. "Arafat and the Anatomy of a Revolt." *Survival* 43 (3): 47–60.

Schmitt, E. 2005. "The Struggle for Iraq: In New Manual, Army Limits Tactics in Interrogation." *New York Times*, April 28, p. 1.

Schulze, K. E. 2001. "Camp David and the Al-Aqsa Intifada: An Assessment of the State of the Israeli-Palestinian Peace Process, July–December 2000." *Studies in Conflict and Terrorism* 24: 215–233.

Secretary of the Navy. 2002. Instruction 1850.4E. http://neds.daps.dla.mil/directives/1850_4e.pdf

Seeley, R. A. 1988. *Advice for Conscientious Objectors in the Armed Forces.* 5th ed. Philadelphia: Central Committee for Conscientious Objectors.

Selgelid, M. J. 2003. "Smallpox Revisited?" *American Journal of Bioethics* 2003, 3(1). http://www.bioethics.net/journal/j_articles.php?aid=91

Shamgar, M. 1977. "The Observance of International Law in the Administered Territories." In J. N. Moor, ed., *The Arab-Israeli Conflict*, 489–507. Princeton, NJ: Princeton University Press.

Sheehan, J. C. 1982. *The Enchanted Ring: The Untold Story of Penicillin.* Cambridge, MA: MIT Press.

Shue, H. 1978. "Torture." *Philosophy and Public Affairs* 7 (2): 124–143.

Sibley, M. Q., and Jacob, P. E. 1952. *Conscription of Conscience: The American State and the Conscientious Objector, 1940–1947.* Ithaca, NY: Cornell University Press.

Sidel, V. W., and Levy, B. S. 2003. "Physician-Soldier: A Moral Dilemma." In T. E. Beam and L. R. Sparacino, eds., *Military Medical Ethics*, vol. 1, 293–312. Textbooks of Military Medicine. Washington, DC: Office of the Surgeon General, Borden Institute.

Sims, N. A. 1987. "Morality and Biological Warfare." *Arms Control* 8 (1): 5–23.

Singer, P. 1972. "Famine, Affluence and Morality." *Philosophy and Public Affairs* 1: 229–243.

Skinner, H., Abdeen, Z., Abdeen, H., Aber, P., Al-Masri, M., Attias, J., and Avraham, K. B. 2005. "Promoting Arab and Israeli Cooperation: Peacebuilding through Health Initiative." *The Lancet* 365: 1274–1277.

Slotten, H. R. 1990. "Humane Chemistry or Scientific Barbarism? American Responses to World War I Poison Gas, 1915–1930." *Journal of American History* 77 (2): 476–498.

Smith, L. 1999. "Quakers in Uniform: The Friends Ambulance Unit." In P. Brock and T. P. Socknat, eds., *Challenge to Mars: Essays on Pacifism from 1918 to 1945*. Toronto: University of Toronto Press.

Spiegelberg, H. 1970. "Human Dignity: A Challenge to Contemporary Philosophy." In R. Gotesky and E. Laszlo, eds., *Human Dignity: This Century and the Next*, 39–64. New York: Gordon and Breach.

Statman, D. 1997. "Question of the Moral Absoluteness of the Prohibition on Torture." *Mishpat vMemshal* [Law and Government, Hebrew] 4: 161–198.

Statman, D. 2001. "Two Concepts of Dignity." *Tel Aviv Law Review* 24 (3): 541–603.

Steinberg, G. 1993. "Israeli Responses to the Threat of Chemical Warfare." *Armed Forces and Society* 20 (1): 85–101.

Steinbock, B., and Norcross, A. 1994. *Killing and Letting Die*. 2nd ed. New York: Fordham University Press.

Stockholm International Peace Research Institute. 1971–1975. *The Problem of Chemical and Biological Warfare*. 6 vols. Stockholm: Stockholm International Peace Research Institute.

Stouffer, S. A., Lumsdaine, A. A., Lumsdaine, M. H., Williams Jr., R. M., Smith, M. B., Janis, I. L., Star, S. A., and Cottrell Jr., L. S. 1949. *The American Soldier: Combat and Its Aftermath*. Vol. 2. New York: Wiley.

St. Petersburg 1868. *Declaration Renouncing the Use, in Time of War, of Explosive Projectiles under 400 Grammes Weight*. Saint Petersburg, November 29/December 11.

Swan, K. G., and Swan, K. G. Jr. 1996. "Triage, the Past Revisited." *Military Medicine*, 161 (8): 448–452.

Swann, S. W. 1985. "Euthanasia on the Battlefield." *Military Medicine* 152: 545–549.

"Symposium on Ethics and Nuclear Deterrence." 1985. Special Issue of *Ethics* 95 (3).

Tarasoff v. Regents of University of California. 1976. 17 Cal. 3d 425, 551 P.2d 334, 131 Cal. Rptr. 14.

Tatum, A. 1970. *Handbook for Conscientious Objectors*, 10th ed. Philadelphia: Central Committee for Conscientious Objectors.

The Laws of War on Land. 1880. Oxford, September 9. http://www.icrc.org/ihl.nsf

Thomson, J. J. 1986. "Self-Defense and Rights." In *Rights, Restitution, and Risk: Essays in Moral Theory*, 33–48. Cambridge, MA: Harvard University Press.

Tindale, C. W. 1996. "The Logic of Torture: A Critical Examination." *Social Theory and Practice* 22: 349–374.

Tuchman, B. 1984. *The March of Folly: From Troy to Vietnam*. London: Little, Brown.

Tucker, J. B. 1984–1985. "Gene Wars." *Foreign Policy* 57: 58–79.

21 Army Group. 1945. *Penicillin Therapy and Control*. London: Director of Medical Services, 21 Army Group.

United Nations. 1982. *Principles of Medical Ethics*. General Assembly Resolution 37/194, December 18. New York: United Nations.

United Nations. 1997. *Report of the Committee against Torture, General Assembly 52nd Session, New York*. Supplement 44 (A/52/54). New York: United Nations.

United Nations. 2004. *A More Secure World: Our Shared Responsibility, Report of the High-Level Panel on Threats, Challenges and Change*. New York: United Nations.

U.S. Department of Defense. 1988. "Sorting of Casualties, Triage." In *2nd U.S. Revision of the Emergency War Surgery NATO Handbook* , 3.12. Washington, DC: U.S. Department of Defense.

U.S. Department of Defense. 2003a. Directive, Number 1300.6, *Conscientious Objectors*, August 20, 1971, certified as current, November 21, 2003. http://usmilitary.about.com/library/milinfo/dodreg/bldodreg1300.6-htm

U.S. Department of Defense. 2003b. *Working Group Report on Detainee Interrogations in the Global War on Terrorism: Assessment of Legal, Historical, Policy and Operational Considerations*, April 4. http://wikisource.org/wiki/Rumsfeld_Torture_Report

U.S. Department of Justice. 2004. *Memorandum for James B. Comey, Deputy Attorney General, Re: Legal Standards Applicable under 18 U.S.C. §§2340–2340A*. http://www.usdoj.gov/olc/dagmemo.pdf

U.S. Food and Drug Administration. 1999. "Human Drugs and Biologics; Determination That Informed Consent Is NOT Feasible or Is Contrary to the Best Interests of Recipients; Revocation of 1990 Interim Final Rule; Establishment of New Interim Final Rule." FDA, *Federal Register* 64 (192), October 5.

U.S. Office of War Information. 1944. *Penicillin*. Washington, DC: U.S. Office of War Information.

U.S. Southern Command. 2003. *Memorandum for the Commander, US Southern Command, April 16, 2003*, Tab B. http://www.gwu.edu/~nsarchiv/NSAEBB/NSAEBB127/03.04.16.pdf

van Courtland Moon, J. E. 1984. "Chemical Weapons and Deterrence: The World War II Experience." *International Security* 84: 3–35.

van Courtland Moon, J. E. 1989. "Project SPHINX: The Question of the Use of Gas in the Planned Invasion of Japan." *Journal of Strategic Studies* 12 (3): 303–323.

van Courtland Moon, J. E. 1999. "US Biological Warfare Planning and Preparedness: The Dilemmas of Policy. " In E. Geissler and J. E. van Courtland Moon, eds., *Biological and Toxin Weapons: Research, Development and Use from the Middle Ages to 1945*, 215–254. SIPRI Chemical and Biological Warfare Studies 18. Oxford: Oxford University Press.

van Creveld, M. 1991. *The Transformation of War*. New York: Free Press.

Vass, A. 2001. "Peace through Health." *British Medical Journal* 323: 1020.

Vastyan, E. A. 1974. "Warriors in White: Some Questions about the Nature and Mission of Military Medicine." *Texas Reports on Biology and Medicine* 32 (1): 327–342.

Veatch, R. M. 1984. "Autonomy's Temporary Triumph." *Hastings Center Report* 14: 38–40.

Vidal-Naquet, P. 1963. *Torture: Cancer of Democracy.* Harmondsworth, Middlesex: Penguin.

von Clausewitz, K. [1832] 1976. Edited and translated by M. E. Howard and P. Paret. Princeton: Princeton University Press.

Wade, N. 2005. "A DNA Success Raises Bioterror Concern," New York Times, January 12. http://query.nytimes.com/gst/health/article-page.html?res=9F00EFDC1638F931A25752C0A9639C8B63

Walzer, M. 1970. "The Obligation to Die for the State." In *Obligations: Essays on Disobedience, War and Citizenship*, 77–98. New York: Simon and Schuster.

Walzer, M. 1977. *Just and Unjust Wars: A Moral Argument with Historical Illustrations*. New York: Basic Books.

Webb, C. 1968. "Medical Considerations in Internal Defense and Development." *Military Medicine* 133: 391–396.

Weissman, F., ed. 2004. *In the Shadow of "Just Wars": Violence, Politics, and Humanitarian Action*. London: C. Hurst and Co.

Wheelis, M. 1999. "Biological Warfare before 1914." In E. Geissler and J. E. van Courtland Moon, eds., *Biological and Toxin Weapons: Research, Development and Use from the Middle Ages to 1945*, 8–34. SIPRI Chemical and Biological Warfare Studies 18. Oxford: Oxford University Press.

White, B., and Gampel, E. 1996. "Resolving Moral Dilemmas: A Case-Based Method." *Healthcare Ethics Committee Forum* 8 (2): 85–102.

White, D. 1968. "Civilian Medical Care in South Vietnam." *Military Medicine* 133: 650–653.

Wicclair, M. R. 2000. "Conscientious Objection in Medicine." *Bioethics* 14 (3): 205–227.

Wilensky, R. J. 2001. "The Medical Civic Action Program in Vietnam: Success or Failure?" *Military Medicine* 166 (9): 815–819.

Williams, R. M., Jr. 1989. "The American Soldier: An Assessment, Several Wars Later." *Public Opinion Quarterly* 53 (2): 155–174.

Wilson, D. 1976. *In Search of Penicillin*. New York: Knopf.

Wilson, L. 1983. "Torture, Doctors and the World Medical Association." *Medical Journal of Australia* 2 (5): 236–239.

Wiltse, C. M. 1965. *The Medical Department: Medical Service in the Mediterranean and Minor Theaters, Chapter XIII, The Italian Communication Zone.* Washington, DC: Office of the Chief of Military History, Department of the Army.

Winslow, G. R. 1982. *Triage and Justice: The Ethics of Rationing Life-Saving Medical Resources*. Berkeley: University of California Press.

World Health Organization. 1970. *Health Aspects of Chemical and Biological Weapons*. Geneva: World Health Organization.

World Health Organization. 2004. *Public Health Response to Biological and Chemical Weapons: WHO Guidance*. Geneva: World Health Organization.

World Medical Association. 1975. *Declaration of Tokyo, Guidelines for Medical Doctors Concerning Torture and Other Cruel, Inhuman or Degrading Treatment or Punishment in Relation to Detention and Imprisonment.* http://www.wma.net/e/policy/c18.htm

World Medical Association. 1990. *Declaration on Chemical and Biological Weapons*. Adopted by the 42nd World Medical Assembly, Rancho Mirage, CA. http://www.wma.net/e/policy/b1.htm

World Medical Association. 1991. *Declaration on Hunger Strikers*. In British Medical Association. 1992. *Medicine Betrayed: The Participation of Doctors in Human Rights Abuses*. London: Zed Books, 212–214.

World Medical Association. 2004. *Regulations In Times Of Armed Conflict*, Adopted by the 10th World Medical Assembly, Havana, Cuba, October 1956. Edited by the 11th World Medical Assembly, Istanbul, Turkey, October 1957, and Amended by the 35th World Medical Assembly, Venice, Italy, October 1983 and The WMA General Assembly, Tokyo 2004. http://www.wma.net/e/policy/a20.htm

Wright, S. 1985. "The Military and the New Biology." *Bulletin of the Atomic Scientists* 41 (5): 10–16.

Wright, S. 2001. "Sub-Lethal Weapons in Human Rights Abuse." *Medicine, Conflict and Survival* 17: 221–233.

Zajtchuk, J. T. 2003. "Military Medicine in Humanitarian Missions." In T. E. Beam and L. R. Sparacino, eds., *Military Medical Ethics*, vol. 2, 773–804. Textbooks of Military Medicine. Washington, DC: Office of the Surgeon General, Borden Institute.

Zamir, I. 1989. "Human Rights and National Security." *Israel Law Review* 23 (2, 3): 375–406.

Zumwalt, J. G. n.d. *Bare Feet, Iron Will.* Sec. 1: Medical Care. (*A working manuscript based on interviews conducted of North Vietnamese medical personnel and soldiers who served in the Vietnam conflict.*)

Zwi, A. B. 1987. "The Political Abuse of Medicine." *Social Science and Medicine* 25 (6): 649–657.

Index